Praise for *The Optimum Nutrition Bible*
and Patrick Holford's work

What the papers say:

'Health guru Patrick Holford addresses the true causes of illness – diet.'

Guardian

'Patrick Holford offers the most informative, easy to read, cutting edge alternative information you can trust.'

HAZEL COURTENEY, winner of 'Health Journalist of the Year'

'If you buy one book about nutrition, this should be it.'

Heat

What the scientists say:

'There have been many dramatic changes in our views about healthcare and Patrick Holford has been right at the forefront.'

DR JOHN MARKS, Life Fellow and former Director of Medical Studies, University of Cambridge

'Optimum nutrition is the medicine of the future.'

DR LINUS PAULING, twice winner of a Nobel Prize

'I am dazzled by the breadth of nutritional knowledge in this book... Areas of complexity and confusion in nutrition are explained in clear, concise terms, understandable by all.'

DR JOHN LEE MD, author of *What Your Doctor Didn't Tell You About the Menopause*

'Patrick Holford is guiding the nutrition revolution.'

DR JEFFREY BLAND, founder of the Institute of Functional Medicine, USA

What readers say:

'I thought my diet was good and that I was fit. My symptoms included energy slumps throughout the day, anxiety, difficulty waking up and going to sleep, night sweats and poor concentration. I also craved sugar, especially after exercise, and in fact only felt alive after exercise or beer. *The Optimum Nutrition Bible* changed my life. I feel more centred, calm, in control, energetic and happy than I can ever remember.'

CHRIS B.

'*The Optimum Nutrition Bible* was recommended to me after I'd been suffering for many years with what doctors described as IBS. I read the book from cover to cover, changed my diet and took the recommended supplements. My energy levels increased within a matter of a week or so and I felt much calmer than usual. For the first time ever found I could tolerate a small amount of wholemeal bread. My husband has also been taking the supplements, plus fish oil, and they have greatly helped his Crohn's Disease. I feel 100 per cent better than I used to.'

CHRISTINE S.

'In mid-April I had my blood checked and found my cholesterol to be 6.5. I do eat really healthily and felt that my condition was due to hereditary cholesterol rather than dietary factors. A friend had reduced theirs through the supplements recommended in your book, so I thought it was worth a try. Five weeks later I went for a second blood test to find my cholesterol had dropped to 5.1. My GP couldn't believe it! He would not wholeheartedly acknowledge the success, but he didn't knock it either, saying whatever you are taking is working – come back in a year!'

MIKE T.

'After reading this book I have been trying to improve my health in the past month by eating better and taking supplements. I was both surprised and pleased to see a rapid reduction in the wrinkly skin under my eyes. My skin is now smooth and 'filled out'. It has shown me that improving your nutrition can have immediate effects. Thanks Patrick, I've finally woken up to the importance of nutrition.'

N.W.

patrick
HOLFORD

THE
OPTIMUM
NUTRITION
BIBLE

patrick
HOLFORD

THE
OPTIMUM
NUTRITION
BIBLE

piatkus

PIATKUS

First published in Great Britain in 1997 by Piatkus Books
This updated and expanded version first published in 2004 as
Patrick Holford's New Optimum Nutrition Bible
Copyright © Patrick Holford 2004

Reprinted 2004, 2005 (twice), 2006 (three times), 2007 (twice), 2008, 2009 (three times)

A CIP catalogue record for this book
is available from the British Library

ISBN 978-0-7499-2552-9

Typeset in ITC Stone Serif by Phoenix Photosetting, Chatham, Kent
Printed and bound in Great Britain by CPI Mackays, Chatham ME5 8TD

Papers used by Piatkus are natural, renewable and recyclable
products sourced from well-managed forests and certified
in accordance with the rules of the Forest Stewardship Council.

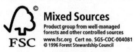

Mixed Sources
Product group from well-managed
forests and other controlled sources
www.fsc.org Cert no. SGS-COC-004081
© 1996 Forest Stewardship Council
FSC

Piatkus
An imprint of
Little, Brown Book Group
100 Victoria Embankment
London EC4Y 0DY

An Hachette UK Company
www.hachette.co.uk

www.piatkus.co.uk

This book is dedicated
to you – the promoter of
your own health

About the author

Patrick Holford BSc, DipION, FBANT, NTCRP is a pioneer in new approaches to health and nutrition, and is widely regarded as Britain's leading spokesman on nutrition and mental health issues. He is also the author of over 30 health books, translated into over 20 languages and selling over a million copies worldwide.

Patrick Holford started his academic career in the field of psychology, and was a student of Dr Carl Pfeiffer and Dr Abram Hoffer, two leading authorities in the field of mental health and nutrition.

In 1984 Patrick founded the Institute for Optimum Nutrition (ION), an independent educational trust for the furtherance of education and research in nutrition, now the largest training school in the UK to offer degree-accredited training in nutritional therapy. During his years at ION, Patrick was involved in groundbreaking research showing that multivitamins can increase children's IQ scores – research that was published in the *Lancet* and the subject of a *Horizon* documentary in the 1980s. He also ran educational campaigns raising awareness of the importance of zinc, antioxidants, essential fats and homocysteine-lowering B vitamins such as folic acid.

He is Chief Executive of the Food for the Brain Foundation, an educational charity, and director of the Brain Bio Centre, the Foundation's treatment centre. He is an honorary fellow of the British Association for Applied Nutrition and Nutritional Therapy, as well as a member of the Nutrition Therapy Council.

Contents

Part 3 The Wonderful World Within

Part 4 The Benefits of Optimum Nutrition

Part 5 Nutrition for All Ages

Part 6 Your Personal Nutrition Programme

Part 7 A to Z of Nutritional Healing

Acne – Alcoholism – Allergies – Alzheimer's and dementia –
Anaemia – Angina and atherosclerosis – Arthritis – Asthma – Breast
cancer – Bronchitis – Burns, cuts and bruises – Cancer – Candidiasis
– Colds and flu – Colitis – Constipation – Chronic fatigue – Crohn's
disease – Cystitis – Depression – Dermatitis – Diabetes –
Diverticulitis – Ear infections – Eczema – Fibromyalgia – Gallstones –
Gout – Hair problems – Hangovers – Hay fever – Headaches and
migraines – Herpes – High blood pressure – HIV infection and AIDS –
Indigestion – Infections – Infertility – Inflammation – Irritable bowel
syndrome – Kidney stones – Menopausal symptoms – Muscle aches
and cramps – Obesity – Osteoporosis – PMS – Prostate problems –
Psoriasis – Schizophrenia – Sinusitis – Sleeping problems – Thyroid
problems – Ulcers – Varicose veins

Part 8 Nutrient Fact File A to Z

Vitamins – Minerals – Essential fats – Semi-essential nutrients

Part 9 Food Fact File

Which Protein Foods? – Which Fats and Oils? – Which
Carbohydrates? – Glycemic Load (GL) of Common Foods – Glycemic
Load (GL) of Common Drinks – How Much Fibre? – Balancing
Acid/Alkaline Foods – Which Foods Are Rich in Phyto-estrogens? –
Which Antioxidant-rich Foods? – The Best Fruit and Vegetables

Acknowledgements

This book would not have been possible without the help and support of many people. Thanks also to Kate Neil for contributing to Part 2, Antony Haynes for contributing to Chapter 24, Natalie Savona for contributing to Chapter 26, Jane Nodder for contributing to Chapter 35, Susannah Lawson for her help with Part 5, Susan Clift, Shane Heaton and Eleanor Burton for their research, Jonathan Phillips, Chris Quayle, Rodney Paull, Dick Vine, Jonathan Phillips and Lynn Alford Burow for their illustrations and charts, Anna Crago, Gill Bailey and Krystyna Mayer for their skilful editing, Charlotte Miller for her editorial help and advice. I'd also like to thank Dr Peter D'Adamo for his research on blood types referred to in Chapter 20. Finally, I'd like to thank Gabrielle, my wife, for putting up with the early mornings and late nights!

Guide to Abbreviations, Measures and References

Abbreviations and measures

1 gram (g) = 1,000 milligrams (mg) = 1,000,000 micrograms (mcg, also written µg).

All vitamins are measured in milligrams or micrograms. Vitamins A, D and E used to be measured in International Units (ius), a measurement designed to standardise the various forms of these vitamins that have different potencies.

6mcg of betacarotene, the vegetable precursor of vitamin A, is, on average, converted into 1mcg of retinol, the animal form of vitamin A. So, 6mcg of betacarotene is called 1mcgRE (RE stands for retinol equivalent). Throughout this book betacarotene is referred to in mcgRE.

1mcg of retinol (mcgRE) = 3.3ius of vitamin A
1mcgRE of betacarotene = 6mcg of betacarotene
100ius of vitamin D = 2.5mcg
100ius of vitamin E = 67mg
1 pound (lb) = 16 ounces (oz) 2.2lb = 1 kilogram (kg)
1 pint = 0.6 litres 1.76 pints = 1 litre
In this book calories means kilocalories (kcals)

References and further sources of information

Hundreds of references from respected scientific literature have been used in the writing of this book. Details of specific studies referred to are listed on pages 534–45. Other supporting research for statements made is available from the library at the Institute for Optimum Nutrition (ION) (see page 525) for members of ION. ION also offers information services, including literature search and library search facilities, for those readers who want to access scientific literature on specific subjects. On pages 521–3 you will find a list of the best books to read, linked to each chapter, to enable you to dig deeper into the topics covered. You will also find many of the topics touched on in this book covered in detail in my feature articles, available at www.patrickholford.com. If you want to stay up to date with all that is new and exciting in this field I recommend you subscribe to my *100% Health* newsletter, details of which are on the website.

Introduction

This book, now available in fifteen languages, is the cutting edge in how to keep yourself looking good, feeling great and living long. First written in 1997 to sum up twenty years' research at the Institute for Optimum Nutrition (ION), an independent educational charity, this edition is revised, expanded and updated.

A lot has happened to our understanding of health, disease and nutrition in the last five years and I wouldn't be doing my job if I didn't let you know about it. Many discoveries have been made – the secret to successful weight loss, preventing Alzheimer's, reversing depression without drugs, why breast and prostate cancer incidence keeps going up and how to do your best to avoid them. Many more propositions have been proven – that 'optimum nutrition' dramatically increases energy, lowers cholesterol better than any drug and halves the recovery time from infections, to name a few. Since the first edition of this book I have received over a thousand exuberant testimonials from people whose lives have literally been transformed through optimum nutrition – people like you.

That's my job – to help you be free of pain and full of health so you can enjoy your life to the full. I spend my time studying literally hundreds of pioneering science and medicine journals, and speaking to the pioneers and trying out new approaches, then turning it all into easy-to-understand language that you can practically apply in your life. When you are 100 per cent healthy and free from pain, discomfort, tiredness and the need for drugs, I've done my job. But first, let me tell you how I got started.

In 1977 I met two extraordinary nutritionists, Brian and Celia Wright. They explained to me, over an enormous bowl of salad and some 'soya sausages', followed by a handful of vitamin pills, how most disease was the result of sub-optimum nutrition. I found this hard to swallow but, being an adventurous spirit, asked them to devise me a diet. There I was, a university student studying psychology, eating a virtually wheat-free, vegetarian diet with masses of fruit and vegetables, and taking a handful of supplements shipped from America since they were not available in Britain at that time. It was a far cry from the usual fish and chips and a pint of bitter! My colleagues, friends and family thought I was crazy. But I persisted.

Within two months I lost fourteen pounds in weight, which has never returned; my skin, which had resembled a lunar landscape, cleared up; my regular migraines virtually vanished; but most noticeable of all was the extra energy I had. I no longer needed so much sleep, my mind was much sharper and my body was full of vitality. I started to investigate this 'optimum nutrition'. Being a psychology student, I looked up research on the greatest problem in mental health today, schizophrenia. There, in the scientific journals, was clear proof that 'optimum nutrition' produced results better than drugs and psychotherapy combined. A pioneer in this field, Dr Carl Pfeiffer, an American doctor and psychiatrist, was claiming an 80 per cent remission rate. So too was Dr Abram Hoffer, a director of psychiatric research in Canada – and the first man ever to carry out a 'double-blind' study in the history of psychiatry. I was fascinated, and before long went to America and Canada to see for myself.

Pfeiffer, a brilliant man who spent most of his life studying the chemistry of the brain, had a massive heart attack when he was fifty. His chances of survival were very slim – ten years at the absolute most, and only then if he had a pacemaker fitted. He decided not to, and spent his next thirty years pursuing and researching optimum nutrition. 'It is my firmly held belief,' he told me, 'that with an adequate intake of micronutrients – essential substances we need to nourish us – most chronic diseases would not exist. Good nutritional therapy is the medicine of the future. We have already waited too long for it.'

Dr Abram Hoffer, who has now treated over 5,000 patients and published forty-year follow-ups, told me he had an 80 per cent cure rate. I asked him to define cure and he said, 'Free of symptoms, socialising with family and friends and paying income tax!' Dr Abram Hoffer, now over ninety years old, is still working, helping and advising people in Vancouver Island, Canada. I was deeply impressed by these two men and became their student.

The optimum nutrition approach is not new: many great visionaries have embraced it. In 390 BC Hippocrates said, 'Let food be your medicine and medicine be your food.' Edison in the early twentieth century said, 'The doctor of the future will give no medicine but will interest his patients in the care of the human frame, diet and the cause and prevention of disease.' In 1960 one of the geniuses of our time, twice Nobel prize winner Dr Linus Pauling, coined the phrase 'orthomolecular medicine'. Linus Pauling was to chemistry what Einstein was to physics. Pauling, who died in 1994, has been voted the second most important scientist of twentieth century. He is the only man to have won two unshared Nobel prizes – he also had forty-eight PhDs! By giving the body the right (ortho) molecules, he asserted, most disease would be eradicated. 'Optimum nutrition,' he said, 'is the medicine of tomorrow.'

In 1984, with Linus Pauling's help and support, I founded the ION in London to research and promote this idea. ION, which is an independent, non-profit educational charity, is now the leading school for training nutritional therapists in Europe. Roughly speaking, we were ten years ahead on most major health issues.

- Our first campaign was to help ban lead in petrol because we knew from the science that it was damaging children's minds.

- In 1986 we helped put zinc on the map and made people 'think zinc' by extolling the virtues of Britain's most commonly deficient mineral.

- In 1987 we helped run the first trial – published in the *Lancet* and filmed by the BBC's *Horizon* – that proved vitamin supplements can boost IQ.

- In the 1990s we showed that increasing your intake of antioxidants helps reduce the risk of cancer and slow ageing.

- In 1993 we went public against hormone replacement therapy (HRT), saying that it causes breast cancer, a fact now well proven.

- In 1995 we said there were better natural remedies for depression than drugs, and that many SSRI anti-depressants increased the risk of suicide and aggression. Last year doctors were rightly advised not to prescribe them to anyone under the age of eighteen.

In recent years I've been explaining why your homocysteine level is your greatest single health statistic, why Alzheimer's disease is preventable, why milk consumption is undeniably linked to breast and prostate cancer risk and why the 'glycemic load' of a food is the best predictor of weight gain. Maybe you haven't heard about the last four, but you will. In short, we've been ten years ahead of what is destined to become public knowledge – knowledge that could add ten years to your life.

The purpose of this book is to show you how to achieve vibrant health and resistance to disease through optimum nutrition. Part 1 explains the principles of optimum nutrition, which necessitates a whole new definition of health, healthcare and medicine. Part 2 defines the perfect diet – not easy to acquire overnight, but good to aspire to. Parts 3, 4 and 5 prove the benefits of optimum nutrition based on the latest breakthroughs in nutritional science. Part 6 shows you how to put optimum nutrition into practice with a step-by-step guide to help you improve your diet and design your own supplement programme. Part 7 is an A to Z guide to specific health problems and how to heal them with optimum nutrition. Part 8 is an A to Z guide to nutrients; what they do, signs and causes of deficiency, what to eat and what to supplement. Part 9 gives you food facts and tables to help put optimum nutrition into practice.

Twenty-five years have passed since I discovered optimum nutrition. In that time thousands of scientific papers have been published proving its potency, and virtually none that negate it. I am now completely convinced that the concept of optimum nutrition is the greatest step forward in medicine for over a century, no less important than Louis Pasteur's discovery of disease-causing 'germs' or the discovery of genes, and that, if applied from an early age, it is a guarantee for a long and healthy life.

Wishing you the very best of health,

Patrick Holford

Part 1

What Is Optimum?

chapter 1

Health – Who Wants to Be Average?

This book is a means to a goal – health. And that means not just an absence of disease, but also an abundance of vitality. Positive health, sometimes called 'functional' health, can be measured in three ways:

- Performance – how you perform physically and mentally

- Absence of ill-health – lack of disease signs and symptoms

- Longevity – healthy lifespan

I believe the experience of a profound sense of well-being can be achieved by everyone. It is characterised by a consistent, clear, high level of energy, emotional balance, a sharp mind, a desire to maintain physical fitness and a direct awareness of what suits our bodies, what enhances our health, and what our needs are in any given moment. This state of health includes resilience to infectious diseases and protection from the major killer diseases such as heart disease and cancer. As a result the ageing process is slowed down and we can live a long and healthy life. At its most profound level health is not merely the absence of pain or tension, but a joy in living, a real appreciation of what it is to have a healthy body with which to taste the many pleasures of this world.

For me, this is not just a belief but an experience that I have had personally and have also witnessed in many other people with whom I have worked over the years since I started to pursue optimum nutrition. Health has not been a static state, but an endless journey of learning about myself from the diseases and imbalances that I have suffered, and a continuing discovery of even higher and clearer levels of energy. From these experiences, and those gained through working with thousands of people suffering from all categories of disease, I am totally convinced that, by means of optimum nutrition, exercise, living in the right environment and being willing to change obsolete beliefs and behaviour patterns that create tension and stress, virtually all disease can be prevented.

Healthcare – the fastest-growing failing business

Nothing in Western culture really teaches us to be healthy. Apart from a little wisdom imparted by our parents, most of whom spend their later years in increasing pain, we are not taught how to be healthy at school, at university or by the media. Government campaigns may advise against smoking and drinking, but there is little real guidance and few results. Each year in the UK alone we consume six billion alcoholic drinks and seventy-five billion cigarettes despite these campaigns.

What we call 'healthcare' is really 'disease care'. Described by Dr Emanuel Cheraskin, Emeritus Professor at the University of Alabama Medical School, as 'the fastest-growing failing business', modern medicine is failing to provide true healthcare and making a lot of money out of it. It is, says Cheraskin, 'primary prevention of health deterioration'.

Take heart disease as an example. Currently, you have a 50 per cent chance of acquiring heart disease during your life. It accounts for a quarter of all deaths before the age of sixty-five, and one in four men has a heart attack before retiring from work – half of these men don't have high cholesterol levels! It is well accepted that high blood pressure is the leading warning of serious cardiovascular problems. Conventional medicine recommends weight loss and drugs to lower high blood pressure and cholesterol, but little heed is paid to the many dietary factors also known to achieve this end. Even 1,000mg of vitamin C can significantly lower blood pressure, yet this is rarely recommended. A mere 500mg of vitamin E reduces the risk of a heart attack in those with cardiovascular disease by 75 per cent, according to a large-scale placebo-controlled trial undertaken at Cambridge University Medical School.[1] Supplementing B vitamins, which lower homocysteine, an often ignored risk factor greater than cholesterol, can also halve the risks of both heart attacks and strokes.[2]

Contrary to popular belief, the risk of death from many common types of cancer is increasing, not declining. Consider breast cancer, which accounts for one-third of all cancers diagnosed in women and around 12,000 deaths each year. If treatment was working, women with breast cancer would live longer and be at less risk of dying. We are told that, in the last thirty years, the survival rate has increased from 60 to 75 per cent. However, the death rate from cancer over the same period has steadily increased. What has happened is that people are being diagnosed earlier, and so appear to survive longer. We are losing the cancer war, not winning it.

According to medical expert Dr John Lee, breast cancer is occurring more frequently and earlier in women's lives than in the mid-1980s. Mammograms show microcalcifications in the breasts that could never have been picked up before. These are not the invasive tumours we need worry about, but they skew the statistics to show better survival rates. The usual treatment is surgery followed by the drug Tamoxifen, yet medicated and non-medicated patients do just as well. Dr Lee believes the major cause of breast cancer is 'unopposed oestrogen' (normally balanced in the body with progesterone), and there are many factors that would lead to this situation. Stress, for example, raises levels of the hormone cortisol, which competes with progesterone. So does insulin resistance, which is the consequence of eating too much sugar and refined carbohydrates. Xenoestrogens from the environment, found in pesticides and plastics among other common sources, can damage tissue and lead to increased cancer risk later in life. Milk, too, is a known promoter of breast and prostate cancer growth.

Clearly there are also nutritional elements to consider. Yet doctors have continued to prescribe unopposed oestrogen for women on hormone-related therapy (HRT) for decades, despite clear evidence of risk back in 1989, when Dr Bergfist's study in Scandinavia showed that if a woman is on HRT for longer than five years she doubles her risk of breast cancer.[3] This was followed by a study by Emery University School of Public Health, which followed 240,000 women for eight years and found that the risk of fatal ovarian cancer was 72 per cent higher in women given oestrogen.[4] However, it was only when the 'million women study' was published in the *Lancet* that HRT started to be phased out. The authors, whose research showed that use of combined oestrogen/progestin HRT increases risk of breast cancer by 66 per cent and risk of death by 22 per cent, estimated that 20,000 women had contracted breast cancer because of HRT in the last decade.[5]

Taking another example, by the age of sixty, nine in every ten people have arthritis. Once the level of pain is unbearable, sufferers are recommended steroidal or non-steroidal anti-inflammatory drugs. While both classes of drugs reduce the pain and swelling, they also speed up the progression of the disease. In the US non-steroidal anti-inflammatory drugs are a $30 billion industry – $17 billion for the drugs and $13 billion for treating the side effects. Thousands of people die from the side effects of these drugs alone. Yet there are proven, safe nutritional alternatives that have as great an anti-inflammatory effect without the harmful side effects.

Put all these and other risks into the health equation and it is easy to understand why the average person today is destined to live a measly seventy-five years and spend the last twenty in poor health, when it is an established fact that a healthy human lifespan should be at least a hundred years. And the sad truth is that the statistics are not getting any better. For all our advances in drugs, surgical procedures and medical technology, a man aged forty-five today can expect to live for only two more years than the same man in 1920; until seventy-four, instead of seventy-two. Conventional approaches to healthcare are clearly barking up the wrong tree. Perhaps what is needed is a new tree.

The new idea of health

Instead of thinking of the body as a machine, and disease as a spanner in the works that must be removed or destroyed with drugs or surgery, medical scientists are now beginning to look at human beings as 'complex adaptive systems', more like a self-organising jungle than a complicated computer. Rather than trying to 'control' a person's health by playing God with hi-tech medicine, a new way of looking at health has emerged that considers a human being as a whole, with an interconnected mind and body designed to adapt to health if the circumstances are right.

Of course, this adaptive capacity is not the same for everyone. We are each born with different strengths and weaknesses and different levels of resilience – some of us have what is popularly called 'good genes' or come from 'good stock', and some of us do not. So, according to this new concept, our health is a result of the interaction between our inherited adaptive capacity and our circumstances. On a physical/chemical level, for example, that interaction would be between our genes and our environment. If our environment is sufficiently hostile (bad diet, pollution, exposure to viruses, allergens, etc.) we exceed our ability to adapt and get sick.

Going back to cancer, we know that the risk is increased if we smoke, regularly drink alcohol, eat beef and dairy produce, take certain drugs and hormones and are exposed to exhaust fumes and other pollutants – to name a few. The risk, on the other hand, is lower if we have a high intake of certain vegetables, fibres, antioxidants such as betacarotene and vitamins C and E, and live in an unpolluted environment. Evidence shows that, when the pluses significantly outweigh the minuses, health can be improved.

Genes and the environment are like the chicken and the egg. Science is proving that our genes are influenced by the environment in which we have evolved. Similarly, how we interact with our environment – for example, our ability to digest certain nutrients – depends on our genetics.

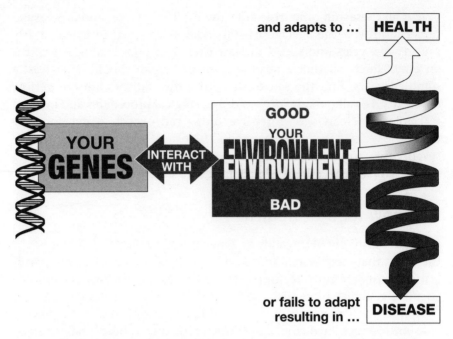

The new model of health. Your genes interact with your environment (every-thing you eat, drink and breathe) to create you. If you have good nutrition the result is that you have the capacity to adapt to the stresses of life. That's health. If your total environmental load exceeds your genetic capacity to adapt, you may develop disease.

I believe that the future of medicine will focus primarily on genetics and on environmental medicine, of which nutrition plays a major part, as the means to influence health. Genes, however, are harder to change than diet, so it is likely that nutrition will form the major part of the new approach to healthcare, along with strategies to reduce 'anti-nutrients' – substances such as environmental pollutants, pesticides and chemical food additives, which all interfere with the action of nutrients.

Remember, we are always being challenged – be it as the result of the neighbour's cold, or unavoidable exhaust fumes. What we take into our bodies – be it healthy food, drink, drugs or junk – can dramatically affect our ability to stay healthy.

chapter 2

Defining Optimum Nutrition

M ost of us are unwitting students of the Breakfast Cereal School of Nutrition. Morning after morning we stare at the cereal packet, reading, '... RDAs ... one serving provides thiamine, riboflavin, niacin', and, together with other clever advertising, this assures us that our reasonably well-balanced diet will give us everything we need. This is, however, the greatest lie in healthcare today – a belief based on wrong information and a complete misconception of the nature of the human body.

Man as machine

The concept of the body as a machine is a product of the thinking of philosophers such as Newton and Descartes and of the industrial revolution, which envisioned a clockwork universe and man as a thinking machine. Until a couple of hundred years ago our ancestors had spent millions of years being hunter-gatherers and ten thousand years being peasant farmers, only to be propelled, as many country people were, into the new towns and cities to fuel the need for labour during the industrial revolution.

The diet that the new industrial workers were fed consisted of fat, sugar and refined flour. A biscuit or cake is a good example. Flour was refined so that it would not support weevils and, like refined sugar and saturated fat, did not go off. These cheap, energy-providing foods were considered 'fuel' in the same way that a car needs petrol. Not surprisingly, health declined. By about 1900 people had started to be smaller than in earlier generations. This led to the discovery of protein – the factor in food needed for growth. Sugar for energy, protein for muscle. With this concept the Western diet of high sugar, fat and protein was born.

Yet people were still sick and, one by one, the classic vitamin-deficiency diseases such as scurvy and rickets were solved as new vitamins were discovered. The importance of minerals was also established, but all these vital nutrients were still dealt with in a very mechanical way. All each person needed was the Recommended Daily Allowance (RDA) of each nutrient, a level considered to be sufficient to protect the body against deficiency diseases. Yet, according to Dr Jeffrey Bland, world-renowned nutritional biochemist, former professor of chemistry and founder of the Institute of Functional Medicine, 'the RDAs have absolutely no relevance to individual nutritional assessment. They are standards of identity to meet the needs of practically all healthy people to prevent the known nutrition disorders beriberi, pellagra, scurvy, kwashiorkor, rickets and marasmus. They have nothing to do with the common disorders of Western society.'

Food, genes, environment and disease

Your body is composed entirely of molecules derived from food. In a lifetime you will eat 100 tons of food, which is broken down by enzyme-rich secretions in the digestive tract produced at a rate of about ten litres per day. Macronutrients (fat, protein, carbohydrate) and micronutrients (vitamins, minerals) are absorbed through the digestive tract, whose health and integrity depends fundamentally on what you eat. Your nutritional status determines, to a substantial extent, your capacity to adapt and maintain health. Biochemical imbalances resulting from sub-optimum nutrition experienced over generations are recorded and expressed genetically as strengths and weaknesses of specific body processes. Your genes express themselves in your environment (food, air, water and so on.) If your environment is too hostile for them, you cannot adapt and disease results. If your environment is nourishing, you have a greater resistance to disease and are more likely to experience health and vitality.

What does optimum nutrition mean?

Optimum nutrition is very simply giving yourself the best possible intake of nutrients to allow your body to be as healthy as possible and to work as well as it can. It is not a set of rules. For example, you do not have to be vegetarian or take supplements, or to avoid eating any particular food, although for some people such advice would be appropriate. Your needs are completely unique and depend on a whole host of factors, from the strengths and weaknesses that you were born with right up to the effects that your current environment has on you. You only have to look at the tremendous variation in the way we look, and in our talents and personalities, to realise that our nutritional needs are also not likely to be identical. No one diet is perfect for everyone, although there are general guidelines that apply to us all.

Your optimum nutrition is the intake of nutrients that:

- Promotes your optimal mental performance and emotional balance.

- Promotes your optimal physical performance.

- Is associated with the lowest incidence of ill-health.

- Is associated with the longest healthy lifespan.

To date, fifty nutrients have been identified as essential for health. Your health can be promoted and maintained at the highest level if you are able to achieve your optimal intake of each nutrient every single day. Gradually, your entire body, including your skeleton, is rebuilt and rejuvenated. Through optimum nutrition you can:

- Improve mental clarity, mood and concentration.

- Increase IQ.

- Increase physical performance.

- Improve quality of sleep.

- Improve resistance to infections.

- Protect yourself from disease.

- Extend your healthy lifespan.

These might sound like bold claims, yet each has been proven by proper scientific research. Recently I rang up two doctors who had been in general practice for many years before discovering the optimum nutrition approach. One told me, 'I'm convinced that nutrition will be a major part of medicine in the foreseeable future. I'm getting substantially better results with diet and supplements than I used to with drugs.' The other, a GP in Dublin, said, 'The evidence for nutritional therapy is becoming so strong that if the doctors of today don't become nutritionists, the nutritionists will become the doctors of tomorrow.'

▪ The fifty essential nutrients

Fats	Amino acids	Minerals	Vitamins	Plus
Linoleic acid	Leucine	Calcium	A (retinol)	Carbohydrate
Linolenic acid	Lysine	Magnesium	B1 (thiamine)	Fibre
	Isoleudne	Phosphorus	B2 (riboflavin)	Light
	Threonine	Potassium	B3 (niacin)	Oxygen
	Tryptophan	Sodium	B5 (pantothenic acid)	Water
	Methionine	Sulphur	B6 (pyridoxine)	
	Valine	Iron	B12 (cyanocobalamine)	
	Phenylalanine	Zinc	Folic acid	
	Histidine	Copper	Biotin	
		Manganese	C	
		Chromium	D	
		Selenium	E	
		Cobalt	K	
		Fluorine		
		Silicon		
		Iodine		
		Molybdenum		
		?Vanadium		
		?Arsenic		
		?Nickel		
		?Tin		

NB: minerals preceded by a question mark are thought to be essential although studies have not yet confirmed this.

Discover your optimum nutrition

Old-fashioned concepts of nutrition assess your needs by analysing what you eat and comparing it with the RDA for each nutrient. This method is very basic since RDAs do not exist for a number of key nutrients; have little relevance to what is needed for optimal health; and do not take into account individual variations in need, or lifestyle factors that alter your needs, such as exposure to pollution, level of stress or exercise.

This book introduces you to the much more useful Optimum Daily Allowances (ODAs) and enables you to assess your optimum nutrition using three proven methods, each of which represents a piece of the jigsaw for calculating your needs. The more methods that can be used, the more effective will be the resultant nutritional plan. In addition, nutritional therapists have access to biochemical tests to find out more precisely what a person's nutritional needs are. The three methods listed below also take into account four key principles – evolutionary dynamics, biochemical individuality, synergy and environmental load – that are fundamental to the optimum nutrition approach and are explained in the following chapters.

Symptom analysis

This enables you to see, from clusters of signs and symptoms (such as lack of energy, mouth ulcers, muscle cramps, easy bruising, poor dream recall, and so on) which nutrients you may be lacking.

Lifestyle analysis

This helps you to identify the factors in your life that change your nutritional needs (such as your level of exercise, stress, pollution, and so on).

Dietary analysis

This compares your diet not with RDAs but with optimal levels of nutrients, and takes into account your consumption of 'anti-nutrients' – substances that rob the body of nutrients.

3.

From Monkeys to Man – Nutrition and Evolution

You are much older than you think. The human body you walk around in is the result of millions of years of evolution, the vast majority of which was spent living in an environment and eating a diet very different from those of today. Understanding the dynamics of our evolution can provide essential clues for promoting health.

To C or not to C?

Take the case of vitamin C. Practically all animals make it in their bodies, so they do not have to eat it. The exceptions are guinea pigs, fruit-eating bats, the red-vented bulbul bird and primates, including man. Most animals produce the equivalent of 3,000 to 16,000mg per day – a little different from the RDA of 60mg and more consistent with the levels known to boost immunity and minimise the risk of cancer. In fact, vitamin C-producing animals are immune to most cancers and viral diseases.

Linus Pauling postulated that we used to make vitamin C but, through eating a fruit-rich diet, lost the ability because we could get enough from our food. Indeed, one characteristic shared by us and other species that have lost this ability is our previously high fruit diet. Now, however, most humans live in a concrete jungle and are prone to vitamin C deficiency, as illustrated by the high incidence of infections and diseases that are associated with poorly functioning immune systems. While a gorilla can eat up to 3,000mg a day (the equivalent of sixty-six supermarket oranges), many children eat, on average, one piece of fruit a week, giving 30mg of vitamin C, while the average adult intake of vitamin C is around three pieces of fruit, or 90mg. This low level contradicts our evolutionary design and is simply not enough for optimal health. Since humans in all age groups are smaller than gorillas, eating twenty-two oranges might be more appropriate – but taking a 1 gram vitamin C tablet is certainly a lot easier!

Homo aquaticus

One of the great mysteries of human evolution concerns how we became upright and developed complex brains, manual dexterity and the ability to use language. We have a brain that is ten times larger, in relation to body mass, than the brains of almost all other animals alongside which we have evolved. While it is accepted that we share many characteristics with tree-dwelling primates, for example the 'gripping' reflex of infant chimps and humans that is good for swinging on branches, how did we develop the characteristics that make us human?

One theory that is rapidly gaining credence in scientific circles is that our early ancestors may have picked the best neighbourhood as far as nutrition was concerned. According to Professor Michael Crawford and David Marsh, authors of *Nutrition and Evolution*, the environment in which a species develops is a major factor in determining its evolution. Derek Ellis, Professor of Biology at the University of Victoria in Canada, believes that for a critical period in our ancestors' evolution they exploited the nutrient-rich environment of the water's edge, eating shellfish, crustaceans and fish, and therefore consumed the high levels of essential fats and nutrients needed to develop modern man's complex brain and nervous system, which is paralleled only in aquatic mammals.[6]

This would certainly explain the one big chemical difference between human brains and those of other animals – the high concentration of complex essential fats that make up a large part of the human brain. These authors believe that early man may have needed to wade in water to access the food supply. This may also explain why we became upright, lost our hair and developed a layer of subcutaneous fat, making humans one of the few species prone to obesity.[7] In the course of time these characteristics would have allowed us to survive better in a semi-aquatic environment.

This theory can also explain the extraordinary 'diving reflex' of an infant in the first six months of life. If dropped into water an infant will submerge, stop breathing, slow down its heart rate, then re-emerge, turn its head to the side, breathe and dive again. This reflex is similar to that of aquatic mammals like dolphins – whose flippers, incidentally, contain every single bone that we have in our arms and hands. The evidence suggests that they evolved on land, then returned to the sea to stay there. Ever wondered what it is you love about being in water?

Clues from the past – hope for the future

While these theories are now starting to gain scientific acceptance, supporters of the *Homo aquaticus* theory, such as Professor Michael Crawford, a zoologist now specialising in brain biochemistry, have shown that, for proper mental development, infants need a very high level of the essential fats found in fish. These fats, formerly excluded from formula milk for babies, are now being added after recommendations from the World Health Organisation. Other sources of these essential fats are seeds and their oils, vital for both infants and mothers. Breastfeeding mothers who are 'fat-phobic' for fear of gaining weight need to eat seafood or seeds and their oils, both for their own health and to support the development of their children's brains. If they don't their children's mental development will suffer. Remarkably, the amount of DHA, a type of Omega 3 fat, in the umbilical cords of newborn babies correlates with their mental abilities at age eight, while supplementing either mother during pregnancy or child in early infancy has clear benefits on subsequent mental development.[8]

Out of sync with nature

In many ways modern living goes against the grain of millions of years of evolution. For instance, if you jolt into action in the morning to the sound of the alarm clock and head on remote control for the kitchen, with neither brain nor body responding, to make a strong cup of coffee or smoke a cigarette, followed by two pieces of toast with marmalade and a glass of orange juice, you, like most people, are living out of line with your natural design. The result can be poor concentration, insomnia, fluctuating 'highs' and 'lows', energy drops, food cravings, uneven weight, feelings of stress and, inevitably, life-threatening illness.

Our ancestors had no alarm clocks. At dawn, light enters through the eyes and translucent portions of the skull to stimulate the pineal and pituitary glands, which in turn stimulate the adrenal glands to release adrenalin into the bloodstream. As adrenalin levels rise we wake up naturally, refreshed and alert. Not so if we wake in the dark to the sound of the alarm clock. Instead of allowing the body to respond naturally we load in a stimulant like caffeine or nicotine. The effect on the body is adrenalin overload. Sure, you wake up – but the body's chemistry scrambles to produce hormones such as insulin and glucagon to restabilise soaring blood sugar levels. So let the light in and get up early if you want to experience more energy.

Grazing or gorging?

Nor are we really designed to eat as soon as we wake up. Little digestion will have occurred when the body was asleep. It is better not to eat until you are totally awake, perhaps an hour after waking. Another way to encourage the body to wake up is to have a brief cold shower after a hot shower, which stimulates circulation and digestion. Even then, most people function better on easy-to-digest carbohydrate-based breakfasts such as fruit or cereal, rather than high-protein cooked breakfasts.

Breakfast – in fact all meals – should be light. We are designed to graze, not gorge. Large meals are hard to digest and can result in indigestion and sleepiness. Our ancestors ate when hungry, not at set times or as emotional compensation. Studies comparing the effects of eating little and often with those of eating two or three large meals a day have consistently shown that better health is the result of small, frequent meals.[9] Just as our jungle ancestors did, this means snacking on fresh fruit – three to four pieces a day between (smaller) meals. Doing this also helps to keep our blood sugar levels even, resulting in more consistent energy, moods and concentration.

Exercise is another great appetite stabiliser. People with sedentary lifestyles tend to have poor appetite control and will actually eat more calories compared to their expenditure than those with active lifestyles. Physical activity appears to be essential to balance appetite in line with body needs.

Against the grain

Modern humans' pattern of eating has totally changed, and so too has the food we select. Primates are designed to run on carbohydrates and have a naturally sweet tooth. However, we have learnt to cheat nature and isolate the sweetness from foods, as well as choosing foods with concentrated sweetness such as juice, dried fruit and honey. These foods are too sweet for the body to deal with.

One of the most common ways we now eat carbohydrates is in grains, especially wheat. Since wheat is such a staple food in our diet, with 600 million tons eaten annually making up about half of the calorie intake of the average person's diet, the idea that it isn't good for you may be difficult to swallow. Yet two top medical experts, Dr James Braly and Ron Hoggan, say just that in their groundbreaking book *Dangerous Grains*.[10]

The old view was that about one in a thousand people had coeliac disease, a digestive disorder caused by sensitivity to gluten. What Braly's research now shows is that coeliac disease affects almost one in a hundred people, while gluten sensitivity affects possibly as many as one in ten, often with no digestive symptoms at all. For some, gluten sensitivity means feeling tired all the time, for others, feeling depressed.

What are the symptoms? The table below gives the most common symptoms of gluten sensitivity. While digestive problems are common among those sensitive to gluten, more gluten-sensitive people have no digestive symptoms at all. If you have a number of these symptoms, or risk factors, I strongly advise you to get tested.

Common symptoms of gluten sensitivity

Upper respiratory tract problems like sinusitis and 'glue' ear.

Malabsorption problems causing fatigue, anaemia, osteoporosis, weight loss.

Diarrhoea, constipation, bloating, Crohn's disease, diverticulitis.

Depression, behavioural problems in children, chronic fatigue syndrome, attention deficit disorder.

Why would this be? Well, our distant ancestors ate almost no gluten grains. Grains started to be cultivated only 10,000 years ago, and even then, only in some parts of the world. The American continent, for example, had no gluten grains until they were introduced a few hundred years ago. This is far too short a time to go from hunter-gatherer to 'canary' and expect the body to genetically adapt. Many of us have simply not yet adapted to tolerate grains, unlike ruminant animals that live off grasses and grains.

This may explain why grain allergy is so widespread. Of all the grains, wheat is the number-one culprit. Modern wheat is also very different from the wheat that grew in the Bronze Age and before. A substance called gluten constitutes 78 per cent of the total protein in modern wheat. There is now plenty of research that shows that it is the specific 'sub-set' of gluten, gliadin, that is an intestinal irritant and causes allergic reactions. The body literally reacts to it as if it were an invader. When yeast reacts with sugar it produces bubbles of gas that expand more easily the more gluten there is in the dough. So the higher the gluten content, the 'lighter' the loaf, but the harder it is on our intestines. Adverse reactions to bread are far more common than to pasta, which is often made from 'hard' wheat with a lower gluten content. This may also be because bread contains yeast (which pasta doesn't), which is another common allergen.

While gluten is the key protein in wheat, it's also found in rye, spelt, barley and oats. Generally, people who are gluten-sensitive should start by avoiding all gluten grains. Gliadin is not found in oats. Therefore, if you feel much better off all grains it's worth reintroducing oats and seeing what happens.

The same story could be told for dairy products. Our ancestors certainly weren't milking buffaloes. (More on this in Chapter 8.)

Raw or cooked?

Another relatively recent addition to the kitchen is heat. Humans discovered fire 400,000 years ago, but even then still ate most of their food raw. For millions of years before then, everything was eaten raw. Cooking changes the molecules in food and destroys many valuable nutrients and the enzymes that break food down into components that can be used by the body, so a natural diet includes a lot of food that is raw or only very lightly cooked. Raw food requires more chewing than cooked food. This not only breaks down food, mixing it with digestive enzymes in the mouth, but also sends signals to the digestive tract to enable the right cocktail of digestive enzymes to be produced, depending on what is in the mouth. Most fast food is soft food that requires minimal chewing; as a result, the jaws of modern humans are smaller than those of our ancestors.

The evolutionary diet

What you have just read are a few examples of the principle of evolutionary dynamics, which is fundamental to the optimum nutrition approach. They also illustrate clearly how we are digging our own graves with a knife and fork, choosing high-sugar, high-fat, highly processed and synthetic food. By investigating what our ancestors ate and how our bodies have adapted to these foods, we can pick up vital clues about the kind of nutrition that is likely to promote our health.

Current theories suggest that early primate evolution took place in the jungle, which provided a carbohydrate-rich diet of fruit and other vegetation. This diet would have yielded substantially larger amounts of vitamins and minerals than our modern diet does. For example, the estimated intake of vitamin A in those times, principally from betacarotene, was above 9,000mcg a day, more than twenty times today's average. The meat our ancestors ate was also fit and organic, not fat and full of anti-biotics, hormones and pesticide residues.

In addition, through the study of evolution it becomes clear that the environment we choose determines our diet, which alters our design and prospects for future survival. Humans now have the ability to manipulate the environment in ways never before possible, and we can choose exactly what we eat. Will we choose to nourish ourselves in a way that does not plunder the resources of the earth? Or will we continue to pollute, overpopulate and plunder the earth? If we choose the latter option the earth and those species best adapted to the changes will continue to exist, but humanity may not. If we opt for the former choice, what a wonderful world this could be. Good planets are, after all, hard to find!

Here are a few simple tips to help you conform to your natural design:

- Get up earlier in summer and later in winter, in line with natural sunlight hours. Don't eat late at night, or before you're fully awake.

- Eat when you are hungry, not out of habit. Graze rather than gorge. Eat little and often, with plenty of fruit as snacks in between.

- Eat a mainly vegan diet, with half your intake of food consisting of fruit, vegetables, seed sprouts, nuts and seeds. If you do eat meat, avoid the intensively reared kind. Choose fish or organic game instead. Eat these foods only with vegetables.

- Eat food as raw and unprocessed as possible. Avoid synthetic chemicals.

- Avoid concentrated foods such as sugar and sweeteners. Dilute fruit juices. Drink plenty of water.

- Minimise your intake of dairy foods, refined wheat and grains.

- Take frequent exercise and keep active.

chapter 4

You Are Unique

There is nobody quite like you. There are many principles that apply to us all as members of the human race – for example, we all need vitamins; but the actual amount we need for peak performance varies from individual to individual. It depends on the evolutionary dynamics that you have inherited from your parents, together with genetically inherited strengths and weaknesses, and the interaction of your genetics with your environment right through foetal development and early infancy. The complex interaction of these factors ensures that each individual is born biochemically unique, although clearly similar to other individuals.

This principle, called biochemical individuality, was first succinctly proposed by Dr Roger Williams in 1956. Dr Williams also discovered vitamin B5 (pantothenic acid) and helped isolate folic acid. He was one of the grandfathers of optimum nutrition. True to form, he was actively teaching, writing and researching into his nineties. In his book *Biochemical Individuality* he showed how in each one of us our organs are different shapes and sizes, how we have different levels of enzymes and different needs for protein, vitamins and minerals. A ten-fold difference in the requirement for vitamins from one person to the next is not at all uncommon. For example, a comparison of the level of vitamin A in the blood of ninety-two individuals, most of whom were on a very similar diet, found a thirty-fold difference. Repeated testing revealed that individuals' blood level of vitamin A stayed remarkably consistent, although the levels from individual to individual varied considerably.[11] This suggests a wide range of need for vitamin A – a fact ignored by today's RDAs.

Some of us have difficulty digesting protein or fat, or need more of a particular vitamin than the average diet can supply. This is well illustrated by the vitamin-deficiency disease pellagra, whose symptoms include mental illness, sometimes accompanied by digestive and skin problems. For most people a mere 10mg a day of vitamin B3 (niacin) will prevent pellagra. That is the amount you would find in a serving of rice or a handful of peanuts. Yet Dr Abram Hoffer, psychiatric research director for the province of Saskatchewan in Canada, found that many patients diagnosed with schizophrenia got better and stayed better only when given 1,000mg or more a day.[12] These people needed a hundred times more than the average level to stay healthy.

Once again this kind of information makes a mockery of RDAs, nicknamed 'Ridiculous Dietary Arbitraries' by Dr Stephen Davies, a leading nutrition researcher in London. How do you know if these government-set averages, which vary from country to country, are the right amounts for you? I guarantee they are not.

From the cradle to the grave

What happens during pregnancy and early childhood has a profound effect on health in later life. In fact the risk of cardiovascular disease increases substantially for those whose birth weight is low, according to research by Professor David Barker at the Medical Research Council Environmental Epidemiology Unit in Southampton.[13] Professor Derek Bryce-Smith from the University of Reading found that, simply by analysing the level of lead, cadmium and zinc in placental tissue, he could predict with remarkable accuracy the birth weight and head circumference of a newborn baby.[14] That means that if your mother was exposed to exhaust fumes containing lead, or to cigarette smoke that contains cadmium, or was zinc-deficient, it will have taken its toll on you. Professor Bryce-Smith concluded from his research that any child born below a weight of 6.9lb should be investigated for sub-optimum nutrition.

One man's food . . .

According to the Royal College of Physicians, one in three people suffer from allergies at some point in their lives, with foods being the most common provokers of allergic symptoms. As Lucretius said in 50 BC, 'One man's food is another man's poison.'

Most of the symptoms do not occur immediately after eating an offending food, but creep up on you over a twenty-four-hour period, so it is easy to live for years without knowing that a particular food does not suit you. What is more, many people may never have felt truly healthy, so do not even know that how they feel is under par.

These are just a few examples that illustrate how each person's optimum nutrition is likely to be slightly different from anyone else's. This book will give you the opportunity to investigate the major lifestyle factors that shape your nutritional needs and to assess your personal nutritional needs on the basis of your symptoms, not according to some arbitrary general guideline. From then on it is a matter of educated trial and error, and noticing which foods make you feel good and which ones take your energy away.

Symptoms linked to food allergy

Anxiety	Diarrhoea
Arthritis	Ear infections
Asthma	Eczema/dermatitis
Attention deficit	Hay fever
Bedwetting	Headaches
Bloating	Inflammatory bowel disease
Bronchitis	Insomnia
Chronic fatigue syndrome	Learning disorders
Coeliac disease	Multiple sclerosis
Colitis	Rhinitis
Crohn's disease	Sleep disorders
Depression	Tonsillitis
Diabetes	Weight gain

Here are a few simple tips to help you work with your biochemical individuality:

● Notice after which meals you feel worse. Look for the common foods, eliminate for two weeks, then see how you feel.

● Just because others can tolerate a certain food does not mean that you can.

● Assess your own nutritional needs (see Part 6) and supplement the recommended nutrients until you are feeling healthy, full of energy and symptom-free.

● Find out what lifestyle works best for you and adjust your life accordingly.

● If you have a family history of particular health problems, pay particular attention to the prevention tips in this book and adjust your nutrition accordingly.

● Listen to your body. It will tell you more than all the experts will.

chapter 5

Synergy – the Whole Is Greater

The science fiction of the 1960s envisaged a future in which humans would simply eat pills or powder containing the finite number of nutrients proved to be essential for the human machine to function. Yet, as each decade passes, we learn more and more about the complexities of the human body and nutrition. Of the fifty currently known essential nutrients (see page 14), all interact with other nutrients and can be said to work in synergy.

Knowing this, it would be unrealistic to deprive a body of one nutrient, for experimental purposes, or to prescribe one nutrient for the treatment of disease. For example, deficiencies of vitamin B6, B12, folic acid, iron, zinc and manganese can all contribute to anaemia. Indeed, in some circumstances prescribing one nutrient can exacerbate deficiency of another. Iron is, for example, a zinc antagonist. Both are frequently deficient. Prescribing excessive amounts of iron exacerbates an undiagnosed or untreated zinc deficiency. Since zinc is a critical nutrient for foetal development, this could have serious detrimental effects during pregnancy.

Greater than the sum of the parts

Some nutrients simply will not work without their synergistic mates. Vitamin B6, pyridoxine, is useless in the body until it is converted into pyridoxal-5-phosphate, a job done by a zinc- and magnesium-dependent enzyme. If you are zinc or magnesium deficient and take a vitamin B6 supplement to help relieve pre-menstrual syndrome (PMS), it may not make any difference. Studies have shown that giving women zinc, magnesium and B6 relieves the symptoms of PMS much more effectively.

The vast majority of research in nutrition, however, has looked at the effects on health of a single nutrient. The results are not comparable with the effects of giving a person optimum nutrition, the right balance of all essential nutrients. For instance, there is little evidence that individual vitamins or minerals can increase IQ scores in children. However, the combination of all vitamins and minerals, even if given only at RDA levels, has consistently been shown to produce a four- to five-point increase in children's IQ scores.[15] Similar combinations of vitamins, minerals and essential fats have produced massive reductions in aggression in prison inmates, compared with placebo, in only two weeks.[16] These kinds of results are simply not seen with individual nutrients.

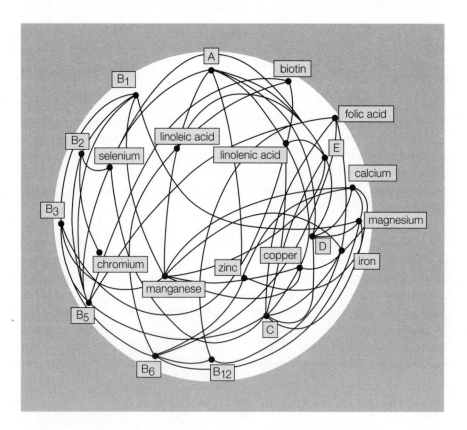

Many nutrients work together to keep you healthy

There are now hundreds of studies that show that the right nutrients in combination can produce improvements in health of a different league from those provided by individual nutrients. A classic example is the combination of B vitamins needed to lower homocysteine. This toxic protein in the blood is an incredible predictor of disease risk, not only for cardiovascular disease, but also for depression, Alzheimer's disease, miscarriage and the risk of birth defects and many more conditions (see Chapter 16). Lowering homocysteine, and hence lowering risk, is easy if you know how. You need an optimal intake of vitamins B6, B12 and folic acid, plus B2, zinc, magnesium and trimethyl glycine (TMG).

Few medical studies, however, have taken this on board. Most just indicate that folic acid should be taken. This, by the way, is why folic acid is given during pregnancy – to lower homocysteine and reduce the risk of birth defects. So, let's take a look at what happens if you give one, two, three or all of these nutrients together. In a research study in Japan, patients with kidney disease, a condition strongly linked to high homocysteine, were divided into four groups: one was given folic acid alone, another B12 alone, another folic acid and B12 together, and another folic acid, B12 and B6 together. The trial lasted for three weeks.[17]

Here are the results of this remarkable study:

Supplement group	Homocysteine change
Folic acid alone	17.3% reduction
B12 alone	18.7% reduction
Folic acid plus B12	57.4% reduction
Folate, B12 and B6	59.9% reduction

Notice that this extraordinary study revealed two very important principles:

- That the more nutrients were provided, the greater was the reduction in homocysteine.

- That the right combination of nutrients at the right dose can more than halve your hymocysteine level, and your risk for homocysteine-related conditions such as heart attack and stroke, in as little as three weeks!

Notice also that no group was given *all* the nutrients that lower homocysteine, including B2, zinc, magnesium and TMG. So we took six volunteers with raised homocysteine levels and gave them these nutrients. Their homocysteine levels dropped by 77 per cent – more than four times as effective as the conventional medical prescription of folic acid to lower homocysteine. That is the power of synergy and that is why the results provided by 'optimum nutrition' are in a different league from those you read about in 'single-nutrient' trials designed by 'pill for an ill' medics.

Another example of this is provided by the interplay of 'antioxidant' nutrients such as vitamins C and E, betacarotene and others such as glutathione, co-enzyme Q10, lipoic acid and anthocyanidins, which are rich in berries. They have some effect in isolation but are much more effective when they work together. They, like all nutrients, are team players.

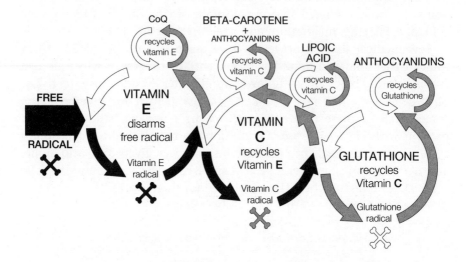

How antioxidants work together. A free radical, for example from a French fry/chip, is disarmed by vitamin E, which is recycled by vitamin C, which is recycled by glutathione, which is recycled by anthocyanidins. Co-enzyme Q10, betacarotene and lipoic acid also help. These are the essential antioxidants and they work together.

In the figure above you can see why. Free-oxidising radicals, sometimes called 'free radicals' or 'oxidants', are the bad guys produced from anything burnt, be it a cigarette, exhaust fumes, fried fat or burnt meat. The free radicals are like red-hot sparks that can damage your body. The antioxidants are like flame-proof gloves that pass these hot potatoes along the line, gradually dissipating their potentially damaging properties. You need all of them to do the job properly and that's why I pay less attention to studies just using one nutrient than to multi-nutrient approaches.

The principle of synergy is a fundamental aspect of the optimum nutrition approach. This book enables you to assess your own needs taking into account the principle of synergy. You may achieve better results by eating the right foods and taking the right combination of nutrients at lower doses than those you have supplemented before. Such is the power of the synergistic effect of nutrients.

Here are a few tips to bear in mind:

- There is no substitute for 'whole foods' (any unrefined and unprocessed foods), which contain hundreds of health-promoting substances, the importance of many of which we have yet to discover.

- Eat a varied diet, choosing from a wide range of different kinds of food.

- Do not supplement your diet with individual nutrients without also taking a good all-round multivitamin and mineral supplement.

- Do not take a large amount of an individual B vitamin without also taking a B complex or a multivitamin.

- Do not supplement your diet with a large amount of an isolated antioxidant nutrient (e.g. vitamin C, E or betacarotene) without also taking a good all-round multivitamin or antioxidant formula.

chapter 6

Anti-nutrients – Avoiding the Vitamin Robbers

O ptimum nutrition is not just about what you eat – what you do not eat is equally important. Since the 1950s over 3,500 man-made chemicals have found their way into manufactured food, along with pesticides, antibiotics and hormone residues from staple foods such as grains and meat. Many of these chemicals are 'anti-nutrients' in that they stop nutrients being absorbed and used, or promote their excretion.

Gone are the days when healthy eating meant simply getting the right balance of nutrients from your food. Now an equally important part of the equation is avoiding harmful chemicals and protecting yourself against those that cannot be avoided. Many of today's diseases are caused just as much by an excess of anti-nutrients as by a deficiency of nutrients. Take cancer, for example. Three-quarters of all cancers are associated with an excess of anti-nutrients, be it cancer-causing chemicals or excessive free radicals as a result of smoking. Many health problems, from arthritis to chronic fatigue, can follow from an overload of anti-nutrients exceeding the body's capacity to detoxify itself. Once this threshold is exceeded, toxins such as pesticide residues accumulate in fat tissue, common drugs from alcohol to painkillers become increasingly toxic, and even the otherwise harmless by-products of the body making energy from carbohydrates start to accumulate, bringing on muscle aches and fatigue.

Nowadays in the UK alone we get through every year a staggering quarter of a million tons of food chemicals, 6 billion alcoholic drinks,

75 billion cigarettes, 80 million prescriptions for painkillers and 50 million prescriptions for antibiotics. In addition, 50,000 chemicals are released into the environment by industry and 400 million litres of pesticides and herbicides are sprayed on to food and pastures. Together, this constitutes a staggering onslaught of man-made chemicals and pollutants, with undeniable global health and environmental repercussions.

Making up the deficit

Even refined food that is free from artificial additives is not neutral. Any food you eat that requires more nutrients for the body to make use of it than the food itself provides is effectively an anti-nutrient. Living on these foods gradually robs the body of vital nutrients. In fact, two-thirds of the calories in the average person's diet in the Western world comes from these foods. That leaves one-third of the diet to provide not only enough nutrients for general health, but also enough to make up the deficit resulting from nutrient-deficient food and to combat other anti-nutrients from car pollution to pesticides.

Exactly what extra quantities of key nutrients we need to combat these anti-nutrients is not known, but it is certainly well in excess of RDA levels. Take vitamin C, for example. How much does a smoker need to consume every day to have the same blood level of vitamin C as a non-smoker, assuming they both start with the same dietary intake equivalent to the RDA level? The answer is in excess of 200mg, roughly quadruple the RDA, according to research by Dr Gerald Schectman and colleagues at the Medical College of Wisconsin.[18] The same is true if you compare heavy drinkers with teetotallers. A heavy drinker needs to take in at least 500mg a day, six times the RDA, to have the same vitamin C blood level as a non-drinker. And what about pollution? If you live or work in an inner city, what is your need for antioxidant protection? Certainly it will be higher than the RDA and, in the case of vitamin C, which detoxifies over fifty undesirable substances including exhaust fumes, a daily intake of 1,000mg (1 gram) is more likely to be optimal.

Chemical self-defence

To a large extent man-made chemicals have been allowed into the food chain as long as they have not been associated with any health risks. Their 'anti-nutrient' status has never been an issue. Tartrazine or E102, one of the more common food-colouring agents, is a case in point. It has long been known to cause allergic reactions and hyperactivity in sensitive children, and Dr Neil Ward and his team from the University of Surrey wanted to know why.[19] They gave two groups of children identical-looking and -tasting drinks, except that one contained tartrazine. They measured the children's mineral levels before and after they consumed the drink. Those who had the drink containing tartrazine became hyperactive and exhibited a decrease in their blood levels of zinc and an increase in the amount of zinc excreted in the urine. What the researchers had found was that tartrazine robbed the children of zinc, a deficiency of which is associated with increased risk of behavioural and immune-system problems.

This is only one of hundreds of food chemicals to be tested in this way and, of course, it begs the question as to what safety criteria a chemical must meet before being allowed to enter the food chain. Or are new chemicals simply innocent until proven guilty? While the legislation on 'novel foods' is becoming more stringent, the concept of testing for anti-nutrient effects is not yet on the checklist.

The pesticide problem

Labelling on food does not tell you everything. Unless you eat only organic food, one in three of all the foods you eat contains traces of pesticides.[20] In fact, the amount of fruit and vegetables consumed by the average person in a year has the equivalent of up to one gallon of pesticides sprayed on it.

The first family of pesticides were organochlorines. These proved so toxic and non-biodegradable that most have been banned in Europe (though not in many exporting developing countries). They were replaced by organophosphates, and in the UK alone more than twenty-five tonnes of pesticides are now applied to crops every year. Many of these compounds are known to be carcinogenic, linked to birth defects or decreased fertility, and toxic to the brain and nervous system. Pesticide exposure is associated with depression, memory decline, aggressive outbursts and Parkinson's disease. According to Professor William Rea, director of the Environmental Health Center in Dallas, Texas, it is also linked with asthma, eczema, migraine, irritable bowel syndrome and rhinitis. We are exposed to pesticides not just in our food but also in our homes via pest control, as well as in the wider environment, especially if we live in or near agricultural areas, where there are now numerous campaigns to ban pesticide sprays drifting over neighbouring communities.

You may be wondering why the government allows pesticides in foods, if they are so harmful. The argument given is that at very low levels they are not harmful to humans, yet the tests used to establish the safety levels are done only on individual pesticides. No one has tested or can test the infinite number of combinations of pesticides we are all regularly exposed to. In 1998 three of every four lettuces tested carried more than one pesticide residue, and up to seven different compounds were found on individual lettuces.[21] Multiple residues on other foods including apples, pears, carrots, oranges, celery and strawberries are common, and of course several different foods are usually eaten at any given meal. It all adds up to a cocktail of pesticide residues, the combined toxicity of which is almost completely unknown.

Studies have shown that pesticides may be hundreds of times more toxic in combination than the same compounds alone.[22] Also, individuals with poor detox function, the young, the elderly and the stressed are far more susceptible to toxins than the average healthy adult, so 'safety levels' are relatively meaningless for many. Washing produce with water has little effect on these residues as most are formulated to resist being washed off by the rain. Tests with potatoes, apples and broccoli have shown that between 50 and 93 per cent of residues remained on produce after washing with water.[23] You should aim to reduce your exposure to pesticides in your diet by choosing organic foods as often as you can.

Genetically engineered food

The long-term consequences on the eco-system and on our health of genetically modified (GM) foods are also unknown. One of the main aims of the genetic engineers is to make crops such as soya or corn resistant to particular types of herbicide. In other words, the crop can be sprayed, all weeds will die, the plant will be contaminated and the yield will be increased. Guess who profits from the increased sales of the herbicides and the GM seeds?

The biotechnology industry asserts that GM technology will reduce the use of herbicides on crops, yet analyses of the US agricultural industry show that the use of herbicides has actually increased significantly since GM planting started in 1996. Although herbicide use decreased slightly in the first three years of GM crop-growing, use increased subsequently. During 2002 and 2003 in the US, an average of 29 per cent more herbicide was applied per acre on GM herbicide-tolerant corn than on non-GM corn. Dr Charles Benbrook of the Northwest Science and Environmental Policy Center in Idaho, USA, points out that GM 'herbicide tolerant crops have increased pesticide use an estimated 70 million pounds over the first eight years of cultivation'.[24]

We, the consumers, pay the price, while the farmers and agrochemical companies (who own both the patent for the new strain of soya and the herbicide to which it is resistant) profit – and we are told that this technological advance is for the benefit of humanity! Consumer groups are campaigning for clear labelling to state when a food contains genetically engineered ingredients, and consumers are advised to avoid these products. Because pollen is carried by bees, insects and the wind, contamination of other crops, including organic ones, will be inevitable if GM crops become widely grown.

The implications for human health and the environment remain unknown, though there are concerns that GM food could pose a serious health risk, with possible health problems involving antibiotic resistance, the creation of new toxins and unexpected allergic reactions. The reality is that these concerns remain largely speculative because no one can predict what the outcome of the introduction of GM food into the food chain will be. No adequate safety tests have been carried out and no one is monitoring the impact of GM food on the diets of those countries now selling significant quantities of GM products for human consumption. Far too little is known about genes and DNA to predict what the possible unexpected effects of genetic engineering will be.

The only known trial of GM food on humans was commissioned by the UK government's Food Standards Agency and carried out by the University of Newcastle in 2002. Seven people were given a meal containing GM soya. It was found that in at least three people the GM material moved out of the food and entered their gut bacteria after only one meal! A Faustian feast, no less. Our gut bacteria perform an important role in digestion and any changes to their characteristics are a cause for concern.

Is your water fit to drink?

Water is not simply H_2O. Natural water provides significant quantities of minerals: a typical spring water, for instance, provides 100mg of calcium per litre. The recommended daily intake of water is at least 1.5–2 litres a day (that's eight glasses), while for calcium it is 600mg. So natural mineral water can provide a sixth of your calcium requirements. However, not all bottled water is the same. In the European Union (EU) only water that comes from an uncontaminated spring that has a consistent level of minerals across the seasons and the years (which means the source of the water is very deep and hence the water is very old) can be called 'natural mineral water'. Other bottled water is not as reliable.

Tap water in a soft-water area provides as little as 30mg of calcium a day. In addition, tap water contains significant levels of nitrates, trihalomethanes, lead and aluminium, all anti-nutrients in their own right. In much of Britain and the US the levels of these anti-nutrients exceed safety limits. Approximately a quarter of all British tap water contains pesticides at levels above Maximum Admissible Concentrations set by the EU for our safety. Concerns over pollutants in water have led many people to switch to bottled, distilled or filtered water. However, filtering or distilling water removes not only the impurities, but also many of the naturally occurring minerals. This again pushes up the need for minerals from food.

Out of the frying pan

What we do to food in the kitchen can alter the balance between nutrients and anti-nutrients. Frying food in oil produces what are known as free radicals, highly reactive chemicals that destroy essential fats in food and can damage cells, increasing the risk of cancer, heart disease and premature ageing, as well as destroying the very nutrients, such as vitamins A and E, that protect us from these dangerous substances.

The damaging effects of frying depend on the oil type, the temperature of the oil and the length of time the food is fried. Ironically, it is the good polyunsaturated oils (see page 69) that oxidise most rapidly, becoming undesirable 'trans' fats. Frying with butter or coconut (saturated fat) or olive oil (monounsaturated fat) is therefore safer. Deep-frying is much worse than a two-minute sauté, followed by adding a water-based sauce and putting a lid on the pan so that the food 'steam-fries' at a much lower temperature. Grilling, steaming, boiling or baking, however, are better cooking methods than any form of frying. Finally, any form of overcooking will increasingly reduce the nutrient content of the food.

We used to think that the main danger of frying was that fats cooked at high temperatures produce oxidants that are powerful cancer-promoting chemicals, hence the very strong association with burnt meat, rich in fat, whether fried or barbecued. However, alarming research has found another cancer-promoting substance, acrylamide, in foods cooked at high temperatures, with or without fat. While the safe limit set for acrylamide in food is ten parts per billion (ppb), chips and crisps have been found to contain more than 100 times this amount!

The worst foods are fast-food-chain chips, crisps and crispbread. According to UK research Walkers crisps averaged 1,250ppb and Pringles 1,480ppb in surveys conducted in 2003. Ryvita contained between 1,340 and 4,000ppb. In America, McDonald's French fries, followed by Burger King's, came out worst. However, even home-cooked chips were found to be high. Acrylamide is produced by frying, barbecuing, baking and even microwaving.

Anything browned or burnt, or cooked or processed using high heat, is therefore likely to be bad for you. The bottom line is: eat more raw food, and steam-fry or boil it, rather than cook it at a high heat. To steam-fry foods rather than stir-fry them, add a very small amount of olive oil to a pan and sauté the ingredients for literally a minute, just enough to generate enough heat so that you can then add a water-based sauce, such as one-third soya sauce, lemon juice and water. This then steams the food when you put on the lid, and gives you hot, steamed food, full of flavour, but not full of oxidants or acrylamide because nothing is burnt.

■ Acrylamide in your food

Ross frying chips – overcooked	12,000
Ryvita – dark, wholemeal rye	4,000
Ross frying chips – cooked	3,500
Home-made deep-fried chips	3,500
Ryvita – rye	2,400
Pringles	1,500
Walkers crisps	1,250
Kellogg's Special K	250
Kellogg's Rice Krispies	150

Source: Food Standards Agency – see
www.foodstandards.gov.uk/news/newsarchive/65268

It is not just what is in your food that matters – what your food is in is also important. The mid-1990s scare concerning phthalates, substances used to soften plastics, being found in nine brands of infant food begged the question as to how significant quantities of such hormone-disrupting chemicals are finding their way into the food chain. Inspection of an average shopping trolley will tell you how. Not only is fresh produce usually wrapped in soft plastics, but so also are drinks in cartons, which contain an inner plastic lining. An analysis of twenty brands of food in cans, now also lined with plastic, found significant levels of Bisphenol-A – some twenty-seven times higher than levels known to cause breast cancer cells to proliferate.

Unfortunately, plastics manufacturers are not required to state which chemicals are present in their products. Also, while the list of hormone-disrupting chemicals is growing, there is as yet no definitive list of what we should be avoiding and what is safe. For now, the best advice is to minimise the amount of food, especially wet or fatty food, that you buy in direct contact with soft plastic. Hard plastic is less likely to be a problem. So store cheese, for example, in a plastic container rather than wrapping it in plastic film, although you can now get 'non-PVC' cling film.

■ What's your anti-nutrient load?

Score 1 point for each 'yes' answer

☐ Do you drink tap water?

☐ Is more than half the food you eat not organic?

☐ Do you spend an hour or more a day in traffic?

☐ Do you live in a city?

☐ Do you smoke, or live or work with smokers?

☐ Do you often eat fried food?

☐ Do you eat non-organic meat or fish or large fish like tuna or swordfish?

☐ Do you take more than twenty painkillers in a year?

☐ Do you take, on average, one course of antibiotics each year?

☐ Is most of the food you eat or drink in contact with soft plastic or cling film?

☐ Do have an alcoholic drink on most days?

The ideal score is **0**. A score of **5** or more means you are likely to be taking in a significant quantity of anti-nutrients. Any 'yes' answer highlights areas in your diet and lifestyle that warrant attention.

Minimise pharmaceutical drugs

Many common medicines are also anti-nutrients. In the UK alone 650 million prescriptions are written every year, and the total cost has doubled in the last ten years to £7 billion. The US annual drug bill is a staggering $200 billion.

In the UK £260 million is spent each year on painkillers such as aspirin and paracetamol.

Salicylic acid, the active ingredient in aspirin and other painkillers, is a gastrointestinal irritant, increasing the permeability of the gut wall. This in turn upsets the absorption of nutrients, allowing incompletely digested foods to pass into the bloodstream, alerting the immune system and triggering allergy responses to common foods. In the long term this weakens the immune system, encourages inflammation and burns up vital vitamins and minerals needed for healthy immunity, as well as triggering intestinal bleeding.

The alternative is paracetamol, of which four billion tablets are taken worldwide every year. While paracetamol does not irritate the gut like aspirin, it is bad news for the liver. As a result, in the UK alone 30,000 people a year end up in hospital as a result of taking paracetamol. In 1994 in the UK 115 paracetamol-related deaths were reported. According to Professor Sir David Carter of Edinburgh University, one in ten liver transplants is made necessary because of damage caused by paracetamol overdose. While twenty paracetamol can kill you, even one is extra work for the liver. If a person takes six a day and lacks the nutrients that help the liver to detoxify, this can reduce their ability to deal with other toxins such as alcohol. The combination of alcohol and paracetamol is particularly dangerous; paracetamol produces a toxic by-product that can be broken down by the liver only if the body contains sufficient stores of the amino acid glutathione. If you run out, the result is trouble.

Many common drugs have direct or knock-on effects on your nutritional status. Antibiotics, for example, wipe out the healthy gut bacteria that manufacture significant amounts of B vitamins. They also pave the way for unfriendly bacteria to multiply, which increases the risk of infection, thereby stressing the immune system. This can then lead to nutrient deficiency. Meanwhile the US National Institutes of Health estimate that more than 50,000 tons of antibiotics are used every year throughout the world.

In summary, the twentieth century has fundamentally changed the chemical environment of every species. Let us hope that the twenty-first century will pursue, with equal fervour, cleaning up the mess. As far as nutrition is concerned we will all need to consider what 'optimum nutrition' is, in the light not only of what our bodies need to be healthy, but also of what extra they need for anti-nutrient protection. There are also simple changes that we can make to our diets and lifestyles to reduce our *environmental load*, which is a fundamental principle of optimum nutrition.

Here are some tips to help decrease your environmental load:

- Invest in a good-quality, plumbed-in water filter and replace the cartridge every six months. Jug filters are also good, if you replace the cartridge as instructed. On drink natural mineral water.

- Buy organic. When not possible, wash or peel fruit and vegetables.

- Never deep-fry foods, and switch to steam-frying instead of sautéeing.

- Don't use cling film unless it states 'non-PVC'.

- Rearrange your daily schedule to minimise time spent in traffic.

- Drink alcohol very infrequently, and avoid smoky places.

- Avoid medical drugs unless they are the only viable option for treating a health problem. If you get frequent infections or aches, investigate the underlying cause rather than relying on painkillers or antibiotics.

Part 2

Defining the Perfect Diet

chapter 7

The Myth of the Well-balanced Diet

A human being is made up of roughly 63 per cent water, 22 per cent protein, 13 per cent fat and 2 per cent minerals and vitamins. Every single molecule comes from the food you eat and the water you drink. Eating the highest-quality food in the right quantities helps you to achieve your highest potential for health, vitality and freedom from disease.

Today's diet has drifted a long way off the ideal intake and balance of nutrients. The pie charts below show the percentage of calories we consume that come from fat, protein and carbohydrate. While little overall change has occurred throughout 99 per cent of humanity's history, in the last hundred or so years, particularly the last three decades, we have started eating much more saturated fat and sugar and less starch (complex carbohydrates) and polyunsaturated fats. Even the government guidelines fall a long way short of our ancestors' diets or what are generally considered to be ideal dietary guidelines.

Part of the problem is propaganda. We are led to believe that as long as you eat a well-balanced diet you get all the nutrients you need. Yet survey after survey has shown that even those who believe that they eat a well-balanced diet fail to get anything like the ideal intake of vitamins, minerals, essential fats and complex carbohydrates. It is not easy in today's society, in which food production is inextricably linked to profit. Refining foods makes them last, which makes them more profitable but at the same time deficient in essential nutrients.

The food industry has gradually conditioned us to buy sugar-sweetened foods to the tune of 2,300,000,000 kilograms of sugar a year – that's 38 kilograms per person per year! The US consumption of sugar now approaches 25 per cent of total calories. The UK government recommends that no more than 10 per cent of calories come from sugar, but does little to discourage us from eating it. Sugar sells, and the more of it we eat the less room there is for less sweet, 'slow-releasing' carbohydrates. As our lives speed up we spend less time preparing fresh food and become ever more reliant on ready meals from companies more concerned about their profit than about our health.

Since 1984 the Institute for Optimum Nutrition has been researching what a perfect diet would be. Our conclusions to date are shown in the top ten daily diet tips on page 51. While for many people this kind of balance of foods is not going to be achievable overnight, it does give a clear indication of where your diet should be heading. The general guidelines, which are substantiated in later chapters, are as follows.

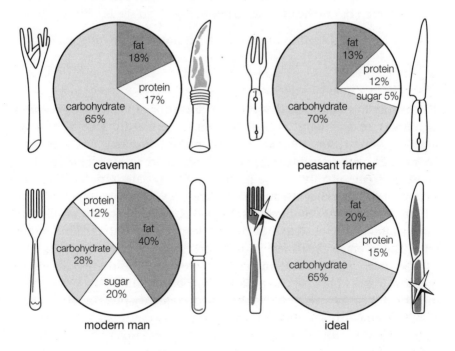

Ancient and modern diets

Fat

There are two basic kinds of fat: saturated (hard) fat and unsaturated fat. It is neither essential to eat saturated fat, nor ideal to eat too much. The main sources are meat and dairy products. There are also two kinds of unsaturated fat: monounsaturated fats, of which olive oil is a rich source; and polyunsaturated fats, found in nut and seed oils and fish.

Certain polyunsaturated fats, called linoleic acid and alpha-linolenic acid or Omega 6 and Omega 3 oils, are essential for the brain and nervous system, immune system, cardiovascular system and skin. A common sign of deficiency of these substances is dry skin. The optimal diet provides a balance of these two essential fats. Pumpkin and flax seeds are rich in linolenic acid (Omega 3), while sesame and sunflower seeds are rich in linoleic acid (Omega 6). Linolenic acid is converted in the body into DHA and EPA, which are also found in mackerel, herring, salmon and tuna. These essential fats are easily destroyed by heating or exposure to oxygen, so having a fresh daily source is important. Processed foods often contain hardened or 'hydrogenated' polyunsaturated fats. These are worse for you than saturated fat and are best avoided.

Eat one tablespoon of cold-pressed seed oil (sesame, sunflower, pumpkin, flax seed, etc.) or one heaped tablespoon of ground seeds a day.

Avoid fried food, burnt or browned fat, saturated and hydrogenated fat.

Protein

The twenty-five amino acids – different forms of protein – are the building blocks of the body. As well as being essential for growth and the repair of body tissue, they are used to make hormones, enzymes, antibodies and neurotransmitters, and help transport substances around the body. Both the quality of the protein you eat, determined by the balance of these amino acids, and the quantities you eat are important.

The government recommends that we obtain 15 per cent of our total calorie intake from protein, but gives little guidance as to the kind of protein. The average breast-fed baby receives just 1 per cent of its total calories from protein and manages to double its birth weight in six months. This is because the protein from breast milk is of a very good quality and easily absorbed. Assuming good-quality protein, 10 per cent of calorie intake, or around 35 grams of protein a day, is an optimal intake for most adults, unless pregnant, recovering from surgery or undertaking large amounts of exercise or heavy manual work.

The current diet trend towards high protein (30 per cent of calories), high fat (50 per cent of calories) and low carbohydrate (20 per cent of calories) provides way more protein than the body needs, let alone fat, and taxes the kidneys heavily.

The best-quality protein foods in terms of amino-acid balance include eggs, quinoa, soya, meat, fish, beans and lentils. Animal protein sources tend to contain a lot of undesirable saturated fat. Vegetable protein sources tend to contain additional beneficial complex carbohydrates and are less acid-forming (see page 516) than meat. It is best to limit meat to three meals a week. It is difficult not to take in enough protein from any diet that includes three meals a day, whether vegan, vegetarian or meat eating. Many vegetables, especially 'seed' foods like runner beans, peas, corn and broccoli, contain good levels of protein and help to neutralise excess acidity, which can lead to losses of minerals, including calcium – hence the higher risk of osteoporosis among frequent meat-eaters.

Eat two daily servings of beans, lentils, quinoa, tofu (soya), 'seed' vegetables (such as peas, broad beans) or other vegetable protein, or one small serving of meat, fish or cheese or a free-range egg.

Avoid too much animal protein.

Carbohydrate

The main fuel for the body, carbohydrate comes in two forms: 'fast releasing', as in sugar, honey, malt, sweets and most refined foods, and 'slow releasing', as in whole grains, vegetables and fresh fruit. The latter foods contain more complex carbohydrate and/or more fibre, both of which help to slow down the release of sugar. Fast-releasing carbohydrates tend to give a sudden burst of energy followed by a slump, while slow-releasing carbohydrates provide more sustained energy and are therefore preferable.

Refined foods like sugar and white flour lack the vitamins and minerals needed for the body to use them properly and are best avoided. The perpetual use of fast-releasing carbohydrates can give rise to complex symptoms and health problems. Some fruit, like bananas, dates and raisins, contain faster-releasing sugars and are best kept to a minimum by people with glucose-related health problems. Slow-releasing carbohydrate foods – fresh fruit, vegetables, pulses and whole grains – should make up two-thirds of what you eat, or around 65 per cent of your total calorie intake. Every day, aim to:

Eat three or more servings of dark green, leafy and root vegetables such as watercress, carrots, sweet potatoes, tenderstem, broccoli, Brussels sprouts, spinach, green beans or peppers, raw or lightly cooked.

Eat three or more servings of fresh fruit such as apples, pears, bananas, berries, melon or citrus fruit.

Eat four or more servings of whole grains such as rice, millet, rye, oats, wholewheat, corn, quinoa as cereal, breads, pasta or pulses.

Avoid any form of sugar, foods with added sugar, white or refined foods.

Fibre

Rural Africans eat about 55 grams of dietary fibre a day, compared with the UK average intake of 22 grams, and have the lowest incidence of bowel diseases such as appendicitis, diverticulitis, colitis and bowel cancer. The ideal intake is not less than 35 grams a day. It is easy to take in this amount of fibre – which absorbs water in the digestive tract, making the food contents bulkier and easier to pass through the body – by eating whole grains, vegetables, fruit, nuts, seeds, lentils and beans on a daily basis. Fruit and vegetable fibre helps slow down the absorption of sugar into the blood, helping to maintain good energy levels. Cereal fibre is particularly good at preventing constipation and putrefaction of food, which are underlying causes of many digestive complaints. Refined diets that are orientated towards meat, eggs, fish and dairy produce will undoubtedly lack fibre.

Eat whole foods – whole grains, lentils, beans, nuts, seeds, fresh fruit and vegetables.

Avoid refined, white and overcooked foods.

Water

Two-thirds of the body consists of water, which is therefore our most important nutrient. The body loses 1.5 litres of water a day through the skin, lungs and gut and via the kidneys as urine, ensuring that toxic substances are eliminated from the body. We also make about a third of a litre of water a day when glucose is 'burnt' for energy. Therefore our minimum water intake from food and drink needs to be more than 1 litre a day. The ideal daily intake is around 2 litres. This is best achieved by drinking eight glasses of water a day, including hot drinks.

Fruit and vegetables consist of around 90 per cent water. They supply it in a form that is very easy for the body to use, at the same time providing the body with a high percentage of its vitamins and minerals. Four pieces of fruit and four servings of vegetables, amounting to about 1.1kg of these foods, can provide a litre of water, leaving a daily 1 litre to be taken as water or in the form of diluted juices or herb or fruit teas. Alcohol acts as a diuretic and causes considerable losses of vitamins and minerals so it doesn't count in this regard.

Drink six to eight glasses of water a day as water or in diluted juices, herb or fruit teas.

Minimise your intake of alcohol, coffee and tea.

The nutritional benefits of water are explained more fully in Chapter 18.

Vitamins

Although needed in much smaller amounts than fat, protein or carbo-hydrate, vitamins are no less important. They 'turn on' enzymes, which in turn make all body processes happen. Vitamins are needed to balance hormones, produce energy, boost the immune system, make healthy skin and protect the arteries; they are vital for the brain, nervous system and just about every body process. Vitamins A, C and E are antioxidants: they slow down the ageing process and protect the body from cancer, heart dis-ease and pollution. B and C vitamins are vital for turning food into mental and physical energy. Vitamin D, found in milk, eggs, fish and meat, helps control calcium balance. It can also be made in the skin in the presence of sunshine. B and C vitamins are richest in fresh fruit and veg-etables. Vitamin A comes in two forms: retinol, the animal form found in meat, fish, eggs and dairy produce; and betacarotene, found in red, yellow and orange fruit and vegetables. Vitamin E is found in seeds, nuts and their oils, and helps protect essential fats from going rancid.

Eat three or more servings of dark green, leafy and root vegetables, and three or more servings of fresh fruit plus some nuts or seeds, every day.

Supplement a multivitamin containing at least the following: vitamin A 1,500mcg, vitamin D 5mcg, vitamin E 67mg, vitamin B1 25mg, vitamin B2 25mg, vitamin B3 (niacin) 50mg, vitamin B5 (pantothenic acid) 50mg, vitamin B6 50mg, vitamin B12 10mcg, folic acid 200mcg, biotin 50mcg. Also supplement 1,000mg of vitamin C a day.

The nutritional benefits of vitamins are explained more fully in Chapter 12.

Minerals

Like vitamins, minerals are essential for just about every body process. Calcium, magnesium and phosphorus help make up the bones and teeth. Nerve signals, vital for the brain and muscles, depend on calcium, mag-nesium, sodium and potassium. Oxygen is carried in the blood by an iron compound. Chromium helps control blood sugar levels. Zinc is essential for all body repair, renewal and development. Selenium and zinc help boost the immune system. Brain function depends on adequate magne-sium, manganese, zinc and other essential minerals. These are but a few of thousands of key roles that minerals play in human health.

We need large daily amounts of calcium and magnesium, which are found in vegetables such as kale, cabbage and root vegetables. They are also abundant in nuts and seeds. Calcium alone is found in large quantities in dairy produce. Fruit and vegetables provide lots of potassium and small amounts of sodium, which is the right balance. All 'seed' foods – which include seeds, nuts, lentils and dried beans, as well as peas, broad beans, runner beans and whole grains – are good sources of iron, zinc, manganese and chromium. Selenium is abundant in nuts, seafood, seaweed and seeds, especially sesame.

Eat one serving of mineral-rich foods such as kale, cabbage, root vegetables, low-fat dairy products such as yoghurt, seeds or nuts, as well as plenty of fresh fruit, vegetables and whole foods such as lentils, beans and whole grains.

Supplement a multimineral containing at least the following: calcium 100mg, magnesium 100mg, iron 10mg, zinc 10mg, manganese 2.5mg, chromium 25mcg, selenium 25mcg.

The nutritional benefits of minerals are explained more in Chapter 13.

Pure food

Organic, unadulterated wholefoods have formed the basis of the human diet through the ages. Only in the twentieth century did we begin to be subjected to countless man-made chemicals in food and in the environment.

One foundation for health is to eat foods that provide exactly the amount of energy required to keep the body in perfect balance. A good deal of energy is wasted in trying to disarm these alien and often toxic chemicals, some of which cannot be eliminated and so accumulate in body tissue. It is now impossible to avoid all these substances, as there is nowhere on this planet that is not contaminated in some way as a result of the by-products of our modern chemical age. Choosing organic foods whenever possible is the nearest we can get to eating a pure diet today. By supporting the movement back to these kinds of food we are helping to minimise the damage of chemical pollution, which poses a real threat to the future of humanity.

Eating raw, organic food is the most natural and beneficial way to take food into the body. Many foods contain enzymes that help digest them once chewed. Raw food is full of vital phytochemicals (see Chapter 17), whose effects on our health may prove as important as those of vitamins and minerals. Cooking food destroys enzymes and reduces the activity of phytochemicals.

Eat organic as much as you can. Make sure that at least half your diet consists of raw fruit, vegetables, whole grains, nuts and seeds.

Avoid processed food with additives, and cook food as little as possible.

1

Take one heaped tablespoon of ground seeds or one tablespoon of cold-pressed seed-oil

2

Eat two servings of beans, lentils, quinoa, tofu (soya), or 'seed' vegetables

3

Eat three pieces of fresh fruit such as apples, pears, bananas, berries, melon or citrus fruit

4

Eat four servings of whole grains such as brown rice, millet, rye, oats, wholewheat, corn, quinoa as cereal, breads and pasta

5

Eat five servings of dark green, leafy and root vegetables such as watercress, carrots, sweet potatoes, broccoli, spinach, green beans, peas and peppers

6

Drink six glasses of water, diluted juices, herb or fruit teas

7

Eat whole, organic, raw food as often as you can

8

Supplement your diet with a high-strength multivitamin and mineral preparation and 1000mg of vitamin C a day

9

Avoid fried, burnt and browned food, hydrogenated fat and excess animal fat

10

Avoid any form of sugar, also white, refined or processed food with chemical additives, and minimise your intake of alcohol, coffee or tea – have no more than one unit of alcohol a day (e.g. a glass of wine, half a pint of beer or lager, or a spirit)

Top ten daily diet tips

chapter 8

The Protein Controversy

What words do you associate with protein? ... Meat, eggs, cheese, muscles, growth. You have to eat these foods to get enough protein to grow big and strong. The protein in meat is more usable than the protein in plants. If you do muscle-building exercise you need more protein ... Right or wrong? Many myths abound about protein, how much you need and the best food sources.

The word protein itself is derived from *protos*, a Greek word meaning 'first', since protein is the basic material of all living cells. The human body, for example, contains approximately 65 per cent water and 25 per cent protein. Protein is made out of nitrogen-containing molecules called amino acids. Some twenty-five types of amino acid are pieced together in varying combinations to make different kinds of protein, which form the material for our cells and organs in much the same way that letters make words that combine to form sentences and paragraphs.

From the eight basic amino acids most of the remaining seventeen can be made. These eight are termed essential amino acids and the body cannot function without them, although others are semi-essential under certain conditions.

Each of the basic eight deserves its own Optimal Daily Amount, although these have yet to be set. The balance of these eight amino acids in the protein of any given food determines its quality or usability. So how much protein do you need, and what is the best-quality protein?

Protein – are you getting enough?

Estimates for protein requirement vary depending on who you speak to. This is not so surprising, since there may be widespread 'biochemical individuality'. In some countries the estimate is as low as 2.5 per cent of total calorie intake. The World Health Organisation estimates that we need 4.5 per cent of total calories from protein, while the US National Research Council adds a safety margin and regards 8 per cent as adequate for 95 per cent of the population. The World Health Organisation builds in a safety margin and recommends around 10 per cent of total calories from protein, or about 35 grams of protein a day. The estimated average daily requirement, according to the UK Department of Health, is 36 grams for women and 44 grams for men. If the quality of protein is high, less needs to be eaten. At the other end of the spectrum are very high-protein diets, unwisely recommended for weight loss. These often contain 100 to 200 grams of protein a day. This is much too high.

So which foods provide more than 10 per cent of their calories from protein? You may be surprised to learn that virtually every lentil, bean, nut, seed and grain and most vegetables and fruit provide more than 10 per cent protein. In soya beans 54 per cent of the calories come from protein, compared with 26 per cent in kidney beans. Grains vary from 16 per cent for quinoa to 4 per cent for corn. Nuts and seeds range from 21 per cent for pumpkin seeds to 12 per cent for cashew nuts. Fruit goes from 16 per cent for lemons down to 1 per cent for apples. Vegetables vary from 49 per cent for spinach to 11 per cent for potatoes.

What this means is that if you are eating enough calories you are almost certainly getting enough protein, unless you are living off high-sugar, high-fat junk food. This may come as a surprise, contradicting all we are taught about protein. Yet the fact of the matter is, to quote a team of Harvard scientists investigating vegetarian diets, 'It is difficult to obtain a mixed vegetable diet that will produce an appreciable loss of body protein.' But surely animal protein is better quality than plant protein?

Animal or vegetable?

Once again, there are a few surprises. Top of the class is quinoa (pronounced keenwa), a high-protein grain from South America that was a staple food of the Incas and Aztecs. Soya too does well. Most vegetables are relatively low in the amino acids methionine and lysine; however, beans and lentils are rich in methionine. Soya beans and quinoa are excellent sources of both lysine and methionine.

Early theories, such as those first expounded by Frances Moore Lappe in her groundbreaking vegetarian cookbook *Diet for a Small Planet*, suggested that vegetable proteins had to be carefully combined with complementary proteins in order to match the quality of animal proteins. However, we have since learnt that careful combining of plant-based proteins is quite unnecessary. As Lappe says in the revised edition of her book, 'With a healthy, varied diet, concern about protein complementarity is not necessary for most of us.'

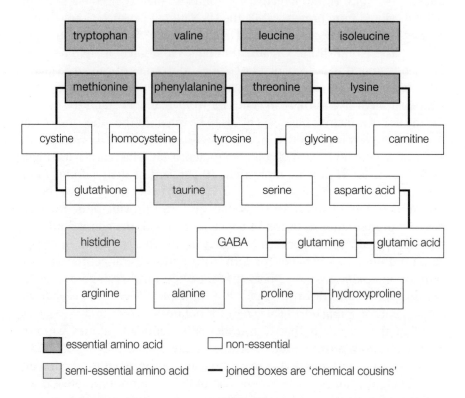

The amino acid family. For a protein food source to contain 'complete' protein it must contain the eight essential amino acids. This is what you find in meat, fish, eggs, soya and quinoa. The semi-essential amino acids are also found in these foods. Taurine appears to be essential in infancy.

Even so, you can increase the effective quality of the protein you eat by combining foods from different groups so that low levels of certain amino acids in one food group are made up by high levels in another. Over a forty-eight-hour period aim to eat a varied diet across the food groups shown in the illustration below. The combination of rice with lentils, for example, increases the protein value by a third. This is, of course, the basis of the diet in the Indian subcontinent.

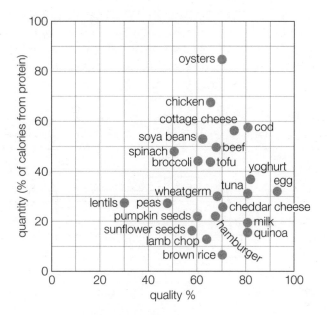

Protein quality and quantity

The best protein foods

The best foods to eat for protein are not necessarily those that are highest in protein. The pros and cons of a food's other nutritional constituents have to be taken into account. A lamb chop, for example, provides 25 per cent of total calories as protein and 75 per cent as fat, much of which is saturated fat. Half the calories in soya beans come from protein, so it is actually a better source of protein than lamb, but its real advantage is that the rest of the calories come from desirable complex carbohydrates. It also contains no saturated fat. This makes foods made from soya ideal, especially for vegetarians.

The easiest way to eat soya is in the form of tofu, a curd made from beans. There are many kinds of tofu – soft, hard, marinated, smoked and braised. Soft tofu can be used to give a creamy texture to soups. Hard tofu can be cubed and used in vegetable stir-fries, stews and casseroles. Since tofu is quite tasteless it is best to use it with well-flavoured foods or sauces.

Quinoa has been grown in South America for 5,000 years and has a long-standing reputation as a source of strength for those working at high altitudes. Called the 'mother grain' because of its sustaining properties, it contains protein of a better quality than that of meat. Although known as a grain, quinoa is technically a seed. Like other seeds it's rich in essential fats, vitamins and minerals, providing almost four times as much calcium

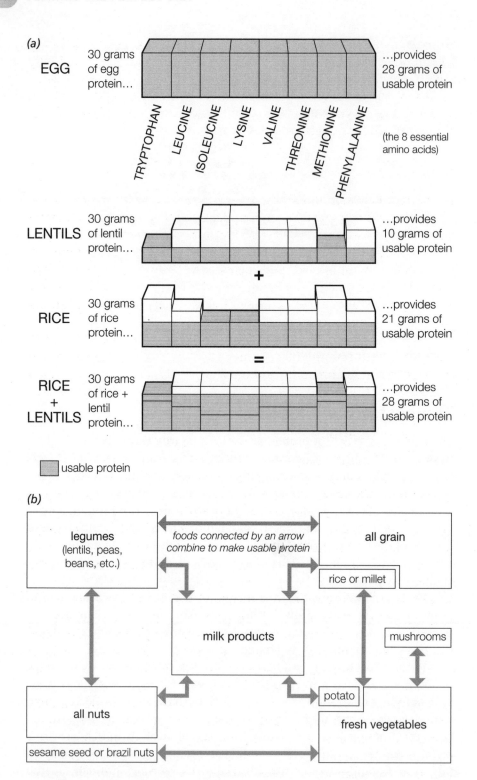

Combining foods for more complete protein

as wheat, plus extra iron, B vitamins and vitamin E. Quinoa is also low in fat: the majority of its oil is polyunsaturated, providing essential fatty acids. As such, quinoa is about as close to a perfect food as you can get.

Quinoa can be found in many health food stores and used as an alternative to rice. To cook it, rinse well, then add two parts water to one of quinoa and boil for fifteen minutes.

Meat

The average person in Britain eats over 2lb/900g of meat a week. The traditional view is that meat is good for you, being high in protein and iron. But the recent BSE ('mad cow disease') scare has fuelled a growing concern that modern farming methods have gone too far. Meat consumption is going down as more and more people are becoming vegetarian and vegan. Leaving moral considerations aside, there are a number of safety issues that give cause for genuine concern: they include the use of antibiotics, growth hormones and pesticide dips.

Described by the microbiologist Professor Richard Lacey as 'fake meat', much of what is on offer in supermarkets and butcher's shops contains growth hormones, antibiotics and pesticide residues and, at worst, could be infected with BSE.

BSE – is it a serious risk?

The infectious agent thought to be responsible for BSE is called a prion. It latches on to proteins in the brain, changing them and thereby triggering disease. It is now proven to pass from species to species, and into humans.

At the time of writing over 130 people have died of new-variant Creutzfeldt-Jakob disease (vCJD) in the UK, and the leading theory as to the source of vCJD is that it results from eating infected beef. The amount of infected meat that needs to be eaten to get vCJD is unknown, as is the incubation period in humans. Some models have estimated that up to 100,000 people may eventually fall victim to vCJD, though increasingly, as time goes by, these estimates are being revised downwards, and Dr James Ironside, a member of the UK CJD Surveillance Unit, whose paper was published in the *Lancet* in 1997, believes that 'a total number of cases over the whole course of the disease will be in the hundreds, rather than thousands'.

With considerable uncertainty persisting about the nature of both BSE and its link to vCJD in humans, it's worth noting that there has never been a case of BSE in an organically born and reared cow. Organic farmers stopped the unnatural practice of feeding cows to cows long before the BSE epidemic began in the 1980s, and are also prohibited from the conventional practice of pouring warble-fly insecticide along the animals' spines, which is also thought to make cattle more susceptible to BSE. Only time will tell how big a health problem BSE and vCJD will eventually be, and in the meantime the safest option is to eat only organic beef.

Hormones – a growing problem

Most meat today, whether chicken, beef, pork or lamb, has received hormone treatment of one kind or another. Milk, too, is a rich source of hormones, particularly oestrogen. Some hormones used widely in the US are banned in Europe, although there are commercial pressures to rescind the ban. These hormones, including synthetic oestradiol and testosterone, are used to force growth rates and increase milk yields. These are the same chemicals that are at the centre of the concern about 'oestrogen dominance', an increasingly common syndrome found in men and women with hormone-related disease. So far, breast cancer, fibroids, ovarian cancer, cervical cancer, prostate and testicular cancer and endometriosis have all been linked to excessive oestrogen levels.

Of course, it is not easy to find out what long-term effects the introduction of hormones into our food is having. Dr Malcolm Carruthers, a specialist in male hormone-related disease, investigated 1,000 cases of patients exhibiting symptoms of the 'male menopause' over seven years. The most common symptoms are fatigue, depression, loss of libido, testicular atrophy, impotence and breast enlargement. Of these 1,000 cases the highest occupational risk group was farmers, the 'front-line' troops in the agrochemical arms race.

According to Carruthers, 'For some the causative agent appeared obvious. They had worked on farms caponizing chickens or turkeys with oestrogen pellet implants, to make the birds plumper and more tender. Unfortunately, though it might be considered poetic justice, they must have taken in large amounts of oestrogen which caused them to become partly caponized themselves.' Farmers less directly exposed to hormones – and to pesticides, which are also known to interfere with male hormone balance – were also at high risk of 'male menopause' symptoms.

Is your meat bugged?

Antibiotics are in widespread use in both humans and animals. Over 500 tons are dished out every year in Britain alone. Unlike human medicines, which are given for a limited period for the treatment of an infection, antibiotics are routinely added to animal feed to prevent infection and enhance growth: the aim is higher profits faster. The consumer, however, is being hit with a double whammy.

Antibiotic residues are frequently found in samples of meat, fish and eggs. So are infectious agents that have become resistant to antibiotics – superbugs. There is growing concern about a strain of enterococci faecium, a dangerous bacterium found in chickens which is resistant to Vancomycin, one of the strongest 'last resort' antibiotics. Fortunately, infection with enterococci is rare compared with salmonella or campylobacter. With 350,000 cases of salmonella and 400,000 cases of campylobacter infection from meat and eggs per year in the UK, it's potentially a huge problem that these common strains of bacteria causing food poisoning are becoming resistant to antibiotics.

The World Health Organization has called for a reduction in the use of antibiotics in agriculture because of the risk to human health, while the British Medical Association has warned that 'The risk to human health from antibiotic resistance developing in micro-organisms is one of the major public health threats that will be faced in the twenty-first century.'[1]

Too much meat could be bad for your health and your bones

Meat-eaters have a low health rating. The risk of heart disease and cancer, particularly cancer of the stomach and colon, is directly related to meat consumption. So too are other diseases of the digestive system such as diverticulitis, colitis and appendicitis. Even more likely to result in cardiovascular disease is a high consumption of milk and dairy products. Overall, a meat-eater is likely to visit the doctor, or be admitted to hospital, twice as often as a vegetarian, and is likely to suffer from degenerative diseases ten years earlier than a vegetarian, according to a survey by Professors John Dickerson and Jill Davies from the University of Surrey.[2]

Most people are in more danger of eating too much protein than too little. Excess protein is a contributor to osteoporosis, over-acidity and many other common health problems. Protein-rich foods – including calcium-packed dairy foods – produce acid when broken down (or metabolised) by your body. But we cannot tolerate substantial changes in the acid pH of blood, so our bodies neutralise or 'buffer' this effect through two main alkaline agents – sodium and calcium. When body reserves of sodium are used up, calcium is taken from the bone. Therefore the more protein you eat the more calcium you lose.

The negative effects of too much protein have also been clearly demonstrated in people with osteoporosis. This disease is reaching epidemic proportions – the rate of hip fractures has more than doubled in the last fifty years, even after you take into account the ageing population. Yet the traditional risk factors – menopause (when oestrogen, the hormone that assists the retention of calcium in the bone, ceases to be produced), lack of calcium in the diet and a couch-potato lifestyle –

account for less than half of all hip fractures. This data has been collected by the Study of Osteoporotic Fractures, which is the largest research project of its kind to date and has followed nearly 10,000 elderly women since 1986. 'Dietary acid load is probably up there at the top of the list of risk factors,' says Uriel Barzel, an endocrinologist at the Albert Einstein College of Medicine in New York.

Of course, this begs the question as to whether eating a lot of dairy produce, high in both protein and calcium, would be protective or contribute to osteoporosis risk. A twelve-year study that involved over 120,000 women throughout the US found that women who drink two or more glasses of milk per day actually had a 45 per cent higher risk of hip fractures and a 5 per cent higher risk of forearm fractures than women who drank less.[3] The director of the study, Diane Feskanich, says, 'I certainly would want women to have adequate calcium in their diets, but I would not rely on that as the prime prevention against osteoporosis.'

Why high-protein, high-fat diets are dangerous

Kidney problems

Protein produces breakdown products that are hard work for the kidneys. If your kidneys are healthy and your protein excess isn't too high, no problem. But, how far can you push it? US researchers tested 1,624 women aged between forty-two and sixty-eight and found that almost one in three had less than ideal kidney function. In the women who had normal kidney function, high-protein intakes caused no decline in renal function. However, those who already had a mild kidney problem who ate a high-protein diet, particularly one high in meat protein, showed a further deterioration.[4] Dairy or vegetable protein was not associated with worsening kidney function. The Atkins diet involves even higher protein intakes than were used in these studies, so you can see the problems it may cause.

Bone problems

Protein is acidic. Too much in the blood has to be neutralised. The Nurses' Health Study recently found that women who consumed 3oz (95g) of protein a day compared with those who consumed less than 2oz (68g) a day had a 22 per cent greater risk of forearm fractures.[5]

'Consumption of a low-carb/high-protein diet for six weeks delivers a marked acid load to the kidney, increases the risk for stone formation, decreases estimated calcium balance, and may increase the risk for bone loss,' said Dr Shalini T. Reddy from the University of Chicago, Illinois, who conducted a six-week study on ten healthy adults on a low-carb diet.[6] Volunteers lost an average of 9 pounds, that's 1.5 pounds a week, but most developed ketones – compounds that are formed when the body uses its own fat as fuel and can raise acid levels in the blood. Acid excretion, a marker of acid levels in the blood, rose by 90 per cent in some volunteers. There was also a sharp rise in urinary calcium levels during the diet despite only a slight decrease in calcium intake. Urinary citrate, a compound that inhibits kidney-stone formation, decreased. While it is not clear from the study whether bone mass was affected, the findings indicate that such diets may increase the risk of bone loss over the long term.

The meat muscle myth

Whether you eat steak, of which 52 per cent of the calories comes from protein, or spinach (the reputed source of Popeye's strength), of which 49 per cent of the calories comes from protein, surely you need more to make strong muscles? According to Dr Michael Colgan, Sylvester Stallone's former nutritionist and adviser to many US Olympic athletes, this is a myth. He points out that, with hard training, the maximum amount of extra muscle you could build in a year would be less than 8lb (3.6kg). That represents a gain of 2.5oz (70g) a week, or 0.3oz (9.5g) a day. Muscle is only 22 per cent protein, so an increased consumption of less than a tenth of an ounce, or 2.8g a day, equivalent to a quarter of a teaspoonful, is all that is needed to bring about the greatest possible muscle gain! So instead of loading in unnecessary protein, which taxes the body more than it helps it, follow the rules of optimum nutrition to ensure that you make proper use of the protein in your diet.

Fish

While there is no doubt about the immense value of protein and essential fats in fish, fish is contaminated with man-made non-biodegradable toxins that tend to accumulate up the food chain (from plankton to small fish to bigger fish that eat the small fish, and so on). The same, of course, is true for animals that eat animals that ate pesticide-laden feed. A survey of salmon, published in 2004 in *Science* magazine, showed that all salmon have some contamination with PCBs and dioxins – industrial pollutants that don't biodegrade, and with dieldrins and toxaphene, which are pesticides/herbicides. Fish caught in the Pacific have consistently lower levels than fish caught in the Atlantic. The survey also showed that farmed salmon consistently had higher levels than wild salmon.

While I generally recommend eating more fish, it's easy to get confused by recommendations to avoid fish because of contamination with PCBs, dioxins and other toxic chemicals. In the case of dioxins and PCBs these contaminants are in the food chain, and both wild fish and farmed fish eat fish, or fish feed. Toxaphene, dieldrin and other pesticide residues are likely to accumulate more from feed fed to farmed fish. You can buy 'organic' fish, which are fed less-contaminated feed, though at least half the feed must be of aquatic origin, meaning other fish, which may also be contaminated to some degree with PCBs and dioxins, depending on the sea in which they swim.

Then there's the mercury question. All fish contain mercury, and generally the larger the fish, the more the mercury. So, for example, the highest content is found in shark (1.5mcg per kilogram), followed by swordfish (1.4), marlin (1.1) and tuna (0.4). Salmon and trout tend to be very low (around 0.05mcg). Where does the mercury come from, you might wonder. Contrary to popular opinion, most of it isn't from man-made pollution. Humans have always been exposed to mercury from volcanoes, and there are plenty on the ocean bed. We all consume, on average, 1mcg of mercury a day from food, water and air. Researchers from Harvard School of Public Health in Boston, Massachusetts, studied children in the Faroe Islands, north of Scotland, who eat large amounts of fish and mercury-laden whale meat. At age seven they had a slower transmission of electrical signals along a particular circuit in their brain than normal, and it had worsened further by the age of fourteen.[7]

The problem of mercury is substantial only if either you are eating a lot of large, carnivorous fish, or you are already mercury toxic, possibly from a mouthful of amalgam fillings, which can further add to your load. In this case you should decrease your large-fish consumption and double or triple my recommendations for supplementing zinc and selenium – and consider having your mercury amalgam fillings removed.

So what's the bottom line on fish? Given that it's a great source of protein and essential fats my advice is to limit large fish such as tuna and swordfish (by eating them only twice a month), and where possible, eat wild Pacific salmon, followed by wild Atlantic salmon, followed by organic farmed salmon or other, smaller carniverous fish three times a week. Sardines are an excellent choice – because they're small they are less likely to have accumulated toxins than other, larger fish.

Milk

Milk and other dairy products are the mainstay of the British diet. Although the UK represents only 20 per cent of the EU population, we consume 40 per cent of its dairy products with an average weekly intake of four pints of milk. It is considered an essential source of protein, iron and calcium. So beneficial is it to our health, said the now-defunct Milk Marketing Board, that you may wonder how we ever existed without it. So why do some authorities not encourage milk-drinking, if it is such a good source of minerals?

Ignore the hype

The truth is that milk is not a very good source of many minerals. Manganese, chromium, selenium and magnesium are all found in higher levels in fruit and vegetables. Most important is magnesium, which works alongside calcium. The ideal calcium to magnesium ratio is 2:1 – you need twice as much calcium as magnesium. Milk's ratio is 10:1, while cheese is 28:1. Relying on dairy products for calcium is likely to lead to magnesium deficiency and imbalance. Seeds, nuts and crunchy vegetables like kale, cabbage, carrots and cauliflower give us both these minerals and others, more in line with our needs. Milk is, after all, designed for young calves, not adult humans.

Not recommended for babies

Another common myth is that a breastfeeding mother needs to drink milk in order to make milk. This, of course, is nonsense. The move away from breastfeeding led to the substitution of human milk with cow's milk. Cow's milk is designed for calves, and is very different from human milk in a number of respects, including its protein, calcium, phosphorus, iron and essential fatty acid content. Early feeding of human babies on cow's milk is now known to increase the likelihood of developing a cow's milk allergy, which affects close to one in ten babies. Common symptoms include diarrhoea, vomiting, persistent colic, eczema, urticaria, catarrh, bronchitis, asthma and sleeplessness. The American Society of Micro-biologists has suggested that some cot deaths may be attributable to cow's milk allergy. Cow's milk should not be given to infants under four months.

Conversely, breast milk is nothing but good news. A breast-fed baby has, on average, a 4-point higher IQ.[8] This advantage can be doubled by giving the pregnant and breastfeeding mother a supplement of Omega 3 fish oils.

Milk, heart disease and breast cancer

Milk consumption is strongly linked with increased risk for cardiovascu-lar disease and also breast and prostate cancer. The higher a country's intake of milk, the higher its incidence of cardiovascular disease.[9] Why is this? Well, contrary to popular opinion it may not be because of the fat content in milk. A candidate for why milk increases heart disease is its poor calcium to magnesium ratio – more than any other mineral, magne-sium protects against heart disease. Another candidate is the discovery of a link between heart-disease risk and the presence of an anti-milk anti-body in the blood. Our bodies actually produce an antibody against milk, which certainly suggests it isn't an ideal food. On top of that 70 per cent of people stop producing lactase, the enzyme to digest milk sugar, once they've been weaned. Is nature trying to tell us something?

Even more insidious than the link to heart disease is new research suggesting that dairy consumption may be the main reason that people in the West have a massive risk of breast and prostate cancer, while Asians don't. The figures for the chances of women in China dying from breast cancer are 1 in 10,000, as opposed to close to 1 in 10 for the UK. For prostate cancer the difference is even greater. In rural China the incidence is 0.5 in 100,000, yet it is estimated that, by 2015, 1 in 4 men in the UK will have a diagnosis of prostate cancer at some point in their lives. Why is a disease that is virtually non-existent in China ruining and often prematurely ending the lives of so many men in Britain? Is it genes, diet or environment? It is obviously not genetics since Chinese men emigrating to Europe soon end up with similar risk. Is China more rural, with less urban pollution? This too is unlikely to be the main reason, although it may be part of the problem. In highly urbanised Hong Kong, the rate of breast cancer rises to 1 in every 300 women, but that's still along way off 1 in 10 in the West. So, is it diet and, if so, what is it about our Western diet and lifestyle that is tipping us towards breast and prostate cancer?

If you asked me to take an educated guess I'd put my money on hormone-disrupting chemicals, both because of the evidence that's emerging and because of the logic. Prostate and breast cells are stimulated to grow by hormonal messages. Ask any oncologist and they'll tell you that these hormone-sensitive cells go into overgrowth when exposed to too much oestrogen or oestrogen-like chemicals. The late Dr John Lee argued eloquently in favour of 'oestrogen dominance' being a primary cause of breast cancer. He explained in his excellent book *What Your Doctor May Not Tell You about Breast Cancer* that oestrogen is the hormone that makes things grow and that progesterone keeps cells healthy. Too much of the former and not enough of the latter could tip the scales to abnormal cell growth. Too much stress and sugar, leading to insulin resistance, exposure to environmental hormone-disrupting chemicals, from DDT to dioxins, and pesticides to PCBs, or oestrogen and synthetic-progestin HRT could swing the balance, but there's another growth promoter. It's called Insulin Growth Factor (IGF). There are different types – IGF-1, IGF-2 and so on, although much of the focus is on IGF-1.

IGF-1 is very rich in milk. It's doubly rich in modern milk, partly because cows have been selectively reared to produce milk during pregnancy. This milk is especially rich in oestrogen. On top of that, in the US cows are treated with bovine growth hormone (BGH), which is a growth hormone capable of further increasing milk yield by about 12 per cent. All this means a cow's daily milk production has gone from 3 to 30 litres. Not surprisingly, this milk has two to five times the amount of IGF-1, while the beef from a BGH-treated animal has about double the IGF. Casein, the protein in milk, helps to carry the IGF into us.

We do make IGF, but produce very little in adulthood. It's produced mainly in childhood to stimulate growth. When levels in the blood increase by 8 per cent, risk for prostate cancer increases seven times. Levels of IGF are, on average, 9 per cent higher in meat-eating omnivores and dairy-eating vegetarians than in vegans. Recent research from Shangai, China, has found that the higher a woman's IGF-1 levels the higher her risk for breast cancer. This study found that women in the top 25 per cent of IGF-1 scores had two to three times the risk of women in the bottom 25 per cent of IGF-1 levels.[10] A study from York University in the UK on the link between IGF and prostate-cancer risk in men found a similar result. Men in the top 25 per cent of IGF levels had three times the risk of prostate cancer.[11] These are just two of a dozen trials finding a strong link between circulating levels of IGF-1 and cancer. There are just as many showing a direct correlation between dairy consumption and breast- and prostate-cancer risk.

What does IGF-1 do, and why is it a strong candidate for increasing risk of cancer? Normally, it is produced by the liver, especially during puberty. In girls it stimulates the growth of breast tissue, encouraging cells to divide and grow. In boys it stimulates growth of the prostate. There's nothing wrong with IGF-1. It's a perfectly normal hormone. It's just that we aren't designed to be eating sources of it in adulthood.

In countries such as the US where cows are treated with BGH, milk from these cows develops raised levels of an insulin-like growth promoter (IGF-1), found in both the cow and those who drink the milk. This growth factor makes oestrogen more potent in the body, and research is increasingly showing that it could increase the risk of breast and colon cancer. University of Illinois toxicologist Dr Samuel Epstein says that 'all women from conception to death will now be exposed to an additional breast-cancer risk due to milk from cows treated with BGH'.

While milk naturally contains small amounts of oestrogen, changes in farming practices now make it possible to milk cows continuously, even while they are pregnant. These pregnant cows produce milk with much higher levels of oestrogen. If you drink milk, my advice is to stick to organic milk, which disallows this practice and the use of BGH. On top of that, cows eating pesticide- or herbicide-sprayed feed tend to accumulate residues in their meat and fat. For a consumer of meat or milk products, choosing the organic rather than non-organic varieties reduces the risk of exposure to pesticide and herbicide residues as well as BGH.

Allergy and its effects

Milk allergy or intolerance is very common among both children and adults. Sometimes this is the result of lactose intolerance, since many adults lose the ability to digest lactose (milk sugar). The symptoms are bloating, abdominal pain, wind and diarrhoea, which subside on giving lactase, the enzyme that breaks down lactose. Probably equally common is an allergy to dairy produce. The most common symptoms are blocked nose and excessive mucus production, respiratory complaints such as asthma, and gastrointestinal problems. These are inflammatory reactions produced by the body when it doesn't like what you're eating. Such intolerances are most likely to occur in people who consume dairy products regularly, in large quantities. Few people who are allergic to milk can tolerate yoghurt. Some can tolerate goat's milk or sheep's milk. Most can't.

Milk and infant-onset diabetes

Growing evidence is linking child-onset diabetes to allergy to bovine serum albumin (BSA) in dairy products.[12] This type of diabetes, which tends to strike in the early teenage years and accounts for 8,000 deaths per year in the UK, starts with the immune system destroying the cells in the pancreas that produce insulin. Why this occurs has long been a mystery.

While there is a genetic predisposition to insulin-dependent diabetes (IDD), this is only part of the picture. Genetically susceptible children who had been breast-fed for at least seven months or exclusively breast-fed for at least three or four months were found to have a significantly decreased incidence of IDD, which suggested another factor. Children who have not been given cow's milk until they are four months or older also show the same substantially reduced risk. The highest incidence of IDD is found in Finland, which has the world's highest milk-product consumption.

Animal studies showed that rats bred to be susceptible to diabetes had a much higher risk of contracting the disease if their feed contained either milk or wheat gluten. In one study even the addition of 1 per cent skimmed milk to their diet increased the incidence of IDD from 15 per cent to 52 per cent.

In 1993 Dr Hans-Michael Dosch, Professor of Immunology at Mount Sinai Hospital, New York, identified BSA as the specific factor in dairy produce that increased the risk of diabetes, and showed that it cross-reacted with the cells of the pancreas. He and his fellow researchers theorised that diabetes-susceptible babies introduced to BSA earlier than around four months, before which age the gut wall is immature and more permeable, would develop an allergic response to BSA. As a result their immune cells would mistakenly destroy not only the BSA molecules but also pancreatic tissue. He went on to show that, of 142 newly diagnosed IDD children,

100 per cent had antibodies to BSA, compared with 2 per cent in unaffected children. Dr Dosch believes that the presence of these anti-BSA antibodies indicated future child-onset diabetes in 80–90 per cent of cases.

He believes that keeping children off dairy products for at least their first six months halves the risk. BSA can, however, pass from the mother's diet into her milk. So if breastfeeding mothers avoid beef and dairy products the risk can be completely removed in genetically susceptible children. The current opinion is that about one in four children is genetically susceptible. Avoiding milk may also have benefits for your child's mental development. The vast majority of autistic children and many who suffer from hyperactivity prove allergic to milk.

Milk and meat – the verdict

From the current evidence, given the present state of intensive farming, neither meat (particularly beef) nor milk (especially for young children) should be staple foods if you really want to pursue optimum nutrition. But this is no loss – not only is it possible to have a healthy diet without including dairy produce and meat; it's also almost certainly going to decrease your risk of the common killer diseases. For meat-lovers who feel they do not want to go vegetarian I recommend avoiding British beef and eating meat no more than three times a week, substituting more fresh vegetables and whole foods such as beans, lentils and whole grains and choosing only organic meats and free-range chicken or fish. For milk, substitute soya or rice milk, or buy organic milk. If you suspect you might be allergic, stay off all dairy produce for fourteen days. If it makes no difference, limit your intake of milk to 2 pints a week.

Here are some general guidelines for your protein intake:

- Eat two servings of beans, lentils, quinoa, tofu (soya), 'seed' vegetables or other vegetable protein, or one small serving of meat, fish or cheese, or a free-range egg, every day.

- Reduce your intake of dairy products and avoid them altogether if you are allergic, substituting soya or rice milk.

- Reduce other sources of animal protein, choosing lean meat or fish and eating no more than three servings a week.

- Eat organic whenever possible, to avoid possible contamination with hormones and antibiotics.

chapter 9

The Fats of Life

Fat is good for you! Eating the right kind of fat is absolutely vital for optimal health. Essential fats reduce the risk of cancer, heart disease, allergies, Alzheimer's disease, arthritis, eczema, depression, fatigue, infections, PMS – the list of symptoms and diseases associated with deficiency is growing every year. If you are fat-phobic you are depriving yourself of essential health-giving nutrients and increasing your risk of poor health. The same is true if the fat you eat is hard – this means fat from dairy products, meat and most varieties of margarine.

The human brain is 60 per cent fat and one-third of this should come from essential fats if you want to achieve your full potential for health and happiness. In fact, unless you go out of your way to eat the right kinds of fat-rich foods, such as seeds, nuts and fish, the chances are that you are not getting enough good fat. Most people in the Western world eat too much saturated fat, the kind that kills, and too little of the essential fats, the kinds that heal.

Fat figures

It is considered optimum to consume no more than 20 per cent of your total calories in the form of fat. The current average in Britain is above 35 per cent. Inhabitants of countries that have a low incidence of fat-related diseases, like Japan, Thailand and the Philippines, consume only about 20 per cent of their total calorie intake as fat. For example, Japanese people eat on average 40 grams of fat a day, whereas British people eat 77 grams, almost double.

Saturated and monounsaturated fats are not essential nutrients: you do not need them, although they can be used by the body to make energy. But polyunsaturated fats or oils are essential. Almost all foods that contain fat have a balance of all three. A piece of meat will contain mainly saturated and monounsaturated fat with little polyunsaturated fat. Olive oil has mainly monounsaturated fat. Sunflower seed oil has mainly polyunsaturated fat.

Most authorities now agree that no more than one-third of our total fat intake should be saturated (hard) fat, and at least one-third should be polyunsaturated oils providing the two essential fats: the linoleic acid family, known as Omega 6, and the alpha-linolenic acid family, known as Omega 3. The ideal balance between these two is roughly the same amount of Omega 6 as of Omega 3. So an ideal 'fat profile', based on fat forming no more than 20 per cent of our total calorie intake, might consist of:

- 3.5 per cent Omega 6

- 3.5 per cent Omega 3

- 7 per cent monounsaturated fat

- 6 per cent saturated fat

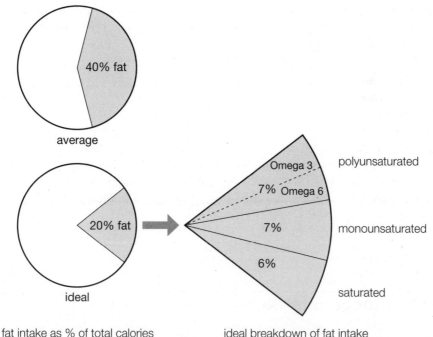

fat intake as % of total calories   ideal breakdown of fat intake

Fat intake

Most people are deficient in both Omega 6 and Omega 3 fats; however, the real change in modern living is a vast increase in saturated fat and a decrease in Omega 3 fats (see figure below). In addition, a lot of the polyunsaturated fats we eat are damaged and become 'trans' fats or processed fats, known as 'hydrogenated' fats. These stop the body making good use of the small quantity of essential fats that the average person eats in a day.

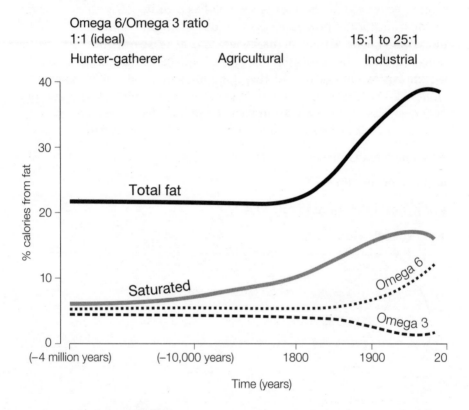

How fat intake has changed. In modern times total fat intake has increased. Saturated-fat intake has increased, although it is now levelling off. Omega 6 fat intake has increased but this is slightly misleading because much of it is 'hydrogenated' vegetable oils, which act like saturated fats. Intake of Omega 3 fats, in fish and seeds, has gone down, leading to widespread deficiency.

Leaf and Weber, Am J Clin Nutr 1987 (45), pp. 1048–53.

The Omega 6 fat family

The grandmother of the Omega 6 fat family is linoleic acid, which is converted by the body into gamma-linolenic acid (GLA). Evening primrose

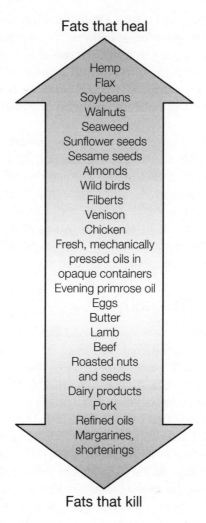

Fats that heal, fats that kill

oil and borage oil are the richest known sources of GLA, and if you take these in supplement form you need less overall oil to obtain enough Omega 6 fats. The ideal intake is around 100mg of GLA a day, equivalent to 1,000mg of evening primrose oil or 500mg of high-potency borage oil – a capsule a day.

GLA has two fats. Some GLA is converted into arachidonic acid. This type of fat is used to build the brain, along with the Omega 3 fat DHA. GLA is also converted into DGLA (di-homo gamma linolenic acid) and from there into prostaglandins, which are extremely active hormone-like substances. The particular kind made from these Omega 6 oils are called series 1 prostaglandins. They keep the blood thin, which prevents clots and blockages, relaxes blood vessels, lowers blood pressure, helps to maintain the water balance in the body, decreases inflammation and pain, improves nerve and immune function and helps insulin to work, which is good for blood sugar balance. And this is only the beginning. Every year more and more health-promoting functions of prostaglandins are being discovered.

Prostaglandins themselves cannot be supplemented, as they are very short-lived; we rely instead on a good intake of their source, Omega 6 fats. This family of fats comes exclusively from seeds and their oils. The best are hemp, pumpkin, sunflower, safflower, sesame, corn, walnut, soya bean and wheat germ oil. About half of the fats in these oils come from the Omega 6 family, mainly as linoleic acid. An optimal intake, if this were your only source of essential fats, would be one to two tablespoons of oil a day, or two to three tablespoons of ground seeds.

The Omega 3 fat family

The modern diet is much more deficient in Omega 3 fats than in Omega 6. This is because the grandmother of the Omega 3 family, alpha-linolenic acid, and her metabolically active grandchildren EPA (eicosapentaenoic acid) and DHA (docosahexaenoic acid), from which series 3 prostaglandin are made, are more unsaturated and more prone to damage in cooking and food processing. Hence, they are often purposely excluded from convenience foods. This, plus the reduced consumption of fish, is fuelling the epidemics of cardiovascular disease and mental health problems since both brain and body depend on Omega 3 fats. As these fats get converted in the body to more 'active' substances they become more unsaturated, and generally the word used for them gets longer (for instance, oleic acid: one degree of unsaturation; linoleic: two degrees of unsaturation; linolenic: three degrees of unsaturation; eicosapentaenoic: five degrees of unsaturation).

You can observe this increasing complexity as we move up the food chain. Plankton, for example, the staple food of small fish, is rich in alpha-linolenic acid. The little fish eat the plankton, then the carnivorous fish, like mackerel or herring, eat the small fish, which have converted some of their alpha-linolenic acid into more complex fats. The carnivorous fish continue the conversion. Seals eat them and have the highest EPA and DHA concentration. Finally Eskimos eat the seals and benefit from a ready-made meal of EPA and DHA. You, if you want to have a healthy brain and body . . . eat Eskimos! Actually, the Inuit people, as they are properly known, have a very low incidence of cardiovascular disease despite a very high intake of fat and cholesterol. This really emphasises that it is the kind of fat you eat, not how much, that is most important.

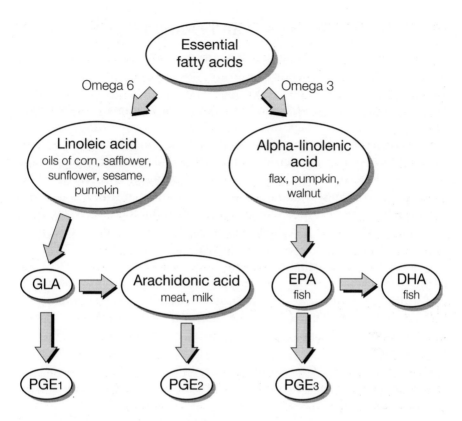

The Omega 3 and 6 fat families. Omega 6 seed oils are processed in the body from linoleic acid into GLA (gamma linolenic acid). GLA is found in evening primrose oil and in borage oil. GLA can also be turned into arachidonic acid, an essential fat found in meat and milk. However, you don't want too much arachidonic acid because it encourages inflammation by making 'series 2' prostaglandins (PGE2). 'Series 1' prostaglandins (PGE1) are anti-inflammatory.

Omega 3 seed oils, found most predominantly in flax seeds, are processed by the body from alpha-linolenic acid into EPA (eicosapentaenoic acid) and then into DHA (docosahexaenoic acid). EPA and DHA are found directly in fish. These, in turn, make 'series 3' prostaglandins (PGE3) which are anti-inflammatory.

The Omega 3 fats EPA and DHA make hormone-like substances called prostaglandins, which are essential for proper brain function, which affects vision, learning ability, co-ordination and mood. Like series 1 they reduce the stickiness of the blood, as well as controlling blood cholesterol and fat levels, improving immune function and metabolism, reducing inflammation and maintaining water balance.

Where to find Omega 3 and Omega 6 fats

The best seed oils for Omega 3 fats are flax (also known as linseed), hemp and pumpkin. While these are certainly good for you, only somewhere between 3 and 10 per cent of these oils gets converted into EPA and DHA. In much the same way as evening primrose oil bypasses the first 'conversion' stage of linoleic acid, if you eat carnivorous fish such as mackerel, herring, tuna and salmon, or their oils, you can bypass the first two conversion stages of alpha-linolenic acid and go straight to EPA and DHA. Fish, especially coldwater fish, are the best *direct* source of these brain-boosters. This is why fish-eaters like the Japanese have three times more Omega 3 fats in their body fat than the average American. Vegans, who eat more seeds and nuts, have twice the Omega 3 fat level of the average American.

The highest concentrations of the Omega 3 fats EPA and DHA are found in mackerel, herring, lake trout, salmon, tuna, sardines, swordfish and white fish, more or less in this order. Mackerel typically contains ten times more EPA and DHA per serving than swordfish or white fish. A 100 gram serving of mackerel could give you as much as 2.5 grams of combined EPA and DHA.

The best seeds for Omega 6 fats are hemp, pumpkin, sunflower, safflower, sesame and maize. Walnuts, soya beans and wheat germ are also rich in Omega 6 fats.

▪ Best foods for essential fats

Omega 3	Omega 6
Flax (linseed)	Corn
Hemp	Safflower
Pumpkin	Sunflower
Walnut	Sesame
EPA & DHA	**GLA**
Salmon	Evening primrose
Mackerel	Borage oil
Herring	Blackcurrant seed
Sardines	
Anchovies	**Arachidonic acid**
Tuna	Meat
Marine algae	Dairy produce
Eggs	Eggs
	Squid

So what should you eat to get an optimal intake of these essential fats? There are three possibilities: eat seeds and fish; eat seed oils, which are more concentrated in essential fats but don't provide other nutrients such as minerals, which are rich in the whole seeds; or supplement concentrated fish oils and seed oils such as flax, evening primrose or starflower oil.

Seeds and fish

If you want to do it with seeds put one measure each of sesame, sunflower and pumpkin seeds, and three measures of flax seeds, in a sealed jar. Keep it in the fridge, away from light, heat and oxygen. Simply adding one heaped tablespoon of these seeds, ground in a coffee grinder, to your breakfast each morning guarantees a good daily intake of essential fatty acids. I'd recommend also eating 100g of oily fish twice a week.

Seed oils

If you want to do it with oils the best place to start is with an oil blend that offers a 1:1 ratio of Omega 3 and Omega 6 fats. You want an oil blend that is cold-pressed, preferably organic and kept refrigerated before you buy it. These are now widely available in health food stores (see Resources, page 530). You need about a dessertspoon a day of such an oil and can add it to salads and other foods (without heating) or just take it neat. Hemp seed oil is the next best thing. It provides 19 per cent alpha-linolenic acid (Omega 3), 57 per cent linoleic acid and 2 per cent GLA (both Omega 6).

Essential fat supplements

As far as supplements are concerned, for Omega 6 your best bet is starflower oil (borage oil) or evening primrose oil. Starflower oil provides more GLA and you need at least 100mg of GLA a day. Fish oils are best for Omega 3 and you need at least 200mg of EPA and 200mg of DHA – or 400mg of these two combined. So, either supplement one GLA capsule and one fish-oil capsule rich in EPA and DHA, or find a supplement that combines EPA, DHA and GLA and take two a day.

Top tip - eat seeds

Smart animals - from parrots to people - eat seeds. Seeds are incredibly rich in essential fats, minerals, vitamin E and protein. You need a tablespoon a day for 100 per cent health. Here's the magic formula:

1. Fill a glass jar with a sealing lid, half with flax seeds (rich in Omega 3) and half with sesame, sunflower and pumpkin seeds (rich in Omega 3).
2. Keep the jar sealed, and place in the fridge to minimise damage from light, heat and oxygen.
3. Put a handful in a coffee/seed grinder, grind up and put on cereals or soups.

The benefits of olive oil

While olive oil contains no appreciable amounts of the essential Omega 3 and Omega 6 oils, much of it is cold-pressed and unrefined. This makes it better for you than refined vegetable oils like the sunflower oil you can buy in the supermarket. Also, while there is a strong association between a high intake of saturated fats, mainly from meat and dairy products, and cardiovascular disease, the reverse is true for olive oil. People in Mediterranean countries, whose diets include large quantities of olive oil, have a lower risk of cardiovascular disease. However, this may be due to a number of positive factors in their diet, including a high intake of fruit and vegetables and relatively more fish than meat. The use of cold-pressed olive oil, which contains tiny amounts of phytochemicals, also results in fewer trans-fats (see page 77) being consumed.

Cook with coconut butter or olive oil

While I've extolled the virtues of the essential polyunsaturated fats in seed and fish oils, these highly active nutrients are very prone to damage and hence are not good for high-temperature cooking such as frying. If you do fry, sauté or bake foods it is best not to use polyunsaturated fats because these generate oxidising free radicals. It is much better to use a saturated fat, the best being coconut butter, or a monounsaturated oil, the best of which is olive oil. These don't generate the harmful free radicals.

Coconut butter is much better for you than regular butter or lard (meat fat). This is because it is what's called a short-chain saturated fat,

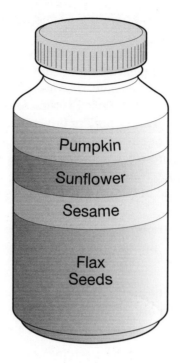

Seed jar

rather than a long-chain saturated fat. While health problems such as increased risk of heart disease have been associated with a diet high in animal fats, the same has not been shown for coconut butter or coconut milk. I use coconut butter and olive oil for sautéing foods, both of which add flavour.

The dangers of trans-fats

Refining and processing vegetable oils can change the nature of the polyunsaturated oil. An example of this is provided by the process used in making margarine. To turn vegetable oil into hard fat the oil goes through a process called hydrogenation. Although the fat is still techni- cally polyunsaturated, the body cannot make use of it. Even worse, it blocks the body's ability to use healthy polyunsaturated oils. This kind of fat is called a trans-fat because its nature has been changed – it is like a key that fits the body's chemical locks but will not open the door. Most margarines contain these so-called 'hydrogenated polyunsaturated oils' and are best avoided. So too are manufactured foods that contain hydrogenated fats, so check ingredients lists on labels carefully. I use pumpkin seed butter instead of butter or margarine as a spread. It tastes delicious.

Frying, as mentioned earlier, is another way to damage otherwise healthy oils. The high temperature makes the oil oxidise so that, instead of being good for you, it generates harmful free radicals in the body (explained fully in Chapter 15). Frying is therefore best avoided as much as possible, as is any form of burning or browning fat. If you do fry, use a tiny amount of olive oil or butter because they are less prone to oxidation than top-quality cold-pressed vegetable oils. The latter should be kept sealed in the fridge, away from heat, light and air, and only used cold in salad dressings or instead of butter on your baked potato or peas.

The general guidelines for getting the right kind and amount of fat in your diet are:

● Eat seeds and nuts – the best seeds are flax, hemp, pumpkin, sunflower and sesame. You get more goodness out of them by grinding them first and sprinkling them on cereal, soups and salads.

● Eat coldwater carnivorous fish – a serving of herring, mackerel, salmon, sardines or, occasionally, fresh tuna two or three times a week provides a good source of Omega 3 fats.

● Use cold-pressed seed oils – choose either an oil blend or hemp oil for salad dressings and other cold uses, such as drizzling on vegetables instead of butter.

● Use pumpkin seed butter as a spread, instead of butter or margarine.

● Minimise your intake of fried food, processed food and saturated fat from meat and dairy produce.

● Supplement fish oil for Omega 3 fats and starflower or evening primrose oil for Omega 6 fats.

In practical terms, you may want to pursue a combined strategy to ensure an optimal intake of brain fats. Here's what I recommend:

A tablespoon of ground seeds	✔ most days (five out of seven)
Cold-pressed seed oil blend	✔ on salad dressings and on vegetables
Pumpkin seed butter	✔ on bread
Coldwater carnivorous fish	✔ twice a week
EPA/DHA/GLA supplement	✔ once a day

chapter 10

Sugar – the Sweet Truth

The human body is designed to run on carbohydrates. While we can use protein and fat for energy, the easiest and most 'smoke-free' fuel is carbohydrate. Plants make carbohydrate by trapping the sun's energy in a complex of carbon, hydrogen and oxygen. Water from the roots provides the hydrogen and oxygen (H_2O), while carbon dioxide (CO_2) from the air provides carbon and more oxygen. Vegetation consists mainly of carbohydrate. We eat the carbohydrate and, in the presence of oxygen from the air, break it down and release the stored solar energy that then provides energy for the body and mind.

When you eat complex carbohydrates like whole grains, vegetables, beans or lentils, or simpler carbohydrates such as fruit, the body does exactly what it is designed to do. It digests these foods and gradually releases their potential energy. What is more, all the nutrients that the body needs for digestion and metabolism are present in those whole foods. Such foods also contain a less digestible type of carbohydrate, classified as fibre, which helps keep the digestive system running smoothly.

While a cat likes the taste of protein, humans are principally attracted to the taste of carbohydrate – sweetness. This inherent attraction towards sweetness worked well for early man because most things in nature that are sweet are not poisonous. It worked well for plants, too. They hid their seeds in their fruit, waiting for animals to pass by, eat the fruit and deposit the seed some distance from the original plant, along with an 'organic manure' starter kit!

But we have discovered how to extract the sweetness and leave the rest – bad news for our nutrition. All forms of concentrated sugar – white sugar, brown sugar, malt, glucose, honey and syrup – are fast releasing, causing a rapid increase in blood sugar levels. If this sugar is not required by the body it is put into storage, eventually emerging as fat. Most concentrated forms of sugar are also devoid of vitamins and minerals, unlike the natural sources such as fruit. White sugar has around 90 per cent of its vitamins and minerals removed. Without vitamins and minerals our metabolism becomes inefficient, contributing to poor energy and poor weight control.

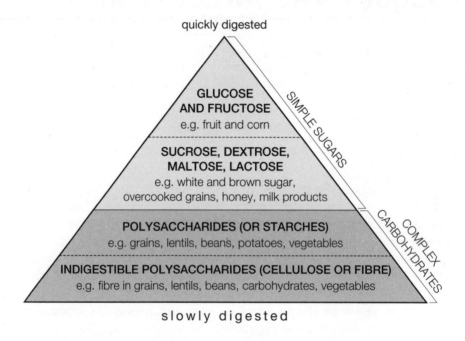

The carbohydrate family

Fruit contains a simple sugar called fructose, which needs no digesting and can therefore enter the bloodstream quickly, like glucose or sucrose. However, unlike them it is classified as slow releasing. This is because the body cannot use fructose as it is, since cells run only on glucose. As a result the fructose first has to be converted by the body into glucose, which effectively slows down this sugar's effect on the metabolism. Lactose, milk sugar, is similar. It is made up of a glucose and galactose. The glucose is fast releasing while the galactose is slow releasing. Some fruit, such as grapes and dates, also contain pure glucose and are therefore faster releasing. Apples, on the other hand, contain mainly fructose and so are slow releasing. Bananas contain both and therefore raise blood sugar levels quite speedily.

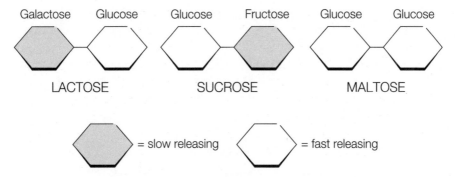

Lactose (milk sugar) versus sucrose (sugar) versus maltose (malt). Galactose and fructose (shown in grey) are slow-releasing sugars while glucose is fast. Hence lactose and sucrose are much slower releasing than maltose, a grain sugar (malt) which is quickly digested into two glucose molecules.

Refined carbohydrates such as white bread, white rice and refined cereals have a similar effect to refined sugar, while oats are more 'complex', and their release of sugar is slower. The process of refining or even cooking starts to break down complex carbohydrates into simple carbohydrates called malt (officially maltose), in effect predigesting them. When you eat simple carbohydrates you get a rapid increase in blood sugar level and a corresponding surge in energy. The surge, however, is followed by a drop as the body scrambles to balance your blood sugar level.

Balancing your blood sugar

Keeping your blood sugar balanced is probably the most important factor in maintaining even energy levels and weight. The level of glucose in your blood largely determines your appetite. When the level drops, you feel hungry. The glucose in your bloodstream is available to your cells to make energy. When the levels are too high the body converts the excess to glycogen (a short-term fuel store mainly in the liver and muscle cells) or fat, our long-term energy reserve. When the levels are too low we experience a whole host of symptoms including fatigue, poor concentration, irritability, nervousness, depression, sweating, headaches and digestive problems. An estimated three in every ten people have impaired ability to keep their blood sugar level even. It may go too high, and then drop too low. The result, over the years, is that they become increasingly fat and lethargic. But if you can control your blood sugar levels the result is even weight and constant energy.

Diabetes is an extreme form of blood sugar imbalance. This condition arises when the body can no longer produce sufficient insulin, a hormone that helps to carry glucose out of the blood and into cells. The result is too

| Glucose | Glucose | Glucose | Fructose |

OATS

| Glucose | Fructose |

SUGAR   GLUCOSE

= slow releasing   = fast releasing

Oats are more complex than glucose. Oats need digesting into single glucose units, which takes time and slows down the release of its sugars. This makes it slower releasing than sugar, which is a molecule of glucose and fructose, which is slower in turn than a glucose molecule, which needs no digesting and directly enters the bloodstream.

much glucose in the blood and not enough for the cells. The early warning signs are similar to those of mild glucose imbalance, but they rarely go away as a result of simple dietary changes. One of the tell-tale signs is a continuous raging thirst as the body tries to dilute the excess blood sugar by stimulating us to drink.

■ Glucose-tolerance check

Answer the questions below, ticking those that you answer 'yes' to. If you tick four or more, there is a strong possibility that your body is having difficulty keeping your blood sugar level even.

- Are you rarely wide awake within twenty minutes of rising?
- Do you need a cup of tea or coffee, a cigarette or something sweet to get you going in the morning?
- Do you often feel drowsy or sleepy during the day, or after meals?
- Do you fall asleep in the early evening or need naps during the day?

◯ Do you avoid exercise because you do not have the energy?

◯ Do you get dizzy or irritable if you go six hours without food?

◯ Is your energy level now less than it used to be?

◯ Do you get night sweats or frequent headaches?

So what makes your blood sugar level unbalanced? The obvious answer is eating too much sugar and sweet foods. However, the kinds of foods that have the greatest effect are not always what you might expect.

The best way to achieve optimal blood sugar balance is to control the glycemic load, or what I call the 'GL', of your diet. This is way superior to 'carbohydrate points' or the 'glycemic index'. Put simply, the glycemic index (GI) of a food tells you whether the carbohydrate in the food is 'fast' or 'slow' releasing. It's a 'quality' measure. It doesn't tell you, however, how much of the food is carbohydrate. Carbohydrate points or grams of carbohydrate tell you how much of the food is carbohydrate, but this doesn't tell you what the particular carbohydrate does to your blood sugar. It's a 'quantity' measure. The glycemic load (GL) of a food is the quantity times the quality. The GL of a food is the best way of telling you how much weight you'll gain if you choose a particular food.

Some foods that you eat a lot of, thinking they are good for you, have a high GL score so be ready for some surprises. Cornflakes and corn chips, for example, are very high, while ice cream and peanuts are not. One single date has the same effect on your blood sugar and weight as a whole punnet of strawberries.

As far as carbohydrates are concerned there are only two rules:

Rule 1   Eat no more than 50 GLs a day, 40 if you want to lose weight (10 per meal and 5 GLs each for two snacks).

Rule 2   For main meals eat low-GL carbohydrates with protein-rich foods.

It isn't just about what you eat, it's also about the quantity you eat, how you prepare it, what you eat it with – and what you drink. Let me give you an example.

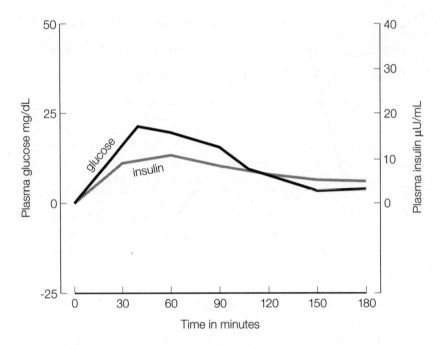

Glycemic response: spaghetti. Within 40 minutes of eating spaghetti, blood sugar levels are at a maximum. The body releases insulin to help get the glucose out of the blood and into body cells. Two hours later both blood glucose and insulin levels have returned to normal.

The first of the graphs above shows how blood sugar levels, and insulin, rise and fall after eating spaghetti. As the blood glucose level rises the body produces insulin, and down it comes again.

In the second graph you can see what happens after eating bread. Now this particular bread and this spaghetti were made from the same flour, using the same amount of flour.[13] So, in this case, the only difference is in the way it has been processed – in rising the bread and cooking it, and what it's mixed with. Bread is risen by feeding yeast sugar, which makes bubbles, hence producing a lighter loaf. The bread is then cooked. Pasta is essentially wheat and some egg. It isn't risen and isn't cooked so long. Both contain the same amount of wheat, but this small difference in preparation makes a big difference in blood sugar response.

Notice that the blood sugar level not only peaks twice as high for bread as for pasta, but also dips twice as low. It's the peaks that damage your arteries, making them less responsive to insulin, and the troughs that leave you tired, sleepy and craving carbohydrates or stimulants. Again, you can see a massive increase in insulin release. In fact, four

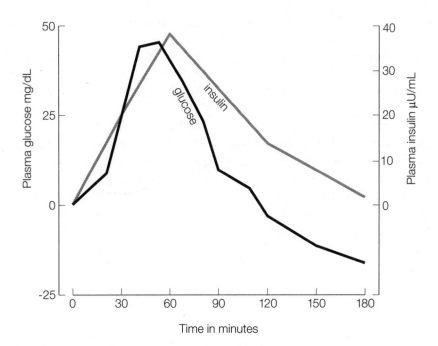

Glycemic response: bread. Within 40 minutes of eating bread, blood sugar levels are almost double those seen with spaghetti. The body produces more than three times as much insulin to bring blood glucose levels under control. The body overreacts and blood glucose goes to low, leading to strong cravings for something sweet or a stimulant such as caffeine, peaking three hours later.

times as much insulin has been produced in the first two hours after eating! What this means is that bread will make you put on weight much more than pasta. It might sound hard to believe, but that is the truth.

Neither fat nor protein has any appreciable effect on blood sugar. Fat and protein can be converted into sugar, but not in the blood, hence their effect on your blood sugar level is negligible. In fact, I recommend you eat some fat and protein with your carbohydrate because this will further lessen the GL score of the carbohydrate you eat.

GL – beyond the glycemic index

It was the discovery that even quite similar foods could have very different effects on blood sugar that led to classifying foods as 'slow-releasing' or 'fast-releasing' carbohydrates. The fast-releasing foods are like rocket fuel, releasing their glucose in a sudden burst. They give a quick burst of energy with a rapid burn-out.

But how do you know what is fast or slow releasing? The very measure of a food's fast- or slow-releasing effect is linked to the degree to which it raises your blood sugar: this can be worked out on the aforementioned scale called the glycemic index (or GI for short). It involves measuring the level to which a food raises your blood glucose in relation to the effect glucose has.

If a food raises blood sugar level significantly, and for some time, the area under the curve made by glucose is great (as for bread, see figure on page 85). Conversely if a food hardly raises blood glucose levels at all, and only for a short time, the area under the curve is smaller (as for pasta, see figure on page 84). The amount of food tested obviously affects how high the blood sugar level will go. The GI of a food is calculated by feeding a person however much of the food is needed to give them 50 grams of carbohydrate. Below you can see the glycemic index for a variety of foods. Generally the high-GI foods are the ones to avoid, while the low-GI foods are the ones to eat. Some examples are given below. Here, apples and oats are slow releasing, while raisins and cornflakes are high.

■ The glycemic index (GI) of common foods

Fast-releasing foods		Slow-releasing foods	
Sucrose	59	Fructose	20
Cornflakes	80	Oats	49
Banana	62	Apple	39
Raisins	64	Pear	38
White bread	70	Whole grain rye bread	41
White spaghetti	50	Wholewheat spaghetti	42
White rice	72	Brown basmati rice	58
Potato (baked)	85	Sweet potato	54
Chocolate	49	Soya beans	15
Rice cake	81	Oatcake	55
Fizzy orange drink	68	Carrots	47
		Apple juice	40

The GI score of a food is very useful, but there's one problem. Compare carrots with chocolate. Why do they have nearly the same scores? Wouldn't you think intuitively that carrots would be good for you? You'd be dead right. The answer is that there is comparatively little carbohydrate in a carrot or a slice of watermelon. In fact, you'd have to eat seven carrots to get the same amount of carbohydrate, and the same effect on your weight, as seven of chocolate would give you. This inconsistency is why the GI score of foods can be misleading.

Forget the GI – it's the GL that counts

The GL score of a food – its glycemic load – solves this inconsistency. It's a calculation based on the amount of carbohydrate in the food *and* its Glycemic Index. It takes both the *quantity* of carbohydrate in the food and the *quality* of the carbohydrate into account. This tells you exactly what a given serving of a food does to your blood sugar. See the chart in Part 9 (pages 501–13) to find out which foods have the lowest GLs.

You'll see that oats are way better than any other cereal; that whole grain rye bread is much better than the others, brown basmati rice is much better than white rice and wholemeal pasta is better than refined. Boiled potatoes are better than baked, while all peas, beans and lentils have very low GLs. The best fruits are berries, plums, apples and pears, while the worst are dates, raisins and bananas.

When you eat carbohydrate foods with a low GL with protein foods you stabilise your blood sugar level even more. An example would be chicken with brown basmati rice, or salmon with wholewheat pasta or a scrambled egg on whole rye toast or oat cakes. The fibre content of a food also lowers its GL, so I'll be recommending high-fibre foods, from beans to brown rice. Lastly, when you eat is very important. It is better to 'graze', eating little and often, rather than to 'gorge', as far as your blood sugar is concerned.

Breaking the habit

The taste for concentrated sweetness is often acquired in childhood. If sweet things are used as a reward or to cheer someone up, they become emotional comforters. The best way to break the habit is to avoid concentrated sweetness in the form of sugar, sweets, sweet desserts, dried fruit and neat fruit juice. Instead, dilute fruit juice and get used to eating fruit instead of having a dessert. Sweeten breakfast cereals with fruit, and have fruit instead of sweet snacks. If you gradually reduce the sweetness in your food you will get used to the taste. Remember, we are designed to eat food that you can pick off a tree or pull out of the ground. Take a look at your average supermarket trolley. Ever seen that stuff grow on trees?

Sugar alternatives

Alternatives to sugar, such as honey or maple syrup, are only marginally better. They both contain more minerals than refined sugar; however, most commercial honey is heated to make it more liquid so that it can be cleaned up and put into jars. The heat turns honey's natural sugar, d-levulose, into another, fast-releasing sugar more like glucose. If you like to eat honey, buy the untreated kind from small local suppliers. Artificial sweeteners are not so great either. Some (admittedly in large quantities) have been shown to have harmful effects on health, and all perpetuate a sweet tooth. One of the best sugar alternatives is xylitol, a vegetable sugar that has a very low GL. It tastes much the same as regular sugar but has little effect on raising blood sugar – half that of fructose. Plums are rich in xylitol, which is part of the reason why they have a very low GL score.

Fibre

Not all types of carbohydrate can be digested and broken down into glucose. Indigestible carbohydrate is called fibre. This is a natural constituent of a healthy diet high in fruit, vegetables, lentils, beans and whole grains, and by eating a high-fibre diet containing these foods you will be at less risk of bowel cancer, diabetes and diverticular disease, and unlikely to suffer from constipation.

Contrary to the popular image of fibre as 'roughage', it can absorb water. As it does so it makes faecal matter bulkier, less dense and easier to pass along the digestive tract. This decreases the amount of time that food waste spends inside the body and reduces the risk of infection or cell changes due to carcinogens that are produced when some foods, particularly meat, degrade. A frequent meat-eater with a low-fibre diet can increase the gut-transit time of food from twenty-four to seventy-two hours, giving time for some putrefaction to occur. So if you like meat make sure you also eat high-fibre foods.

There are many different types of fibre, some of which are proteins and not carbohydrates. Some kinds, such as that found in oats, are called 'soluble fibre' and combine with sugar molecules to slow down the absorption of carbohydrates. In this way they help to keep blood sugar levels balanced. Some fibres are much more water-absorbent than others. While wheat fibre swells to ten times its original volume in water, glucomannan fibre, from the Japanese konjac plant, swells to one hundred times its volume in water. By bulking up foods and releasing sugars slowly, highly absorbent types of fibre can help to control appetite and play a part in weight maintenance.

An ideal intake of fibre is not less than 35 grams a day. Provided the right foods are eaten, this level can easily be achieved without adding extra fibre. Professor of Nutrition John Dickerson from the University of Surrey has stressed the danger of adding wheat bran to a nutrient-poor diet. The reason is that wheat bran contains high levels of phytate, an anti-nutrient that reduces the absorption of essential minerals, including zinc. Overall, it is probably best to get fibre from a mixture of sources such as oats, lentils, beans, seeds, fruit and raw or lightly cooked vegetables.

Much of the fibre in vegetables is destroyed by cooking, so they are best eaten crunchy.

To ensure that you get enough of the right kinds of carbohydrates:

- Eat whole foods — whole grains, lentils, beans, nuts, seeds, fresh fruit and vegetables — and avoid refined, white and overcooked foods.

- Eat five servings a day of dark green, leafy and root vegetables such as watercress, carrots, sweet potatoes, broccoli, Brussels sprouts, spinach, green beans and peppers, either raw or lightly cooked.

- Eat three or more servings a day of fresh fruit, preferably apples, pears and/or berries.

- Eat four or more servings a day of whole grains such as rice, rye, oats, wholewheat, corn, quinoa as cereal, breads, pasta or pulses.

- Avoid any form of sugar, added sugar, and white or refined foods.

- Dilute fruit juices and eat dried fruit only infrequently and in small quantities, preferably soaked.

Dig deeper by reading *The Holford Diet* which shows you how to eat the 'low GL' way.

chapter 11

Stimulants – Are You Addicted?

Sugar is only one side of the coin, as far as blood sugar problems are concerned. Stimulants and stress are the other. As you can see from the figure below, if your blood sugar level dips there are two ways to raise it. One is to eat more glucose, and the other is to increase your level of the stress hormones adrenalin and cortisol. There are two ways in which you can raise adrenalin and cortisol. Consume a stimulant – tea, coffee, chocolate or cigarettes – or react stressfully, causing an increase in your own production of adrenalin.

Knowing this, you can see how easy it is to get caught up in the vicious cycle of stress, sugar and stimulants. It will leave you feeling tired, depressed and stressed much of the time.

Here's how it works. Through excess sugar, stress and stimulants you lose your blood sugar control and wake up each morning with low blood sugar levels and not enough adrenalin to kick-start your day. So you adopt one of two strategies:

- **Either** you reluctantly crawl out of bed on remote control and head for the kettle, make yourself a strong cup of tea or coffee, light up a cigarette or have some fast-releasing sugar in the form of toast, with some sugar on it called jam. Up go your blood sugar and adrenalin levels and you start to feel normal.

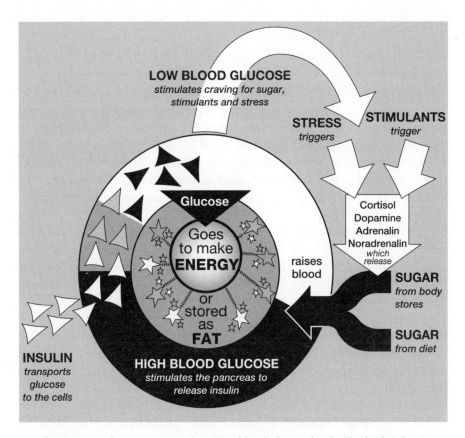

The sugar cycle. Eating sugar increases blood glucose levels. The body releases insulin into the blood to help escort glucose out and into body cells, to make energy or convert into fat. The result is low blood glucose. Either 'real' stress, causing an increase in adrenalin, or stress induced by consuming a stimulant such as caffeine, which raises adrenal hormones, causes breakdown of stores of sugar in the liver and muscles, called glycogen, which raises blood sugar levels. Low blood glucose causes stress or cravings for either something sweet or a stimulant.

- **Or** you lie in bed and start to think about all the things that have gone wrong, could go wrong, will go wrong. You start to worry about everything you've got to do, haven't done and should have done. About ten minutes of this gets enough adrenalin pumping to get you out of bed.

If this sounds like you, you're caught in that vicious circle, with all its negative effects on your mind and mood.

Caffeine makes you tired

Here's the irony. The reason that people get hooked on drinking coffee, particularly in the morning, is because it makes them feel better, more energised and alert. But, wondered Dr Peter Rogers, a psychologist at Bristol University, does coffee actually increase your energy and mental performance, or just relieve the symptoms of withdrawal? When he researched this he found that after that sacred cup of coffee, coffee-drinkers don't feel any better than people who never drink coffee. Coffee-drinkers just feel better than they did when they woke up.[14] In other words, drinking coffee relieves the symptoms of withdrawal from coffee. It's addictive.

Not only is coffee addictive, but also it worsens mental performance. A study published in the *American Journal of Psychiatry* looked at 1,500 psychology students and divided them into four categories depending on their coffee intake: abstainers, low consumers (one cup or equivalent a day), moderate (one to five cups a day) and high (five or more cups a day). The moderate and high consumers were found to have higher levels of anxiety and depression than the abstainers, and the high consumers had the greatest incidence of stress-related medical problems, as well as lower academic performance.[15] A number of studies have shown that the ability to remember lists of words is reduced by caffeine. According to one researcher, 'Caffeine may have a deleterious effect on the rapid processing of ambiguous or confusing stimuli.' That sounds like a description of modern living!

Caffeine blocks the receptors for a brain chemical called adenosine, whose function is to stop the release of the motivating neurotransmitters dopamine and adrenalin. With less adenosine activity, levels of dopamine and adrenalin increase, as does alertness and motivation. Peak concentration occurs thirty to sixty minutes after consumption.

The more caffeine you consume, the more your body and brain become insensitive to its own natural stimulants, dopamine and adrenalin. You then need more stimulants to feel normal, and keep pushing the body to produce more dopamine and adrenalin. The net result is adrenal exhaustion – an inability to produce these important chemicals of motivation and communication. Apathy, depression, exhaustion and an inability to cope set in.

Coffee isn't the only source of caffeine. There's as much in a cup of strong tea as in a cup of regular coffee. Caffeine is also the active ingredient in most cola and other energy drinks such as Red Bull, which sold over 100 million cans last year. Chocolate and green tea also contain caffeine, but much less than these drinks.

■ Caffeine buzzometer

Here are caffeine levels in a number of popular products:

Product	Caffeine content
Coca-Cola Classic 350ml (12fl oz)	46mg
Diet Coke 350ml (12fl oz)	46mg
Red Bull	80mg
Hot cocoa 150ml (5fl oz)	10mg
Coffee, instant 150ml (5fl oz)	40–105mg
Coffee, espresso, cappuccino, latte	30–50mg
Coffee, filter 150ml (5fl oz)	110–150mg
Coffee, Starbucks (grande)	500mg
Decaffeinated coffee 150ml (5fl oz)	0.3mg
Tea 150ml (5fl oz)	20–100mg
Green tea (5 fl oz)	20-30mg
Chocolate cake (1 slice)	20–30mg
Dark (cooking) chocolate 28g (1oz)	5–35mg
Caffeine pills (per pill)	50–200mg

Kicking the habit

If you want to be in tip-top mental health, stay away from stimulants. This is doubly important for those with mental health problems because too much caffeine can, in some, produce symptoms that lead to a diagnosis of schizophrenia or mania. This may happen because high caffeine consumers can become both allergic to coffee and unable to detoxify caffeine. The net effect is serious disruption of both mind and mood.[16]

Here's how you can give up.

Coffee contains three stimulants: caffeine, theobromine and theophylline. Although caffeine is the strongest, theophylline is known to disturb normal sleep patterns and theobromine has a similar effect to caffeine, although it is present in much smaller amounts in coffee. So decaffeinated coffee isn't exactly stimulant-free. As a nutritionist, I have seen many people cleared of minor health problems such as tiredness and headaches just from cutting out their two or three coffees a day. The best way to find out what effect it has on you is to quit for a trial period of two weeks. You may get withdrawal symptoms for up to three days. These reflect how addicted you've become. After this, if you begin to feel perky and your health improves, that's a good indication that you're better off without coffee. The most popular alternatives are Teecino, Caro Extra or Bambu (made with roasted chicory and malted barley) or herb teas.

Tea is the great British addiction. A cup of strong tea contains as much caffeine as a cup of regular coffee and is certainly addictive. Tea also contains tannin, which interferes with the absorption of essential minerals such as iron and zinc. Particularly addictive is Earl Grey tea containing bergamot, itself a stimulant. If you're addicted to tea and can't get going without a cuppa, it may be time to stop for two weeks and see how you feel. The best-tasting alternatives are Rooibosch tea (red bush tea) with milk, and herbal or fruit teas. Drinking very weak tea from time to time is unlikely to be a problem.

Chocolate bars are usually full of sugar. Cocoa, the active ingredient in chocolate, provides significant quantities of the stimulant theobromine, whose action is similar to caffeine's, though not as strong. It also contains small amounts of caffeine. Theobromine is also obtained in cocoa drinks like hot chocolate. As chocolate is high in sugar and stimulants, and delicious as well, it's all too easy to become a chocoholic. The best way to quit the habit is to have one month with *no* chocolate. Instead, eat healthy 'sweets' from health food shops that are sugar free and don't contain chocolate. After a month you will have lost the craving.

Cola and 'energy' drinks contain anything from 46 to 80mg of caffeine per can, which is as much as there is in a cup of coffee. In addition, these drinks are often high in sugar and colourings and their net stimulant effect can be considerable. Check the ingredients list and stay away from drinks containing caffeine and chemical additives or colourings.

Changing any food habit can be stressful in itself, so it is best not to quit everything in one go. A good strategy is to avoid something for a month and then see how you feel. One way to greatly reduce the cravings for foods you've got hooked on is by having an excellent diet. Since all stimulants affect blood sugar levels, you can keep yours even by always having something substantial for breakfast, such as an oat-based, not-too-refined cereal; unsweetened live yoghurt with banana, ground sesame seeds and wheat germ; or an egg. You can snack frequently on fresh fruit. The worst thing you can do is go for hours without eating. Eating a highly alkaline-forming diet can reduce cravings for cigarettes and alcohol. This means eating lots of fresh vegetables and fruit. These high-fibre foods also help to keep your blood sugar level even.

As we saw in Chapters 12 and 13, vitamins and minerals are important too because they help to regulate your blood sugar level, and hence your appetite. They also minimise the withdrawal effects of stimulants and the symptoms of food allergy. The key nutrients are vitamin C, the B complex vitamins, especially vitamin B6, and the minerals calcium, magnesium and chromium. Fresh fruit and vegetables provide significant amounts of vitamin C and B vitamins, while vegetables and seeds such as sunflower and sesame are good sources of calcium and magnesium. For maximum effect, however, it is best to supplement these nutrients as well as eating foods rich in them.

■ Are you dependent on stimulants?

To find out if you are stimulant-dependent, complete the 'stimulant inventory' below, for a week.

	Unit	Sun	Mon	Tue	Wed	Thu	Fri	Sat
Green tea	2 cups							
Tea	1 cup							
Coffee	1 cup							
Cola or caffeinated drinks	1 can							
Caffeine pills (e.g. No-Doz, Excedrin, Dexatrim)	1 pill							
Chocolate	50gm							
Alcohol (units: Glass of wine is 1 Bottle of beer is 1 or 2 Shot of spirits is 1)	1 unit							
Added sugar	1 teaspoon							
Hidden sugar (see sugar contents on ingredients lists)	1 teaspoon/5gm							
Cigarettes	1 cigarette							

Add up your total number of 'units'. The ideal is 5 or fewer per week. If you are having more than 10 stimulant units a week, this is going to have an effect on your mental well-being. If you score 30 or more this could well be contributing to mental health problems. It is strongly recommended that you reduce or avoid all these substances for at least a month and see how this helps your symptoms.

In summary, here are a few simple steps you can take to reduce your intake of and addiction to stimulants and balance your blood sugar:

- Avoid sugar and foods containing sugar.

- Break your addiction to caffeine by avoiding coffee, tea and caffeinated drinks for a month, while improving your diet. Once you are no longer craving caffeine, the occasional cup of weak tea or very occasional coffee is not a big deal.

- Break your addiction to chocolate. Once you are no longer craving it, the occasional piece of chocolate is not a problem, but choose the dark, low-sugar kind.

- Eat breakfast, choosing low-GL foods, lunch and dinner, plus two fruit snacks in between.

- Take a high-strength multivitamin, plus 2,000mg per day of vitamin C and 200mcg of chromium.

chapter 12.

The Vitamin Scandal

Every survey of eating habits conducted in Britain since the 1980s shows that even those who said they ate a balanced diet fail to eat anything like the US, EU or World Health Organisation Recommended Daily Allowances (RDAs). But these RDAs of nutrients are set by governments to prevent deficiency diseases like scurvy; they are certainly not designed to ensure optimal health, and there is a big difference between a lack of illness and the presence of wellness. For example, the average person gets 3.5 colds a year. In a study of 1,038 doctors and their wives, those who took 410mg of vitamin C a day had the least signs of illness and lowest incidence of colds. This intake is roughly seven times the RDA for vitamin C.

RDAs are set by panels of scientists in different countries, based on what is known to prevent classic nutrient-deficiency diseases. The trouble is that the scientists cannot agree. From country to country there is often a ten-fold variation in recommended levels of nutrients. Dr Stephen Davies, a medical researcher, tested blood levels of B vitamins in thousands of people and found more than seven in every ten to be deficient.[17] The RDAs do not take into account an individual's circumstances, nor do they consider the question of what is optimal. For example, if you smoke, drink alcohol, live in a polluted city, are pre-menstrual, menopausal or on the pill, exercise a lot, are fighting an infection or stressed out, your nutrient needs can easily double.

What is more, it is very difficult to eat a diet that meets the RDA levels. What most people conceive of as a well-balanced diet fails to meet RDA requirements. The Bateman Report, published in 1985,[18] found that more than 85 per cent of people who generally thought they ate a well-balanced diet failed to meet RDA levels. At the other end of the scale, 25 per cent of women on income support take in smaller quantities of eight nutrients than the level known to result in serious deficiency diseases (Food Commission, 1992). The latest comprehensive survey of what we eat in Britain, called the National Diet and Nutrition Survey (NDNS), compared with the RDAs, shows just how many of us fail to achieve even these basic RDA levels. In truth, fewer than one in ten people eat a diet that meets even the RDA requirements.

While you might think that our diets are getting better, comparison with a similar survey in 1986–7 shows that our intakes of vitamins A and B12, iron, magnesium and zinc have all fallen. These vitamins and minerals are vital for health and the evidence is that we need more, not less, for optimal health. B12, for example, is often low in older people and helps lower homocysteine thereby reducing risk for heart disease and Alzheimer's disease. Yet if you give older people with raised homocysteine levels 10mcg of B12, which is ten times the RDA, it neither corrects their deficiency nor lowers homocysteine. Only levels of 50mcg, that's fifty times the RDA, bring them back to optimal health.[19]

Empty calories

As much as two-thirds of the average calorie intake is from fat, sugar and refined flours. The calories in these foods are called 'empty' because they provide no nutrients, and are often hidden in processed foods and snacks that usually weigh little but satisfy our appetite instantly. For instance, two sweet biscuits provide more calories than 1lb (0.45kg) of carrots and are considerably easier to eat – but they provide no vitamins or minerals. If a quarter of your diet by weight, and two-thirds by calories, consists of such dismembered foods, there is little room left to accommodate the necessary levels of the essential nutrients. Wheat, for example, has twenty-five nutrients removed in the refining process that turns it into white flour, yet only four (iron, B1, B2 and B3) are replaced. On average, 87 per cent of the essential minerals zinc, chromium and manganese are lost. Have we been short-changed?

This raises three questions. What is 'need'? Are the RDA levels enough? How can we achieve the necessary intake?

Why feeling just 'all right' is not all right

To date the evidence is that most people *are* being short-changed on health, owing to inadequate intakes of vitamins and minerals. Since the

1980s proper scientific studies using multi-nutrient supplements have shown that they boost immunity, increase IQ, reduce birth defects, improve childhood development, reduce colds, stop PMS, improve bone density, balance moods, reduce aggression, increase energy, reduce the risk of cancer and heart disease and basically promote a long and healthy life. Most people are putting up with 'feeling all right' – accepting the odd cold, headache, mouth ulcer, muscle cramp or bout of PMS, mood fluctuations, poor concentration and lack of energy. Back in 1982 at the Institute for Optimum Nutrition we put seventy-six volunteers on a six-month supplement programme.[20] At the end of this time, 79 per cent reported a definite improvement in energy, 60 per cent spoke of better memory and mental alertness, 66 per cent felt more emotionally balanced, 57 per cent had fewer colds and infections and 55 per cent had better skin.

What is optimum?

The RDAs are not enough for optimum health. Thanks to Dr Emanuel Cheraskin and colleagues from the University of Alabama, we are getting closer to defining optimum nutrition.[21] Over a fifteen-year period they studied 13,500 people living in six regions of the US. Each participant completed in-depth health questionnaires and was given physical, dental, eye and other examinations, as well as numerous blood tests, cardiac function tests and a detailed dietary analysis. The object was to find which nutrient-intake levels were associated with the highest health ratings.

The results consistently revealed that the healthiest individuals, meaning those with the fewest clinical signs and symptoms, were taking supplements and eating diets rich in nutrients relative to calories. The researchers found that the intake of nutrients associated with optimal health was often ten or more times higher than the RDA levels. At the Institute for Optimum Nutrition we've continued this research and have identified the kinds of intakes of nutrients that are optimum by looking at studies that prove better health with additional intakes of nutrients above the so-called 'well-balanced diet'.

For example, ninety-six healthy elderly people were given a high-strength multivitamin and mineral supplement or placebo. Those on the supplement had fewer infections and blood tests revealed a stronger immune system; in fact they were healthier overall. Of 22,000 pregnant women, some on supplements, some not, the group taking supplements gave birth to 75 per cent fewer babies with birth defects.[22] In another study, ninety schoolchildren were given a high-strength multivitamin and mineral supplement, placebo or nothing. Seven months later the IQ scores of those on supplements were 10 per cent higher than those of the other two groups.

A similar study was carried out on a group of ninety-six people over the age of sixty-five. They too had dramatic improvements in mental performance and memory.[23] The same research group gave multivitamins to elderly people and found it halved their risk of infection.[24] A professor of medicine examined all studies looking at vitamin C versus the common cold, selecting only those where 1,000mg or more was given, and involving a placebo group (known as double-blind testing).[25] Of these tests, thirty-seven out of thirty-eight concluded that supplementing 1,000mg, twenty times the RDA, had a protective effect. Professor Morris Brown at Cambridge University gave 2,000 patients with heart disease vitamin E or a placebo. Those taking vitamin E had 75 per cent fewer heart attacks.[26]

These are just some of the hundreds of scientific studies published in respected medical journals proving that an intake of vitamins above RDA levels enhances resistance to infection, improves intellectual performance and reduces the risk of birth defects, cancer and heart disease. By reviewing all this research we have established our suggested optimal intakes of nutrients. At ION we call these levels the Optimum Daily Allowances, or ODAs for short, shown below. Also shown below is what you can reasonably be expected to achieve from your diet. The shortfall between this and our ODAs is well worth supplementing.

Despite this, some 'flat-earthers' continue to say that supplements are a waste of money. To quote one anti-supplement survey of people who took supplements, published in the journal *Nutrition Reviews*, 'It is ironic that adults who were not overweight and whose health was good used supplements more frequently than did less healthy individuals.' What a strange coincidence! I think of supplements like clothes – they are not strictly natural, although they are made from natural ingredients. They don't have any downsides if used properly and, as every year passes, have more and more proven benefits. I think soon everyone will be taking them in addition to, I hope, eating a healthy diet.

Vitamin A

This vitamin is essential for reproduction and for the maintenance of epithelial tissue found in skin, inside and out, such as the lungs, gastrointestinal tract, uterus and so on. Betacarotene is the most active precursor of vitamin A, and in high doses, unlike vitamin A itself, is not toxic. Vitamin A is important in cancer prevention and treatment of pre-cancerous conditions. It is also essential for vision. Many autistic children have problems with visual perception and don't look straight at you. This is because there are more receptors for black and white vision – called rods – in the periphery of the

NUTRIENTS	RDA	100% RDA ↓ (Average diet / Good diet)		Shortfall	ODA
Vitamin A (mcg)	800	900▶	1500▶	◀Shortfall 1000▶	2500
Vitamin D (mcg)	5	4▶	7▶	◀Shortfall 4▶	11
Vitamin E (mg)	10	14▶	50▶	◀Shortfall 250▶	300
Vitamin C (mg)	60	100▶	200▶	◀Shortfall 1800▶	2000
Vitamin B1 (mg)	1.4	2▶	5▶	◀Shortfall 30▶	35
Vitamin B2 (mg)	1.6	2.18▶	5▶	◀Shortfall 30▶	35
Vitamin B3 (mg)	18	39.6▶	50▶	◀Shortfall 35▶	85
Vitamin B5 (mg)	6	2.175▶	20▶	◀Shortfall 80▶	100
Vitamin B6 (mg)	2	3.1▶	5▶	◀Shortfall 70▶	75
Folic Acid (mcg)	200	325.5▶	400▶	◀Shortfall 400▶	800
Vitamin B12 (mcg)	1	5.95▶	10▶	◀Shortfall 15▶	25
Biotin (mcg)	150	36.50▶ 120▶		◀Shortfall 105▶	225
GLA* (Omega-6) (mg)	–	20▶	40▶	◀Shortfall 110▶	150
EPA/DHA* (Omega-3) (mg)	–	60▶	100▶	◀Shortfall 600▶	700
Calcium (mg)	800	(800:good diet)▶	912.5▶	◀Shortfall 200▶	1000
Iron (mg)	14	12.8▶	15▶	◀Shortfall 5▶	20
Magnesium (mg)	300	272▶	350▶	◀Shortfall 150▶	500
Zinc (mg)	15	9.3▶ 10▶		◀Shortfall 10▶	20
Iodine (mcg)	150	193.5▶	240▶	◀Shortfall 60▶	300
Selenium (mcg)*	–	40▶	50▶	◀Shortfall 50▶	100
Chromium (mcg)*	–	50▶	75▶	◀Shortfall 50▶	125
Manganese (mcg)*	–	3▶	6▶	◀Shortfall 4▶	10

Key

■ Average diet
▨ Good diet

RDA = Recommended daily allowance
ODA = Optimum daily allowance (diet plus supplements)
* items marked with an asterisk have no RDA

RDAs versus ODAs and dietary intakes. *This chart shows the differences between the RDA, our average intake, and our ideal intake. The grey amounts are the levels we could reach if we ate a good variety of fruit and vegetables daily – i.e. a good diet.*

Using vitamin C as an example, the RDA is 60mg. The average intake is 100mg. If you eat plenty of fruit and vegetables you could achieve 200mg. The optimal intake is somewhere between 1,000 and 3,000mg. The ODA is set at the mid-point of 2,000mg. The shortfall between a good diet (200mg) and the ODA (2,000mg) is 1,800mg. This is the kind of level worth supplementing.

eye. Give these kids natural vitamin A from fish oil and they look straight at you. In regard to cancer, people with low betacarotene intake have a 30–220 per cent higher risk of developing lung cancer, for example. The optimal intake of vitamin A is likely to be at least double the RDA. Even higher levels of betacarotene may confer extra benefits.

Vitamin B complex

This group of vitamins includes eight essential nutrients. These five are most commonly deficient.

- **B1 (thiamine)** is unlikely to be needed at levels more than eleven times the RDA unless you are consuming a lot of refined carbohydrates. A study of 1,009 dentists and their wives found the healthiest to consume on average 9mg of thiamine a day.

- **Vitamin B2 (riboflavin)** is needed in greater quantities by those who take exercise frequently. To date there is insufficient evidence to recommend more than double the RDA.

- **Vitamin B3 (niacin)** is famous for its ability to help remove unwanted cholesterol but notorious for its vasodilatory or blushing effect in high doses. According to one study the healthiest people consume 115mg a day, which is nine times the RDA.

- **Vitamin B6 (pyridoxine)** is another B vitamin that appears to have considerable benefit at levels ten times higher than the RDA. It is essential for all protein utilisation and has been helpful in a variety of conditions from PMS to carpal tunnel syndrome (a strain condition affecting nerves in the wrist) and cardiovascular disease.

- **Folic acid** is now recognised as essential for the prevention of neural tube defects in pregnancy, and the UK government recommends pregnant women take a daily 400mcg supplement. Optimal levels, especially in the elderly, may be much higher. There is one caution, however: folic acid supplementation can mask B12-deficiency anaemia, so it is best to supplement extra folic acid with vitamin B12.

Vitamin C

This one is necessary for a strong immune system, for collagen and bone formation, for energy production and as an antioxidant. In a study of 1,038 doctors and their wives, those with a daily intake of 410mg of vitamin C had the fewest signs of illness or degenerative disease.[24] This intake, roughly ten times the RDA, is close to that of our primitive ancestors. A large number of studies have found a reduced risk of cancer in those with a high vitamin C intake. Vitamin C status and bone density decline from the age of thirty-five. Numerous studies have shown vitamin C to be associated with improved bone density as well as keeping the absorption of iron, giving us good reason to increase our intake as we get older.

The protective role of vitamin C against various cancers, cardiovascular disease and the common cold becomes significant only when the intake is above 400–1,000mg a day. In a large survey in the US, analysed by Dr Paul Enstrom and Dr Linus Pauling, significant reductions in overall mortality and mortality from cancer and cardiovascular disease were reported in those who took vitamin E and C supplements. Since 1,000mg of vitamin C is equivalent to twenty-two oranges, supplementation is essential. The RDA for vitamin C is only 60mg – the equivalent of an orange a day.

Vitamin E

One of the most essential antioxidants, vitamin E helps the body to use oxygen properly. A number of studies have found low vitamin E status to be associated with high cancer incidence. Supplementation of this vitamin has been shown to boost immunity and reduce infections in the elderly as well as halving the risk of cataracts. The optimal intake of vitamin E is thirty times the RDA.

Vitamins D and K

These are not commonly deficient. Vitamin K is made by bacteria in the gut, while vitamin D can be made in the skin on exposure to sunlight. Vitamin D is also found in milk, meat and eggs. Deficiency is likely only in dark-skinned vegans who have little exposure to the sun.

The decline of fruit and vegetables

The sad truth is that food today is not what it used to be. Fruit and vegetables are only as good as the soil in which they are grown. Minerals pass from the soil to the plant, and in turn help the plant to grow and produce vitamins. The trouble is that modern farming, which relies heavily on artificial fertilisers and pesticides, robs the soil of nutrients and does not replace them. Phosphates found in fertilisers and pesticides bind to the minerals in the soil, making them less available to the plant. Through overfarming, the soil becomes nutrient-deficient anyway. However, adding fertiliser (nitrogen, phosphate and potassium) enables plants to go on growing, but without the full complement of minerals.

So the plant does not make its full complement of vitamins and we too end up deficient.

For these reasons, plus the length of time we store foods, there is a staggering range of nutrient content in fruit and vegetables. An orange may provide from 180mg of vitamin C to none at all, the average being around 60mg. Yes, some supermarket oranges contain no vitamin C! A hundred grams of wheat germ (about three cups) provides from 2.1mg to 14mg of vitamin E. A large (100 gram) carrot can provide from 70 to 18,500iu of vitamin A. While it's great to eat lots of fruit and vegetables, the quality is just as important as the quantity. For this reason it is best to buy local produce in season and consume it quickly. The worst thing you can do is to buy fruit shipped in from the other side of the world and leave it hanging around for two weeks before you eat it. Organic food also tends to have much higher levels of both vitamins and minerals and other antioxidants.

■ Variations in nutrient content in common foods

Nutrient	Variation (per 100g of food)
Vitamin A in carrots	70 to 18,500iu
Vitamin B5 in wholewheat flour	0.3 to 3.3mg
Vitamin C in oranges	0 to 116mg
Vitamin E in wheat germ	3.2 to 21iu
Iron in spinach	0.1 to 158mg
Manganese in lettuce	0.1 to 16.9mg

Good food goes off

Food manufacturing, even more than farming practices, is the greatest cause of vitamin loss. Foods are refined so that they last longer. Flour, rice and sugar lose more than 77 per cent of their zinc, chromium and manganese in the refining process. Other essential nutrients, such as essential fats, will not be present in processed foods because these and other nutrients (except antioxidant vitamins A, C and E, which preserve foods) can decrease shelf life. There is an old saying among nutritionists that 'good food goes off' – the trick is to eat it first.

What about cooking?

More than half the nutrients in the food you eat are destroyed before they reach your plate, depending on the food you choose, how you store it and how you cook it. Every process that food goes through, whether boiling, baking, frying or freezing, takes its toll. Think about the life of a runner bean. It is picked, stored, cooked, frozen, stored in the supermarket until you buy it, partially defrosted on the way home, refrozen, boiled and eaten. Just how much goodness is left?

The three main enemies of vitamins and minerals are heating, water and oxidation. Vitamin C is very prone to oxidation, sacrificing itself to harmful oxides that make food go rancid. While it might protect your food, it will not protect you if there is none left by the time you eat it. The longer your food has been stored, and the more surface area is exposed to air and light, the less vitamin C there is likely to be. Orange juice, which is packed using a special process to minimise oxide exposure on packing, suffers a 33 per cent loss of vitamin C in twenty-two weeks, which is a conceivable time lag between orange grove and breakfast glass. Once you open the carton oxidation occurs rapidly, especially if you fail to put it back in the fridge, which also protects it from light. Analyses of rosehip teabags have shown negligible traces of vitamin C or none at all, even before they are immersed in boiling water which is likely to kill off any remaining traces.

Nor is vitamin C the only vitamin susceptible to oxidation: the anti-oxidant vitamins A and E are also prone to damage. Being fat-soluble, they tend to be protected by being in fattier foods. Betacarotene, the vegetable form of vitamin A, is water soluble and highly prone to oxidation. While storing foods in cool, dark places tends to help, oxidation still occurs even in the fridge. Spinach stored in an open container will lose 10 per cent of its vitamin C content every day.

On the whole, frozen foods keep their nutrient content much better. Chilled foods, kept for two weeks in the supermarket and one week in your fridge, will have lost their vitamin vitality, while there is little difference in nutrient loss between frozen peas and fresh peas, once boiled.

Any form of heating destroys nutrients. The degree of destruction depends on the cooking time and on whether the container disperses the heat evenly, but most of all on the temperature. On average, 20–70 per cent of the nutrient content of leafy vegetables is lost in cooking.

Deep-frying produces temperatures in excess of 200°C, which oxidise fat and turn essential fatty acids into trans-fats that are no good for anything. Animals fed such oils develop atherosclerosis. Refined oils, left for weeks on supermarket shelves exposed to light, are already damaged. These oils should not be used for frying as they increase the destruction of antioxidant nutrients like vitamins A, C and E both in the food and later in the body. See page 76 for the best way to fry food if you still want to use this cooking method.

Minerals and water-soluble vitamins leach into cooking water. The more water you use and the longer the cooking time, the more this is likely to occur. If the temperature is above 50°C, cell structures begin to break down, which enables nutrients within them to be leached out. High temperatures can also destroy some of the vitamins, though not the minerals. If you boil or steam food for a short while, the temperature at the core of the food will be much lower than at the outside. Foods can therefore be protected by being cooked whole, or in large pieces. The loss of nutrients in boiled food tends to be around 20–50 per cent. It is a good idea to use the mineral-rich water as stock for soups or sauces.

Microwaving water-based foods such as vegetables generates heat by vibrating the water particles in the food; and vitamin and mineral losses are minimal. However, as far as essential fats are concerned the heat generated by microwaving rapidly destroys them, so never microwave a dish with oils, nuts or seeds in it. And if you do microwave your food, stand well back. You need to be about ten feet away to no longer be exposed to its electromagnetic radiation.

Here are some guidelines for getting the most vitamins out of your food:

- Eat foods as fresh and unprocessed as possible.
- Keep fresh food cool and in the dark in the fridge in sealed containers.
- Eat more raw food. Be adventurous: try raw beetroot and carrot tops in salad.
- Prepare foods cold where possible (e.g. carrot soup) and heat to serve.
- Cook foods as whole as possible, slicing or blending before serving.
- Steam or boil foods with as little water as possible, and keep the water for stock.
- Fry as little food as possible and do not overcook, burn or brown it.
- Supplement your diet to ensure optimum levels of vitamins.

chapter 13

Elemental Health from Calcium to Zinc

More than a hundred years ago a Russian chemist called Mendelyeff noticed that all the basic constituents of matter, the elements, could be arranged in a pattern according to their chemical properties. From this he produced what is known as the periodic table. There were many gaps where elements should be, and sure enough over the years these missing elements have been discovered. All matter, including your body, is made out of these elements.

Some of these are gases, like oxygen and hydrogen; some are liquids; and some, such as iron, zinc and chromium, are solids. Ninety-six per cent of the body is made up of carbon, hydrogen, oxygen and nitrogen, which form carbohydrate, protein and fat, as well as vitamins. The remaining 4 per cent is made from minerals.

These minerals are mainly used to regulate and balance our body chemistry; the exceptions are calcium, phosphorus and magnesium, which are the major constituents of bone. These three, plus sodium and potassium, which control the water balance in the body, are called macro-minerals because we need relatively large amounts each day (300–3,000mg). The remaining elements are called trace minerals because we need only traces each day (30mcg–30mg). But all these minerals are required in tiny amounts compared with carbon, hydrogen and oxygen. For instance, a 10-stone man needs 400 grams of carbohydrate a day but only 40 micrograms of chromium, which is less than a millionth of the amount. Yet chromium is no less important.

Mineral deficiency is widespread

Minerals are extracted from the soil in the first place by plants. Like vitamins, they may be obtained directly from those plants or indirectly via meat. And, again like vitamins, they are frequently deficient in our modern diets. There are three primary reasons for this.

Mineral levels in natural foods are declining

This is partly because soil gradually loses its mineral content through overfarming, unless the farmer replaces the minerals by adding back mineral-rich manure. But many of the minerals that pass from plant to us are not needed to make the plant grow, so there is no incentive for the farmer to add them back. The minerals that are added back in fertiliser (nitrogen, phosphate and potassium) make the plant grow faster and, in the case of phosphate, bind to trace minerals like zinc and make them harder for the plant to take up. Analyses of mineral levels in plants in 1939 compared with those in 1991 show, on average, a drop of 22 per cent. (The accuracy of this data is, however, a little suspect as analytical methods have improved dramatically over this period.)

Essential minerals are refined out of food

Refining food to make white rice, white flour and white sugar removes up to 90 per cent of the trace minerals. Foods like refined cereals must meet a legal minimum nutrient requirement and therefore have some calcium, iron and B vitamins added back. To help sell them the packet says 'enriched' or 'with added vitamins and minerals'. The irony is that vitamins and minerals keep being added. The US now enriches flour with folic acid and the UK is thinking of following suit. This would not be necessary if the food we ate was not refined in the first place.

Our mineral needs are increasing

Dr Stephen Davies from London's Biolab Medical Unit has analysed 65,000 samples of blood, hair and sweat over the past fifteen years. Without exception, the results, when looked at alongside the ages of the patients, show that levels of lead, cadmium, aluminium and mercury are increasing, while those of magnesium, zinc, chromium, manganese and selenium are decreasing. The first group are toxic minerals, anti-nutrients which compete with essential minerals. As we age, these toxic elements accumulate. Today we need more 'good' minerals than ever to protect us from the unavoidable toxic minerals that reach us via polluted food, air and water.

■ Mineral loss caused by food processing

	White flour	Sugar refining	Rice polishing
Chromium	98%	78%	86%
Zinc	95%	88%	89%
Manganese	92%	54%	75%

For these reasons, and because many of us choose to eat foods such as refined bread, pasta and cereal, and avoid the mineral-rich foods such as seeds and nuts, modern humans are mineral-deficient. The average dietary intake of zinc (7.8mg according to one survey) is a lot less than the RDA of 15mg. The recommended intake for a breastfeeding woman is 25mg, more than three times the average intake, leaving breast-fed infants hopelessly deficient in a mineral that is essential for all growth processes including intellectual development.

The average intake of iron is well below RDAs. The average intake is 10mg compared with the RDA of 14mg. While no RDAs exist for manganese, chromium and selenium, dietary intakes are certainly below estimates of what we need for optimal health.

In animals, such a state of mineral malnutrition is a known cause of a wide range of illnesses. For this reason livestock feed is enriched with minerals. Not so with man. Is it any wonder we are not healthy?

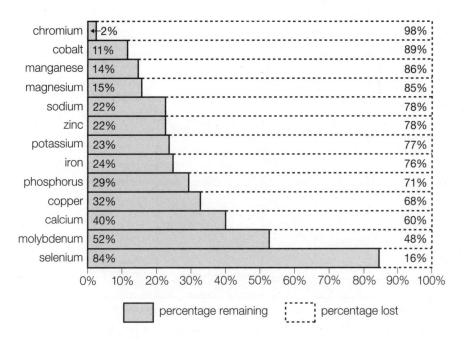

Percentage of minerals lost in refining flour

The macro-minerals

The minerals that are present in the body in relatively large amounts include calcium, magnesium, phosphorus, potassium and sodium.

Calcium – the bone-builder

Nearly 3lb of your body weight is calcium, and 99 per cent of this is in your bones and teeth. Calcium is needed to provide the rigid structure of the skeleton. It is particularly important in childhood when bones are growing, and also in the elderly because the ability to absorb calcium becomes impaired with age. The remaining 10 or so grams of calcium are found in the nerves, muscles and blood. Working together with magnesium, calcium is needed to enable nerves and muscles to 'fire'. It also assists the blood in clotting and helps maintain the right acid–alkaline balance.

The average Western diet provides marginally more than the RDA for calcium. Most of it comes from milk and cheese, which are poor sources. However, vegetables, pulses, nuts, whole grains and water provide significant quantities of both calcium and magnesium, and it is likely that our ancestors relied on these foods for their calcium.

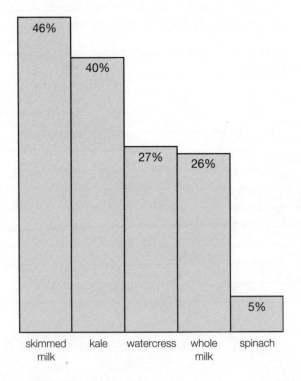

Calcium – how much is absorbed?

The ability to use calcium depends not only on its intake but also on its absorption. The amount absorbed depends on the food, but is normally around 20–30 per cent. The calcium balance of the body is improved by adequate vitamin D intake and by weight-bearing exercise. It is made worse by vitamin D deficiency, exposure to lead, consumption of alcohol, coffee and tea or a lack of hydrochloric acid produced in the stomach. The presence of naturally occurring chemicals called phytates, which are found in grains, and excessive phosphorus or fat in the diet also interferes with absorption. Excessive protein consumption also causes loss of calcium from the bones.

Symptoms of deficiency include muscle cramps, tremors or spasms, insomnia, nervousness, joint pain, osteoarthritis, tooth decay and high blood pressure. Severe deficiency causes osteoporosis. However, this is more likely to be connected with protein and excess hormone imbalances (see Chapters 8 and 20).

Magnesium – calcium's comrade in arms

Magnesium works with calcium in maintaining both bone density and nerve and muscle impulses. The average diet is relatively high in calcium but deficient in magnesium, because milk, our major source of calcium, is not a very good source of magnesium. Both minerals are present in green leafy vegetables, nuts and seeds. Magnesium is a vital component of chlorophyll which gives plants their green colour and is therefore present in all green vegetables. However, only a small proportion of the magnesium within plants is in the form of chlorophyll.

Magnesium is essential for many enzymes in the body, working together with vitamins B1 and B6. It is also involved in protein synthesis and is therefore essential for production of some hormones. It may be its role in hormone production or prostaglandin production that is responsible for its beneficial effects on pre-menstrual problems.

A lack of magnesium is strongly associated with cardiovascular disease: people who die from this cause have abnormally low levels of the mineral in their hearts. Lack of magnesium causes muscles to go into spasm, and there is considerable evidence that some heart attacks are caused not by obstruction of the coronary arteries but by cramping of them, resulting in the heart being deprived of oxygen.

Sodium – for nerve transmission and water balance

Sodium is eaten mainly in the form of sodium chloride, more familiarly known as salt; there is 92g of sodium in the human body. More than half is in the fluids surrounding cells, where it plays a vital role both in nerve transmission and in the maintenance of water concentration in blood and body fluids.

Sodium deficiency is exceedingly rare, because too much is added to foods and also because its excretion is carefully controlled by the kidneys. It is present in small amounts in most natural foods and is mainly supplied in processed foods. There is no need to add it to food, and good reasons not to. Excess sodium is associated with raised blood pressure, although it appears that some people are not salt-sensitive in this way. As sodium levels in the body rise, fluids are made less concentrated by retaining more water. This gives rise to oedema or fluid retention.

Not all salts are bad news. One I sometimes use is Solo salt. This is a type of sea salt that has 46 per cent less sodium, and more potassium and magnesium, than other types of salt. A study in the *British Medical Journal* gave this salt to people with high blood pressure and it lowered it.[27] This is because potassium and magnesium are good news as far as the arteries and your blood pressure are concerned.

Potassium – sodium's partner

This mineral works in conjunction with sodium in maintaining water balance and proper nerve and muscle impulses. Most of the potassium in the body is inside the cells. The more sodium (salt) is eaten, the more potassium is required, and since the average daily intake of potassium is only 4g, relative deficiency is widespread. The same level of intake of these two minerals is more consistent with good health. Fruit, vegetables and whole grains are rich in potassium.

Severe potassium deficiency may result in vomiting, abdominal bloating, muscular weakness and loss of appetite. Potassium deficiency is most likely to occur in people taking diuretic drugs or laxatives or using corticosteroid drugs over a long period.

The trace minerals

Iron – the oxygen carrier

Iron is a vital component of haemoglobin, which transports oxygen and carbon dioxide to and from cells. Sixty per cent of the iron within us is in the form of red pigment or haem. This is the form present in meat, and is much more readily absorbed than the non-haem iron present in non-meat food sources. Non-haem iron occurs in the oxidised or ferric state in food, and not until it is reduced to the ferrous state (for example by vitamin C) during digestion can it be absorbed.

The symptoms of iron deficiency include pale skin, sore tongue, fatigue or listlessness, loss of appetite and nausea. Anaemia is clinically diagnosed by checking haemoglobin levels in the blood. However, symptoms of anaemia can be caused by a lack of vitamin B12 or folic acid. Iron-deficiency anaemia is most likely to occur in women, especially during pregnancy. Since iron is an antagonist to zinc, increasing the requirement for zinc, supplements containing more than 30mg of iron – over twice the RDA – should not be taken without ensuring that enough zinc is also being consumed. Although iron supplements are often given in doses above 50mg, there is little evidence that this is more effective than lower doses in raising haemoglobin levels.

Too much iron may also increase the risk of cardiovascular disease. According to a Finnish study of 1,900 men, those with higher iron stores were more than twice as likely to have a heart attack as those with lower iron stores. Jerome Sullivan, a pathologist at the Veterans' Affairs Medical Center in South Carolina, found a correlation between blood ferritin levels (most iron reserves in the body are stored as ferritin) and cardiovascular risk, and thinks that this might explain why menstruating women, who lose iron each month, have a lesser risk of cardiovascular disease than men until after the menopause.[28] This theory is yet to be proven, but it suggests that meat-eating men should not go overboard on iron supplements. In practice, this means limiting the dose to 10mg a day unless you are deficient.

Zinc – a major role-player

A large part of the population is at risk of being zinc-deficient. With half the population eating less than half the RDA, few people get enough from their diet. Deficiency symptoms are white marks on the nails, lack of appetite or lack of appetite control, pallor, infertility, lack of resistance to infection, poor growth (including hair growth), poor skin including acne, dermatitis and stretch marks, plus mental and emotional problems.

Zinc deficiency plays a role in nearly every major disease, including diabetes and cancer. Zinc is needed to make insulin, to boost the immune system and to make the antioxidant enzyme SOD (superoxide dismutase). It is also required to make prostaglandins from essential fatty acids. These hormone-like substances help to balance hormones and to control inflammation and the stickiness of the blood. Sucking zinc lozenges helps to shorten the life of a cold.

Zinc's main role is the protection and repair of DNA, and for this reason it is found in higher levels in animals and fish than in plants – animals have higher levels of DNA. A vegetarian diet may therefore be low in zinc. Stress, smoking and alcohol deplete zinc, as does frequent sex, at least for men, since semen contains very high concentrations of

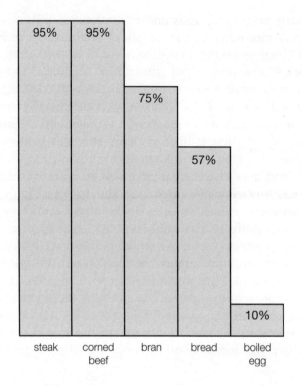

How much iron is absorbed?

zinc. Oysters are popularly said to be aphrodisiacs. They are also the highest dietary source of zinc, providing about 15mg per oyster, and for both men and women zinc is essential for fertility.

Manganese – the forgotten mineral

This mineral is known to be involved in no fewer than twenty enzyme systems in the body. One of the most critical is SOD, which acts as an antioxidant, helping to disarm free radicals. In animals, manganese deficiency results in reduced insulin production. Since diabetics frequently have low manganese levels it is thought to be involved in maintaining blood sugar balance. It is also involved in the formation of mucopolysaccharides, a constituent of cartilage. One of the first signs associated with deficiency is joint pain.

Manganese is also required for proper brain function. Deficiency has been associated with schizophrenia, Parkinson's disease and epilepsy. It is frequently deficient in the diet and the best sources include tropical fruit, nuts, seeds and whole grains. Tea is also a significant source of this mineral and supplies half our daily intake. Little more than 5 per cent of the manganese eaten in the diet is absorbed, though exactly why is unknown. Similarly, supplements are poorly absorbed, the best forms being manganese citrate or manganese amino acid chelate.

Copper – good and bad

Both a nutritional and a toxic element, copper is required by humans in doses as little as 2mg a day. It is rarely deficient for the simple reason that most water supplies are contaminated via copper pipes. It is needed among other things for the formation of the insulating myelin sheath around nerves. Copper and zinc are strongly antagonistic, and zinc deficiency may lead to a greater uptake of copper. Likewise, excessive zinc supplementation can induce copper deficiency.

In reality, excess is a more common problem than deficiency. If you are on a whole-food diet there is no actual need to supplement copper, yet it is often included in multimineral tablets. A good multi should contain roughly ten times more zinc than copper (e.g. zinc 10mg, copper 1mg). Taking the birth-control Pill or HRT also increases your copper stores. All these factors make it relatively easy to accumulate too much copper, which is associated with schizophrenia, cardiovascular disease and possibly rheumatoid arthritis. However, copper deficiency has also been associated with rheumatoid arthritis. Copper is a constituent of an antioxidant enzyme involved in some inflammatory reactions. This may be the reason why too much or too little can result in greater inflammation in sufferers from rheumatoid arthritis. Copper levels rise during pregnancy, and it is speculated that it plays a role in bringing on labour and, in excess, post-natal depression.

Chromium – the energy factor

This is a vital constituent of glucose-tolerance factor, a compound produced in the liver that helps transport glucose from the blood to the cells. Vitamin B3 and the amino acids glycine, glutamic acid and cystine are also required for glucose-tolerance factor. Continued stress or frequent sugar consumption therefore deplete the body of chromium. A diet high in refined foods is also likely to be deficient in this mineral since it is found in whole grains, pulses, nuts, seeds and especially in mushrooms and asparagus. Chromium supplements have been used successfully in the treatment of diabetes and glucose intolerance.

Selenium – the anti-cancer mineral

Deficiency of this mineral was first discovered in China as the cause of Keshan disease, a type of heart disease prevalent in areas in which the soil was deficient in selenium. It has since been associated with another regional disease, this time in Russia, involving joint degeneration. Perhaps the most significant finding is selenium's association with a low risk of certain kinds of cancer.

Selenium is the vital constituent of the antioxidant enzyme glutathione peroxidase. A ten-fold increase in dietary selenium causes a doubling of the quantity of this enzyme in the body. Since many oxides are cancer-producing, and since cancer cells destroy other cells by releasing oxides, it is likely to be selenium's role in glutathione peroxidase production that gives it protective properties against cancer and premature ageing. It may also be essential for the thyroid gland, which controls the body's rate of metabolism. Selenium is found predominantly in whole foods, particularly seafood and sesame seeds. If you grind the seeds the nutrients become more readily available.

The unknown minerals

As research unfolds and analytic techniques improve, we will probably find that many more minerals have an important role to play. Some are already proven, although not widely known. They include boron, which helps the body use calcium and may be beneficial for arthritis sufferers; molybdenum, which helps remove undesirable free radicals, petrochemicals and sulphites from the body and is therefore useful for city dwellers who want protection from pollution; vanadium, proved to be essential in some animals, which may be useful for the treatment of manic depression; and germanium, which has antioxidant potential.

Since the 1970s analytical chemists have moved from being able to detect minerals in food, blood, hair and so on at a level of one part in a million, to being able to detect one part in a quillion – that's a millionth of a million, or the equivalent of dissolving a lump of sugar in the Mediterranean and being able to detect the difference. It is highly likely that we have much more to learn about the magic of minerals.

14.

Toxic Minerals from Aluminium to Mercury

Since optimum nutrition is about both increasing your intake of nutrients and avoiding anti-nutrients it is well worth being aware of the toxic minerals that we are exposed to. These include aluminium, cadmium, copper, lead and mercury. We are also exposed to some arsenic, present in some pesticides and herbicides, although this is most easily avoided by eating organic foods. There are others, but these are the major toxic minerals of concern because just about everybody is being unwittingly exposed to them.

Analyses of hair show that these undesirable elements tend to accumulate with age, suggesting that our exposure generally exceeds our ability to get rid of them. However, with some simple strategies you can dramatically reduce your load and increase your body's ability to detoxify any residues in your body.

Here's how.

Aluminium

Aluminium is in widespread use in food packaging and turns up in many common household products. It's in antacids, toothpaste tubes, deodorants, aluminium foil, pots and pans and water. Not all aluminium will enter the body. Only in certain circumstances will aluminium leach, for example, from a pan. Old-fashioned aluminium cookware, if used to heat something acidic like tea, tomatoes or rhubarb, will leach particles of aluminium into the water. Also, the more zinc-deficient you are the more you absorb.

Like many toxic metals, aluminium binds to essential vitamins and minerals, so seriously compromising nutritional status. Although we know it interferes with brain function and memory, aluminium has also has been linked to kidney problems in babies and behavioural problems and autism in older children.[29]

In areas where there are high levels of aluminium in the water, studies have shown that there is a 50 per cent greater risk of developing Alzheimer's disease (AD).[30] While plenty of studies have shown increased accumulation of aluminium in people with AD, what isn't clear is whether this is a cause or a consequence of the disease. The likelihood is that it's a bit of both and still a significant contributor to memory problems. Numerous epidemiological surveys have linked aluminium intake in water to increased risk of AD. Other sources (food, medicines, toiletries and cosmetics) are less well investigated.

In a study in the 1980s of 647 Canadian goldminers who had routinely inhaled aluminium since the 1940s (this used to be a common practice, thought to prevent silica poisoning), all tested in the 'impaired' range for cognitive function, suggesting a clear link between aluminium and memory loss.[31] A number of recent review papers have kept aluminium firmly on the map of potential contributors to dementia and AD.[32] While the mechanism for action of aluminium in brain degeneration is far from clear, aluminium acts as an oxidant in the brain, especially in combination with excess copper.[33]

Cadmium

Cadmium accumulates in the body and brain when zinc is low, and builds up in the kidneys and liver, where it binds to other essential minerals and vitamins, so preventing their utilisation. In their study on mineral status in new babies, Professor Derek Bryce-Smith and Dr Neil Ward, then at Reading University, found that cadmium levels are higher in the placentae of stillborn babies or those born with spina bifida. Greater accumulation of cadmium is also associated with low birth weight and small head circumference (therefore reduced brain size); and it reduces fertility in both men and women.

Our main sources of cadmium are cigarette smoke (directly or passively inhaled – according to the Health Education Authority, only 15 per cent of the smoke from a cigarette is inhaled by the smoker; the rest goes into the air and is inhaled by those close by) and refined grains found in processed foods. Cadmium is also widely used by the manufacturing industries and has even been found in shellfish from polluted waters.

Copper

Copper is both an essential element and a toxic one. Owing to the widespread use of copper in water pipes, plus exposure from jewellery, kitchen utensils and even swimming-pool anti-fungal agents, we are today more at risk from toxicity than from deficiency. The 2mg we need each day is supplied simply from drinking water that has passed through copper pipes, irrespective of any copper that is absorbed from our food. What's more, long-term use of the contraceptive Pill, IUDs and fertility hormones such as Clomid further increases copper levels in the body. Yet high levels of copper antagonise zinc and can induce deficiency.

Once a woman is pregnant, copper levels in her blood tend to rise dramatically and remain elevated for around a month after her child's birth. The reason is believed to be because copper acts as a stimulus for the uterus. But if there's already a high level to start with, the additional accumulation can cause copper toxicity and this is far more common during pregnancy than at other times. In fact, too much too soon may be a factor in inducing premature babies or miscarriages.

High levels of copper may also be a factor in post-natal depression or mental illness, especially anxiety, paranoia and schizophrenia. Consider this story. On holiday I once met a headmaster of a school for 'problem' children. We got talking about the effects of lead and other toxic metals on behaviour, and decided to set up a challenge. When we returned from holiday, he would send me a dozen hair samples from different students, which I would analyse and use to predict their behaviour.

After receiving the hair samples, I ran the hair-mineral analyses and found three abnormal results. One had a very high lead level. I predicted aggressive behaviour, hyperactivity and poor attention span. I was right. The child in question was the worst-behaved in the school! Two others had high copper levels. I predicted anxiety. They turned out to be a schoolteacher and his wife. They had recently moved into a new house, built in the grounds of the school, with new copper pipes in a soft-water area. The wife had started to become more and more anxious and had been prescribed medication. The husband was apparently free of symptoms.

This story illustrates how easy it is to be copper toxic without knowing it. Copper excess, which can cause extreme fears, paranoia and hallucinations, is rarely checked or tested in those with mental health problems, despite the fact that this link has been often reported in people with schizophrenia.[34] The copper may be the result of drinking water passing through copper pipes, or using copper pots and pans, the contraceptive pill and even copper IUDs. Or it could be the result of a deficiency of zinc, or of vitamin C or B3, which are copper antagonists. It also highlights the importance of drinking filtered or bottled water.

Lead

The first study to shake the status quo on lead toxicity was the Needleman study. Herbert Needleman, an associate professor of child psychiatry, looked at a group of 2,146 children in first- and second-grade schools in Birmingham, Alabama, in the US. He examined lead concentrations in shed baby teeth to obtain more long-term levels than shown by a simple blood test. He then asked the schoolteachers to rate the behaviour of children they had taught for at least two months. This was done using a questionnaire designed to measure the teachers' rating of children for a number of characteristics. He also ran a series of behavioural, intellectual and physiological tests on each child before dividing the children into six groups according to the lead concentration in their teeth.

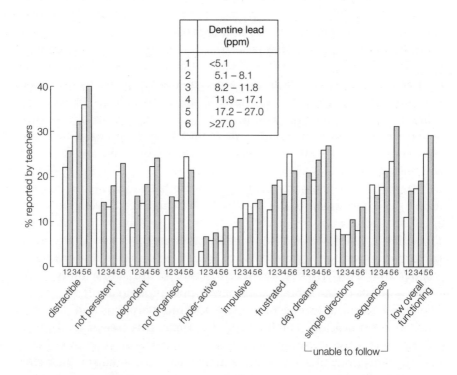

	Dentine lead (ppm)
1	<5.1
2	5.1 – 8.1
3	8.2 – 11.8
4	11.9 – 17.1
5	17.2 – 27.0
6	>27.0

Classroom behaviour in relation to dentine lead concentration: results for 2,146 children. The higher the level of lead in a child's baby teeth, the worse their behaviour and learning ability is likely to be. By comparing 1 and 6 in each category (i.e. the lowest and highest levels of lead) you can see a clear difference in behaviour.

As you can see, his results showed a clear relationship between lead concentrations and bad school behaviour, as rated by the teachers without any knowledge of the children's lead levels. Needleman also found that the average IQ for the high-lead children was 4.5 points below that of the low-lead group. Reaction time (a measure of attention capability) was also consistently worse in those with higher lead levels. EEG readings (which measure brain-wave patterns) showed clear differences, based on lead concentration. Perhaps the most interesting result was that none of the high-lead children had an IQ above 125 points (100 is average), compared with 5 per cent in the low-lead group.[35]

Richard Lansdown, principal psychologist at the London Hospital for Sick Children, and William Yule, psychologist at the University of London, decided to replicate the essentials of Needleman's study on London children using lead levels in the blood instead of teeth. The 160 children involved had blood lead levels from 7 to 33 micrograms per decilitre, averaging 13.5 mcg/dl (35 mcg/dl is the 'safe' level recommended by the Lawther Report *Lead and Health*, 1980). This is similar to other national studies of mean lead levels. Again, the teachers rated the children's behaviour, and IQ and other tests were made. Lansdown's results were even more striking than Needleman's. The difference in IQ score between high- and low-lead children was seven IQ points. Once again, none of the high-lead group children had an IQ above 125, while in the low-lead group, 5 per cent did.[36] His findings have long since been proven by many other researchers and in fact helped bring about the banning of lead in petrol.

Professor Derek Bryce-Smith has also found elevated levels of lead in the placentae of stillborn babies and those born with spina bifida or 'water on the brain' (hydrocephalus).[37] An American study also found higher levels of lead in babies who died of cot death.[38] Perhaps more interesting is the fact that this correlation exists even in mothers whose lead levels would be considered 'normal'. As with many environmental poisons, there appears to be no threshold at which lead can categorically be called safe.

The important lesson to learn from lead is that tiny changes in what we ingest can have vast consequences for our health, which, although invisible to the eye, have been proven by research. Banning lead in petrol was the first campaign of the Institute for Optimum Nutrition, working with Professor Bryce-Smith. There are many others yet to be won.

Although our lead exposure today may be less than it was in previous decades, lead pollution is still present in the atmosphere (it's even been found in the polar ice-caps) and also comes from water contaminated by lead piping and from flaking paint and paint dust, pesticides, cosmetics and industrial exposure. When intakes of the essential minerals calcium, zinc or iron are low, lead becomes that much more toxic. Given that many people are deficient in all three, it's important to redress the balance through diet and supplements.

Mercury

Mercury is the reason nineteenth-century hatters went mad. By polishing top hats with mercury, they became overloaded with this toxic element, which disturbs brain function and makes you crazy. Mercury is very toxic indeed and small amounts reach us from contaminated foods and from tooth fillings. Of particular concern is fish caught in polluted waters.

Mercury is used in a number of chemical processes, and accidents and illegal dumping have led to increased mercury levels in some areas, including the English Channel. Fish, especially larger species like tuna, store the mercury, which we then ingest. Fortunately, tuna is high in selenium, a mercury protector. Mercury has also been used as a constituent of thimerosal, found in diphtheria and hepatitis vaccines. This practice has recently been stopped.

Sadly, owing to widespread pollution, fish are one of our biggest sources of mercury. The larger and fattier, the greater the accumulation – up to nine million times the amount found in the water.[39] One in twelve American women of childbearing age has potentially hazardous levels of mercury in her blood as a result of consuming fish, according to government scientists.[40] As a result, the US Food and Drug Administration recommend that pregnant women don't eat tuna, shark, swordfish, king mackerel and tile fish. In the UK, the Food Standards Agency advises women who intend to become pregnant and those who are pregnant or breastfeeding to limit their consumption of tuna to no more than two medium-size cans or one fresh tuna steak per week. It also advises avoiding shark, swordfish and marlin altogether.

Mercury is also found in water contaminated by industrial processes and in pesticides, but besides fish, our other most common source of this toxic metal is dental fillings. The mercury in teeth is not totally immobile and it's possible to detect traces of mercury in the breath of people with mercury fillings. After fillings have been fitted or removed, urinary mercury may also show a slight increase. Sweden has now banned mercury fillings for pregnant women.

Autopsies on brains from AD patients, compared with those of control patients of the same age, have shown raised levels of mercury.[41] Researchers from the University of Basle, Switzerland, have also found high blood mercury levels, more than double those of the control groups, in AD patients, with early-onset AD patients having the highest mercury levels of all.[42] Trace amounts of mercury can cause the type of damage to nerves that is characteristic of AD, according to recent research at the University of Calgary Faculty of Medicine, strongly suggesting that the small amounts we are exposed to, for example from amalgam fillings, may be contributing to memory loss.[43] Although the research on the link of mercury to AD is in its infancy, it is certainly logical to reduce exposure to this highly toxic metal.

Detoxifying your body

You can easily test your own mineral levels with a hair-mineral analysis (see Tests, Resources, pages 527–8). But what do you do if you have raised levels of toxic minerals?

Once we've ingested toxic minerals they must compete with other minerals for absorption. These minerals are called antagonists and form our first line of defence. Once a mineral has been absorbed, some natural body substances latch on to it and try to take it out of the body. These are called chelators (pronounced key-lay-tors).

It is the latter principle that lies behind the administration of two drugs, penicillamine and EDTA, given to get rid of heavy metals. However, vitamin C is even better. In a study of rats with high concentrations of lead in their brains, administering EDTA resulted in an 8 per cent lowering of lead, while vitamin C decreased levels by 22 per cent.[44] Vitamin C is an all-rounder with the ability to latch on to most heavy metals in the blood and escort them out, sacrificing itself in the process. So high metal burdens call for more vitamin C. It is effective in removing lead, arsenic and cadmium, and is a most important part of any detoxification programme.

Another substance that is known to lower lead levels is zinc, which acts as an antagonist to lead by preventing its absorption in the gut. Zinc also lowers body and brain levels of cadmium. Indeed, most of us could benefit from extra zinc. In addition, calcium is effective at keeping down lead levels, since lead otherwise stores more easily in our bones.

Keeping calcium levels topped up pushes lead out and prevents the rapid rise in toxic minerals that, according to research by Dr Ellen O'Flaherty at the University of Cincinnati College of Medicine, occurs at a rate of 15 per cent following the menopause.[45] Calcium is particularly effective at keeping down cadmium and aluminium levels. Toxic elements such as lead and uranium accumulate in bone tissue over a lifetime of repeated exposure, and are released into the bloodstream as bone tissue breaks down. Bone loss can increase dramatically following the menopause, which explains the rise in blood lead levels found in O'Flaherty's research.

Selenium is specifically a mercury antagonist, and normally protects us from the mercury present in most seafood. Supplementing an extra dose is always a good idea if there are signs of excess mercury. It also has a similar protective effect with arsenic and cadmium, although it is not so pronounced.

Foods that fight heavy metals

In terms of specific foods, there are a few that can help keep your brain clean. Sulphur-containing amino acids are found as the proteins in garlic, onions and eggs. The specific amino acids are called methionine and cystine and protect against mercury, cadmium and lead toxicity. Alginic acid in seaweed, and pectin in apples, carrots and citrus fruits also help chelate and remove heavy metals, thereby promoting your health. One more reason for an apple a day.

In summary, here are a few simple steps you can take to avoid toxic minerals:

- Avoid busy roads and smoky atmospheres where possible.

- Remove outer leaves of vegetables and thoroughly wash all fresh produce in a vinegar solution (just add a dessertspoonful to a bowl of water) to remove pollutants.

- Limit your intake of marlin, swordfish or tuna to no more than twice a month.

- Avoid copper or aluminium cookware and don't wrap food in aluminium foil (or if you do, put a layer of greaseproof paper in between foil and food).

- Cut down on alcohol, as this increases lead and cadmium absorption.

- Avoid antacids, which can contain aluminium salts.

- Check whether your water pipes are made of lead or copper. If they are, don't use a water-softener, as soft water dissolves lead or copper more easily; do not drink or cook with hot tap water; use a water filter or drink distilled or natural water.

- Take a good antioxidant supplement.

- Eat mineral-rich foods such as seeds and nuts.

- Eat fruit rich in pectin and vitamin C.

- Supplement vitamin C every day, as this protects you from toxic minerals, plus a multimineral containing zinc, calcium and selenium.

chapter 15.

Antioxidants – the Power of Prevention

S ince the 1980s more and more research has confirmed that many of the twentieth century's most common diseases are associated with a shortage of antioxidant nutrients, and helped by their supplementation. So important is the role of antioxidants that medical science is beginning to consider the presence of any one of the diseases listed below as a sign of probable antioxidant deficiency, in the same way that scurvy is a sign of vitamin C deficiency.

In the future we may be tested for blood levels of antioxidant nutrients alongside levels of blood sugar and cholesterol and blood pressure. Capable of predicting your biological age and expected lifespan, your antioxidant-nutrient status may prove to be your most vital statistic.

■ Probable antioxidant-deficiency diseases

Alzheimer's disease	Macular (eye lens) degeneration
Cancer	Measles
Cardiovascular disease	Mental illness
Cataracts	Periodontal (tooth) disease
Diabetes	Respiratory tract infections
Hypertension	Rheumatoid arthritis
Infertility	

The common denominator in the process of ageing and its associated diseases is called oxidative damage. This has put the spotlight on the use of antioxidants – nutrients that help protect the body from this damage by preventing and treating disease. So far, over a hundred antioxidant nutrients have been discovered and hundreds, if not thousands, of research papers have extolled their benefits. The main players are vitamins A, C and E, plus betacarotene, the precursor of vitamin A that is found in fruit and vegetables. Their presence in your diet and levels in your blood may prove to be the best marker yet of your power to delay death and prevent disease.

What is an antioxidant?

Oxygen is the basis of all plant and animal life. It is our most important nutrient, needed by every cell every second of every day. Without it we cannot release the energy in food that drives all body processes. But oxygen is chemically reactive and highly dangerous: in normal biochemical reactions oxygen can become unstable and capable of 'oxidising' neighbouring molecules. This can lead to cellular damage that triggers cancer, inflammation, arterial damage and ageing. Known as free oxidising radicals, this bodily equivalent of nuclear waste must be disarmed to remove the danger. Free radicals are made in all combustion processes including smoking, the burning of petrol to create exhaust fumes, radiation, frying or barbecuing food and normal body processes. Chemicals capable of disarming free radicals are called antioxidants. Some are known essential nutrients, like vitamin A and betacarotene, and vitamins C and E. Others, like bioflavonoids, anthocyanidins, pyenogenol and over a hundred other recently identified protectors found in common foods, are not.

The balance between your intake of antioxidants and your exposure to free radicals may literally be the balance between life and death. You can tip the scales in your favour by making simple changes to your diet and by antioxidant supplementation.

Antioxidants in health and disease

Slowing down the ageing process is no longer a mystery. The best results in research studies have consistently been achieved by giving animals low-calorie diets high in antioxidant nutrients – in other words, exactly what they need and no more. This reduces 'oxidative stress' and ensures maximum antioxidant protection. Animals fed in this way not only live up to 40 per cent longer, but also are more active during their lives. Although long-term studies have yet to be completed, there is every reason to assume that the same principles apply to humans. Already, large-scale surveys show that the risk of death is substantially reduced in those with either high levels of antioxidants in their blood or high dietary intakes.

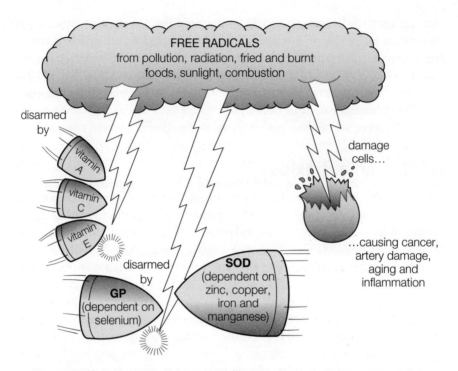

Burnt foods harm the body. Free radicals, or oxidants, from anything burnt, damage the body resulting in ageing and disease, and are disarmed by anti-oxidant nutrients. In this diagram, GP stands for the antioxidant enzyme glutathione peroxidase, and SOD is the antioxidant enzyme superoxide dismutase.

Conversely, a lower level of vitamin A, vitamin C and vitamin E is associated with Alzheimer's disease. The blood levels of vitamin E and betacarotene in sufferers are half those of elderly people who do not have Alzheimer's.[46] A US study gave 633 disease-free sixty-five-year-olds large amounts of either vitamin E or vitamin C. A small number in each group would have been expected to show the signs of AD five years later. None did.[47] Another study published in the *Journal of the American Medical Association* found that the risk of developing AD was 67 per cent lower in those with a high dietary intake of vitamin E than in those with a low intake.[48]

Elderly people with low levels of vitamin C in their blood have eleven times the risk of developing cataracts compared with those with high levels.[49] Similarly, those with low vitamin E blood levels have almost double the risk, while people consuming 300mg of vitamin E a day have half the risk of developing cataracts.[50, 51]

Levels of vitamin A are consistently found to be low in people with lung cancer. In fact, having a low vitamin A level doubles the risk of lung cancer. Similarly, a high intake of betacarotene from raw fruit and vegetables reduces the risk of lung cancer in non-smoking men and women. [52] In one study, giving a 30 mg per day supplement of betacarotene resulted in 71 per cent of patients with oral pre-cancer (leukoplakia) improving, while 57 per cent of patients given 200,000iu of vitamin A per day had complete remission.[53] Betacarotene on its own, however, may not be wise to supplement if you are a smoker (see page 278).

Supplementing vitamins E and C effectively halves the risk of ever having a heart attack, while in a massive study on nurses, those who consumed 15–20mg of betacarotene per day had a 40 per cent lower risk of a stroke and a 22 per cent lower risk of a heart attack compared with those consuming only 6mg per day.[54] Those with high dietary intakes of betacarotene had half the risk of death from cardiovascular disease. Supplementing 1,000mg of vitamin C also reduces blood pressure.[55]

Antioxidants also help boost your immune system and increase your resistance to infection. In children, regular supplementation of vitamin A significantly reduces respiratory tract infections. Antioxidants have been shown to reduce the symptoms of AIDS and, in a small number of cases, to reverse the condition. They increase fertility, reduce inflammation in arthritis and have key roles to play in many conditions including colds and chronic fatigue syndrome. (For more information on specific diseases see Part 7.)

The synergy of antioxidants is vital

As we saw in the chart on page 30 antioxidants are team players. You need a combination of vitamins E and C and betacarotene, as well as glutathione, anthocyanidins, lipoic acid and co-enzyme Q10 to do the job of disarming oxidants properly. Taking only one of these antioxidants not only is unwise, but also could be dangerous. While more than 200 studies have shown that betacarotene reduces your risk for a variety of cancers, three studies have shown that supplementing betacarotene on its own can raise the risk of cancer, although only if you smoke. Why the apparent contradiction?

Let's examine the most recent negative trial, conducted by the National Cancer Institute. They divided people with a history of colorectal tumours into four groups. One group was given 25mg of betacarotene, a second group was given 100mg of vitamin C and 400mg of vitamin E, a third group received the betacarotene and vitamins C and E and the fourth group received a placebo. While there was less recurrence of colorectal tumours in the first three groups, there was a modest *increase* in cancer recurrence among those who took only betacarotene supplements and both smoked and drank alcohol every day.

Does this mean that betacarotene is a moralistic vitamin, adding risk to those who both smoke and drink, but saving those who don't? Of course not. What is almost certainly happening here is that the oxidants in cigarettes are oxidising betacarotene and, in the absence of other synergistic vitamins such as vitamin C and E, this does more harm than good. My advice is to quit the cigarettes, eat foods high in antioxidants including betacarotene and supplement either a multivitamin containing antioxidants or a good, all-round antioxidant formula. I take both.

Testing your antioxidant potential

Your ability to stay free of these diseases depends on the balance between your intake of harmful free radicals and your intake of protective antioxidants. As the scales start to tip away from health, early warning signs start to develop, such as frequent infections, difficulty shifting an infection, easy bruising, slow healing, thinner skin or excessive wrinkles for your age.

Another sign of impaired antioxidant status is a reduced ability to detoxify the body after an onslaught of free radicals. So, for example, if you feel groggy or achy after a burst of exercise or after exposure to pollution (such as being stuck in a traffic jam or a room full of cigarette smoke), your antioxidant potential may need a boost.

A more accurate way to determine your antioxidant status is to have a biochemical antioxidant profile done. This blood test measures the levels of betacarotene, C and E in your blood and determines how well your antioxidant enzyme systems (such as glutathione peroxidase) are functioning. Most nutritional laboratories offer this kind of test. A less expensive and less extensive total reactive antioxidant potential (TRAP) test is also available. But while this will indicate if there is an antioxidant problem, it will not define which nutrients are missing. Ask your doctor or nutritionist about these tests, as they are rarely available direct to the public.

Antioxidants – the best foods

Every year more and more antioxidants are found in nature, including substances in berries, grapes, tomatoes, mustard and broccoli, and in herbs such as turmeric and ginkgo biloba. These substances, such as bioflavonoids, lycopene and anthocyanidins, are not essential nutrients but are highly beneficial. They are classified as phytochemicals and are discussed fully in Chapter 14.

Your Personal Antioxidant Profile

Test your powers of prevention and score 1 point for each 'yes' answer.

Symptom Analysis

- Do you frequently suffer from infections (coughs, colds)?   *yes / no*
- Do you find it hard to shift an infection?   *yes / no*
- Do you have a recurrent infection (cystitis, thrush, earache etc.)?   *yes / no*
- Do you bruise easily?   *yes / no*
- Have you ever suffered from any of the conditions listed on page 126?
  yes / no
- Have your parents collectively suffered from two or more of these conditions?
  yes / no
- Do you easily get exhausted after physical exertion?   *yes / no*
- Does your skin take a long time to heal?   *yes / no*
- Do you suffer from acne, dry skin or excessive wrinkles for your age?
  yes / no
- Are you overweight?   *yes / no*

Your Score

Lifestyle Analysis

- Have you smoked for more than five years of your life, less than five years
  ago?   *yes / no*
- Do you smoke now?   *yes / no*
- Do you smoke more than ten cigarettes a day?   *yes / no*
- Do you spend time most days in a smoky atmosphere?   *yes / no*
- Do you have an alcoholic drink each day?   *yes / no*
- Do you live in a polluted city or by a busy road?   *yes / no*
- Do you spend more than two hours in traffic each day?   *yes / no*
- Are you quite often exposed to strong sunlight?   *yes / no*
- Do you consider yourself unfit?   *yes / no*

● Do you exercise excessively and get easily 'burnt out'?   *yes / no*

Your Score   ◻

Diet Analysis

● Do you eat fried food most days?   *yes / no*

● Do you eat less than a serving of fresh fruit and raw vegetables each day?   *yes / no*

● Do you eat fewer than two pieces of fresh fruit a day?   *yes / no*

● Do you rarely eat nuts, seeds or whole grains each day?   *yes / no*

● Do you eat smoked or barbecued food or grill cheese on your food?   *yes / no*

● Do you supplement less than 500mg of vitamin C each day?   *yes / no*

● Do you supplement less than 100iu of vitamin E each day?   *yes / no*

● Do you supplement less than 10,000iu of vitamin A or betacarotene each day?   *yes / no*

Your Score   ◻

Your Total Score: ◻

0–10   This is an ideal score, indicating that your health, diet and lifestyle are consistent with a high level of antioxidant protection. Keep up the good work.

11–15   This is a reasonable score, although you can increase your power of prevention by converting 'yes' answers into 'no'.

16–20   This is a poor score, indicating plenty of room for improvement. See a nutritionist to upgrade your diet and look at how you can alter your lifestyle for increased antioxidant protection.

20+   This is a bad score, putting you in the high-risk group for rapid ageing. See a nutritionist and ask for an antioxidant profile blood test. You will need to make changes to your diet and lifestyle, plus supplementing antioxidants, to reverse or slow down the ageing process.

The main essential antioxidant vitamins are A, C and E and the precursor of vitamin A, betacarotene. Betacarotene is found in red/orange/yellow vegetables and fruits. Vitamin C is also abundant in vegetables and fruit eaten raw, but heat rapidly destroys it. Vitamin E is found in 'seed' foods, including nuts, seeds and their oils, and vegetables like peas, broad beans, corn and whole grains – all of which are classified as seed foods. The best all-round foods are shown in the table below. Eating sweet potatoes, carrots, watercress, peas and broccoli frequently is a great way to increase your antioxidant potential – provided, of course, that you do not fry them.

Thanks to groundbreaking research at Tufts University in Boston, there's a new way to rate a food's overall antioxidant power. Each food can now be assigned a certain number of ORAC units (short for 'oxygen radical absorbance capacity'). Foods that score high in these units are especially helpful in countering oxidant, or free-radical, damage in your body.

Top-scoring foods include prunes, raisins, blueberries and blackberries. Other top-scoring foods include kale, spinach, strawberries, raspberries, plums, broccoli and alfalfa spouts. These and other fresh fruits and vegetables are the kinds of foods you need to eat every day to keep young and energetic. (See the chart below for the ORAC ratings for several foods. You can find a more comprehensive listing of ORAC ratings in Part 9, on pages 519–20.)

We should all obtain 3,500 ORAC units a day, although 5,000 to 6,000 will give you even more protection against ageing. You'll also be better protected against many diseases, including cancer and heart disease. What this means in practice is eating a cup of blueberries (3,240 ORAC units), a quarter of a cup of raisins, and three prunes; or a half-pint of strawberries and two servings of kale, tenderstem or broccoli. Alternatively, you could eat five servings of fresh fruit and vegetables every day.

▪ Fruits and vegetables with antioxidant power

Per 100 grams	ORAC units	Per item or serving	ORAC units
Prunes	5770	1 pitted prune	462
Raisins	2830	¼ cup	1019
Blueberries	2234	½ cup	1620
Blackberries	2036	½ cup	1466
Kale	1770	½ cup cooked	1150
Strawberries	1536	½ cup	1144
Spinach, raw	1210	1 cup	678
Raspberries	1227	½ cup	755
Tenderstem	1183	½ cup cooked	1159
Plums	949	1 plum	626
Alfalfa sprouts	931	1 cup	307
Spinach, steamed	909	½ cup cooked	1089
Broccoli	888	½ cup cooked	817
Beets	841	½ cup cooked, sliced	715
Avocado	782	½ cup	149

The best fruits are berries. Another great antioxidant fruit is watermelon. The flesh is high in betacarotene and vitamin C, while the seeds are high in vitamin E and in the antioxidant minerals zinc and selenium. You can make a great antioxidant cocktail by blending the flesh and seeds into a great-tasting drink. Seeds and seafood are the best all-round dietary sources of selenium and zinc.

Including vegetables such as tenderstem, broccoli, spinach and avocado in your diet on a regular basis is another great way to up your antioxidant intake. The amino acids cysteine and glutathione also act as antioxidants. They help make one of the body's key antioxidant enzymes, glutathione peroxidase, which is itself dependent on selenium. This enzyme helps to detoxify the body, protecting us against car-exhaust fumes, carcinogens, infections, too much alcohol and toxic metals. Cysteine and glutathione are particularly high in white meat, tuna, lentils, beans, nuts, seeds, onions and garlic, and have been shown to boost the immune system as well as to increase antioxidant power.

Supplementary benefit

Given the unquestionable value of increasing your antioxidant status, it is wise to make sure that your daily supplement programme contains significant quantities of antioxidants, especially if you are middle-aged or older, live in a polluted city or suffer any other unavoidable exposure to free radicals. The easiest way to do this is to take a comprehensive antioxidant supplement. Most reputable supplement companies produce formulas containing a combination of the following nutrients: vitamin A, betacarotene, vitamin E, vitamin C, zinc, selenium, glutathione and cysteine, plus plant-based antioxidants like bilberry or pyenogenol. Also important are lipoic acid and co-enzyme Q10 (CoQ10).

Lipoic acid is a sulphur-containing, vitamin-like substance that has very effective antioxidant properties. As an antioxidant, it is particularly useful because it is one of the few that is both water- and fat-soluble, which means that it can protect a wider range of molecules than, say, just vitamin C or vitamin E. Foods said to be high in lipoic acid are liver and yeast. CoQ10 is a vital antioxidant helping to protect cells from carcinogens and also helping to recycle vitamin E. CoQ10's magical properties lie in its ability to improve the cell's use of oxygen. CoQ10 works by controlling the flow of oxygen, making the production of energy most efficient and preventing damage caused by these oxidants. CoQ10 is found in meat, fish, nuts and seeds.

The kind of total supplementary intake (which may come in part from a multivitamin and extra vitamin C) to aim for is shown below:

Vitamin A (retinol/beta carotene)	2,500µgRE (7500iu)	to	6,600µgRE (20,000iu)
Glutathione (reduced)	25mg	to	75mg
Vitamin E	66mg (100iu)	to	330mg (500iu)
Vitamin C	1,000mg	to	3,000mg
CoQ10	10mg	to	50mg
Lipoic acid	10mg	to	50mg
Anthocyanidin source	50mg	to	250mg
Selenium	30mcg	to	100mcg
Zinc	10mg	to	20mg

Here are some simple tips for improving your antioxidant potential and boosting your power of prevention:

● Eat lots of fresh fruit, especially berries.

● Eat lots of vegetables, especially tenderstem, spinach, avocado, sweet potatoes, carrots, peas, watercress and broccoli.

● Take a multivitamin and/or a good antioxidant supplement daily containing all the above nutrients.

● Do your best to avoid pollution, smoky places, direct exposure to strong sunlight and fried foods.

● Don't over-exercise or exercise beyond your aerobic potential.

chapter 16

Homocysteine – Your Most Important Health Statistic

Forget your blood pressure, your cholesterol, even your weight. There is one factor that can determine better than any other whether you will live long and healthy or die young. It's called homocysteine.

Homocysteine is a type of protein, produced by the body and found in the blood, that, ideally, should be present in very low quantities. However, if you are not optimally nourished homocysteine can accumulate in the blood, increasing the risk for over fifty diseases, including heart attacks, strokes, certain cancers, diabetes, depression and Alzheimer's disease. One in two people in Britain has a high homocysteine level. The good news is that this new and important risk factor can be reversed in weeks.

What is homocysteine?

Homocysteine is produced from the amino acid methionine, which is found in normal dietary protein. Homocysteine in itself isn't bad news – your body naturally turns it into one of two beneficial substances. These are called glutathione (the body's most important antioxidant) and a methyl donor called SAMe (a very important type of 'intelligent' nutrient for both brain and body).

The trouble is, if you don't have optimal amounts of B vitamins in your diet, the enzymes that turn homocysteine into these beneficial substances don't work well enough. Your homocysteine can't be converted, so your level of it rises dangerously (see figure opposite).

To make matters more complex, it has been discovered that one in ten people has an inherited genetic mutation that makes them more prone to a higher homocysteine level than other people. This means that the enzyme that converts homocysteine into SAMe (it's called the MTHFR enzyme) doesn't work so well. Luckily, studies show that larger daily intakes of B12 and folic acid can help to make the deficient enzyme work better.

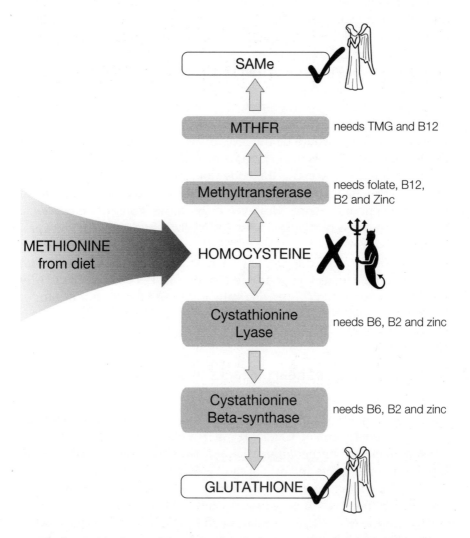

The homocysteine pathway. We all make homocysteine from eating protein. Normally, it is quickly turned into SAMe or glutathione, two very essential and health-promoting substances in the body. But if you lack enough of certain nutrients such as B2, B6, B12, folic acid, zinc or TMG, you end up accumulating toxic homocysteine.

While the importance of antioxidants is now well established, the new buzzword in medicine is 'methylation'. The ability of the body to maintain chemical balance hinges upon its ability to add or subtract molecules called methyl groups. This is how the body turns one thing into another. To make this real, let's say all this talk of 'premature death' is stressing you out. Your body responds by adding a methyl group to noradrenalin to produce adrenalin. On hearing that homocysteine is rapidly reversible you relax. The body responds by removing a methyl group from adrenalin, turning it into noradrenalin. This kind of chemical reaction occurs a billion times every second, keeping everything in balance.

If there was one measure of your antioxidant 'IQ' it would be the level of glutathione inside your cells. All those antoxidants you eat and supplement every day have the greatest effect if they ultimately raise this level of intra-cellular glutathione. Similarly, if there was one measure of your methyl 'IQ' it would be the level of SAMe (s-adenosyl methionine) inside your cells. This is because SAMe can easily donate a methyl group, or accept one back, keeping the body's biochemistry flexible. Normally, both SAMe and glutathione are made from the amino acid methionine in our diet, via homocysteine. However, if the conversion of homocysteine is blocked in any way, the homocysteine level goes up and SAMe and glutathione levels go down.

This is only half of the bad news. The other half is the discovery that homocysteine damages your arteries, brain and DNA itself. That's why your homocysteine level is theoretically the most important indicator of the health and adaptability of your body's total biochemistry, and your risk of degenerative diseases. But where's the hard proof?

Reduce your risk of heart attacks and strokes by 75 per cent

The largest review of ninety-two studies, by David Wald and colleagues from the Department of Cardiology at Southampton General Hospital, recently published in the *British Medical Journal*, examined the association between homocysteine and risk for cardiovascular disease in 20,000 people.

They found that, with every 5-unit increase in homocysteine measured in the blood, the risk for heart disease went up by 42 per cent in those with the MTHFR gene mutation and by 32 per cent in those without it. The risk for strokes went up by 65 per cent in those with the genetic mutation and by 59 per cent in those without it. The researchers concluded that these 'highly significant results indicate strong evidence that the association between homocysteine and cardiovascular disease is causal'.[56]

This means that having a high homocysteine level isn't just associated with higher risk, it actually causes heart disease – a conclusion that is also being reached by other research groups.[57] If, therefore, you can lower your homocysteine level (your H score) you remove the cause, and hence the risk.

While the average homocysteine level is around 10 units, an ideal level is below 6 units. Those with a history of cardiovascular disease often have a level above 15 units. According to this study, lowering a high homocysteine from 16 to 6 units, a 10-point drop, might cut risk by 75 per cent! This is not only a much more substantial reduction than can be made for cholesterol, but it's also more achievable. How? With nutrients, not drugs.

Cancer – cut your risk by a third

Cancer is about 85 per cent preventable. Research published in the *New England Journal of Medicine* describing a study involving 45,000 pairs of twins found that cancer is more likely to be caused by diet and lifestyle choices than by genes. The results of the study showed that identical twins, who are genetically the same, have no more than a 15 per cent chance of developing the same cancer. This suggests that the cause of most cancers is about 85 per cent environmental – that is, down to factors such as diet, lifestyle and exposure to toxic chemicals. The study found that choices about diet, smoking and exercise accounted for 58 to 82 per cent of cancers studied.[58]

Where does homocysteine come into all this? Cancer is triggered by damage to DNA – and having a high homocysteine level makes your DNA more vulnerable to damage, and not easily properly repaired once damaged. At the other end of the scale, high homocysteine has been found to be a very good indicator of whether cancer therapies are working. The homocysteine level rises when tumours grow, and falls when they shrink. Forms of cancer already clearly linked to high homocysteine include cancers of the breast and colon, and leukaemia, among others. Low homocysteine is likely to reduce your risk of these by a third. By lowering your homocysteine level, along with making other dietary and supplement changes, you should be able to cut your cancer risk by substantially more than half.

Diabetes – lower your risk substantially

Type II or adult-onset diabetes is highly preventable, yet more and more young people are developing it. The obesity 'epidemic' in the West has helped fuel this rise. If you are obese, the risk of developing diabetes goes up seventy-seven times! Diabetics are at risk of having high homocysteine because we now know that the abnormally raised insulin seen in most diabetics stops the body from lowering and maintaining a healthier homocysteine level. By following a homocysteine-lowering diet and taking supplements, you will be able to help to reduce your risk of diabetes or, if you are diabetic, you'll be able to help keep the condition under better control and reduce complications.

Alzheimer's disease – halve your risk

The evidence indicates that if you can lower your H score, you will significantly lower your risk of getting Alzheimer's disease. Homocysteine is strongly linked to damage in the brain. Dr Matsu Toshifumi and colleagues at Tohoku University, Japan, conducted brain scans on 153 elderly people and checked them against each individual's homocysteine level. The evidence was crystal clear – the higher the homocysteine, the greater the damage to the brain.[59]

A recent study in the *New England Journal of Medicine* charted the health of 1,092 elderly people without dementia, measuring their homocysteine levels. Within the next eight years, 111 were diagnosed with dementia. Eighty-three of this group were diagnosed with Alzheimer's. Those with a high blood homocysteine level (in this study, above 14 units) had nearly double the risk of Alzheimer's. All this strongly suggests that following a homocysteine-lowering regime should, at the very least, halve your risk of developing Alzheimer's in later years.[60]

Halve your risk of death from all causes

One of the best ways to extend your healthy lifespan is by reducing your homocysteine level. This is because, with every five-point increase in your H score, you gain:

- A 49 per cent increased risk of death from all causes.

- A 50 per cent increased risk of death from cardiovascular disease.

- A 26 per cent increased risk of death from cancer.

- A 104 per cent increased risk of death from causes other than cancer or heart disease.

These are the extraordinary findings of a comprehensive research study at the University of Bergen in Norway, published in 2001 in the *American Journal of Clinical Nutrition*.[61] The researchers measured the homocysteine levels of 4,766 men and women aged 65 to 67 back in 1992, and then recorded any deaths over the next five years, during which 162 men and 97 women died. They then looked at the risk of death in relation to the individuals' homocysteine levels. Remarkably, they not only reconfirmed the relationship between heart attacks, strokes and high homocysteine, but also found that 'a strong relation was found between homocysteine and *all* causes of mortality'. In other words, homocysteine is an accurate predictor of how long you are going to live, whatever the eventual cause of death may be!

If you are already in your fifties or sixties, you might be tempted to view all this news with gloom. But with a guaranteed solution the news is all good, because you can begin to do something about it right now.

Measuring your homocysteine

Your homocysteine level is easy to measure at home (see Resources, page 527). Homocysteine is measured in mmol/l. We used to think a 'high' level was above 15 units (mmol/l). This is what increases your risk of a heart attack and doubles your Alzheimer's risk. Now, however, levels as low as 7 units are being linked to increased disease risk. Basically, there's no official safe level and no guarantee that the diet and supplements you are currently taking are keeping homocysteine at bay. Up to 30 per cent of people with a history of heart disease have a homocysteine level above 14 units. The average level in Britain is 10.5. However, experts believe that a level below 6 units is ideal. If you have any of the associated risk factors below it's especially important to get tested.

High homocysteine risk factors

These include:

- Genetic inheritance, meaning family history of heart disease, strokes, cancer, Alzheimer's disease, schizophrenia or diabetes

- Folate intake of less than 900 mcg/day

- Increasing age

- Male sex

- Oestrogen deficiency

- Excessive alcohol, coffee or tea intake

- Smoking

- Lack of exercise

- Hostility and repressed anger

- Inflammatory bowel diseases (coeliac, Crohn's, ulcerative colitis)

- *H. pylori*-generated ulcers

- Pregnancy

- Being a strict vegetarian or vegan

- High-fat diet with excessive red meat, high-fat dairy intake

- High salt intake

Lowering your homocysteine

The good news is that, whatever your homocysteine level is, you can lower it with the right combination of nutrients and dietary changes, together with lifestyle changes designed to reduce your risk. Follow the H Factor Diet below.

The H Factor Diet

Eat less fatty meat, more fish and vegetable protein
Eat no more than four servings of lean meat a week; fish (but not fried) at least three times a week; and if you're not allergic or intolerant, a serving of a soya-based food, such as tofu, tempeh or soya sausages, or beans, such as kidney beans, chickpea hummus or baked beans, at least five times a week.

Eat your greens
Have at least five servings of fruit or vegetables a day. This means eating two pieces of fruit every single day, and three servings of vegetables. Vary your selections from day to day. Make sure half of what's on your plate for each main meal is vegetables.

Have a clove of garlic a day
Either eat a clove of garlic a day, or take a garlic supplement every day. You can take garlic oil capsules or powdered garlic supplements.

Don't add salt to your food
Don't add salt while you're cooking or to the food on your plate. The only salt I consider healthy is Solo salt, which has half the sodium of ordinary salt and lots of potassium and magnesium. Use this in moderation instead.

Cut back on tea and coffee

Don't drink more than one cup of caffeinated or non-caffeinated coffee, or two cups of tea, in a day. Instead choose from the wide variety of herbal teas and grain coffees available.

Limit your alcohol

Limit your alcohol intake to no more than half a pint of beer, or one glass of red wine, in a day. Ideally, limit your intake to two pints of beer or four glasses of wine a week.

Reduce your stress

If you are under a lot of stress, or find yourself reacting stressfully much of the time, make a decision to reduce your stress load by changing both the circumstances that are giving you stress and your attitude. Simple additions to your life, such as yoga, meditation and/or exercise, or seeing a counsellor if you have some issues to resolve, can make all the difference.

Stop smoking

If you smoke, make a decision to stop, and seek help to do it. There is simply no safe level of smoking as far as homocysteine and your health is concerned. Smoking is nothing less than slow suicide. The sooner you stop the longer you'll live.

Correct oestrogen deficiency

If you are post-menopausal, or have menopausal symptoms or other menstrual irregularities, check your oestrogen- and progesterone-levels with a hormone saliva test. If you are oestrogen- or progesterone-deficient, you can correct this with 'natural progesterone' HRT in the form of a transdermal skin cream. Natural progesterone has none of the associated risks of HRT and your body can make its own oestrogen from progesterone.

Supplement a high-strength multivitamin every day

Take a high-strength multivitamin and mineral supplement providing at least 25mg of the main B vitamins, 200mcg of folate and 10mcg each of vitamins B12 and B6, plus A, D and E, and the minerals magnesium, selenium, chromium and zinc. Also supplement 1g of vitamin C for general health, as well as the specific homocysteine-lowering nutrients indicated below.

Take homocysteine supplements

The most powerful and quickest way to restore a normal H score, below 6 units, is to supplement specific homocysteine-lowering nutrients. These include vitamins B2, B6, B12, folic acid, trimethyl glycine (TMG) and zinc. Here are the guidelines:

Nutrient	No risk Below 6	Low risk 6–9	High risk 9–15	V. high risk Above 15
Folate	200mcg	400mcg	1,200mcg	2,000mcg
B12	10mcg	500mcg	1,000mcg	1,500mcg
B6	25mg	50mg	75mg	100mg
B2	10mg	15mg	20mg	50mg
Zinc	5mg	10mg	15mg	20mg
TMG	500mg	750mg	1.5–3g	3–6g

The current vogue is to recommend folic acid. However, this alone is far less effective than the right nutrients in combination. The amount you need also depends on your current homocysteine level. One study found that homocysteine scores were reduced by 17 per cent on high-dose folic acid alone; 19 per cent on vitamin B12 alone; 57 per cent on folic acid plus B12; and 60 per cent on folic acid, B12 and B6.[62] All this was achieved in three weeks!

However, even better results would have been achieved by including trimethyl glycine (TMG). TMG is the best 'methyl donor' to supplement, better than SAMe. This is because only it can immediately donate a methyl group to homocysteine, thus detoxifying it (see figure opposite).

In a study in New Zealand, the homocysteine scores of patients with chronic kidney failure and very high homocysteine levels were reduced by a further 18 per cent when 4g of TMG was given, along with 50mg of vitamin B6 and 5,000mcg of folate, compared with the levels of patients taking just B6 and folate.[63] Some companies produce combinations of these nutrients (see www.thehfactor.com). These are the most cost-effective supplements for restoring a healthy homocysteine level.

The combination of the diet and supplements recommended above has the potential to half your homocysteine score in weeks. The goal is to bring your score to below 6. Mine is 4.5. Your homocysteine score is probably the best objective measure of whether you are achieving optimum nutrition for *you*.

Dig deeper by reading my book, co-authored with Dr James Braly, *The H Factor*.

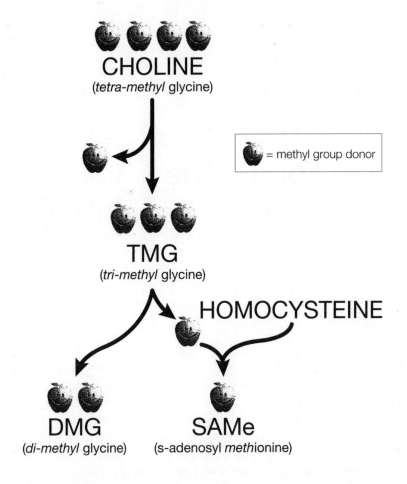

The methyl donors. The body needs 'methyl groups'. Choline, found in eggs and in lecithin, contains these, as does TMG (also called betaine), found in sugar beet and other vegetables. TMG is the best source because it can donate one methyl group (DMG) and turn toxic homocysteine into SAMe, the body's best methyl-group carrier.

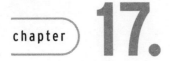

chapter 17

Living Food – the Phytochemical Revolution

Every time you eat a natural food, for example a piece of broccoli, you are receiving a cocktail of a vast number of active compounds that will influence your health for the better. Some of these, as we've seen, are classified as vitamins, minerals, essential fats or amino acids. However, there are many more substances that play a very important part in your health. These are called phytochemicals (*phyton* means plant in Greek) and have a major impact on our body systems, helping to promote health and prevent disease.

Phytochemicals are biologically active compounds in food; they are not classified as nutrients, in that our lives do not depend on them as they do on vitamins. However, they do play a vital role in the body's biochemistry in ways that affect our health as significantly as vitamins and minerals. In this sense they are best thought of as semi-essential nutrients. As they are not stored in the body it is best to eat foods rich in phytochemicals on a regular basis. Over a hundred phytochemicals have been identified, some of which act as antioxidants, immune-system boosters and hormone stabilizers. Listed below are those with proven health benefits.

■ Phytochemicals found in common foods

Allium compounds	Dithiolthiones	Phenols
Anthocyanidins	Ellagic acid	Phytoestrogens
Bioflavonoids	Genistein	Phytosterols

Boswellic acid	Glucosinolates	Piperine
Capsaicin	Indoles	Probiotics
Carotenoids	Isothiocyanates	Quercetin
Chlorophyll	Lentinan	Proanthocyanidins
Coumarins	Lignans	Saponins
Chlorogenic acid	Lutein	Sulforaphane
Curcumin	Lycopene	Zeanxanthin

Now let's take a look at how some of these phytochemicals can support your health.

Phytochemicals – nature's pharmacy

Allium compounds Members of the *Allium* genus include garlic, onions, leeks, chives and shallots. Garlic has long been renowned as a health food, with many benefits attributed to it. Though it is rich in many vitamins and minerals, the main active ingredients seem to be sulphur compounds. These include allicin, allixin, diallyl disulphide and diallyl trisulphide.

Studies from China show that people who eat a lot of garlic are protected against stomach cancer.[64] This may be because garlic is able to block the conversion of nitrites and nitrates (found in many preserved foods) into cancer-causing nitrosamines. Garlic can also inhibit the action of aflatoxins, which are naturally occurring substances found in peanuts, which can cause cancer. The results of a large study involving 41,837 women from Iowa, USA, aged between fifty-five and sixty-nine, indicated that garlic was the most protective type of vegetable against colon cancer. Women who said they ate garlic at least once a week were 50 per cent less likely to contract colon cancer than those who said they never ate it.[65] By acting as an antioxidant, garlic helps to prevent both cancer and heart disease.

Garlic significantly lowers cholesterol in the blood and prevents atherosclerosis. A three-year study at Tagore Medical College in India divided over 400 patients who had already suffered heart attacks into two groups. One group were given garlic supplements (equal to six to ten cloves per day) – they suffered fewer heart attacks and had significantly lower cholesterol counts than those who did not take garlic.[66] Garlic also helps prevent blood clots – probably a safer way to maintain thin blood than taking an aspirin a day, which can cause stomach bleeding.

Anthocyanidins and proanthocyanidlns These are particularly rich in berries and grapes. These are types of bioflavonoids (see overleaf), reputedly good against gout and certain types of arthritis.

Bioflavonoids   These have a number of beneficial roles. They act as potent antioxidants; they can bind to toxic metals and escort them out of the body; they have a synergistic effect on vitamin C, stabilising it in human tissue, they have a bacteriostatic and/or antibiotic effect, which accounts for their anti-infection properties; and they are also anti-carcinogenic. They are used to deal with capillary fragility, bleeding gums, varicose veins, haemorrhoids, bruises, strain injuries and thrombosis. Bioflavonoids include rutin (lots in buckwheat) and hesperidin, found particularly in citrus fruits. The best food sources are rosehips, buckwheat leaves, citrus fruit, berries, broccoli, cherries, grapes, papaya, cantaloupe melon, plums, tea, red wine and tomatoes. There are also special bioflavonoids in cucumbers that stop cancer-causing hormones from binding to cells.

Boswellic acid   This is a powerful anti-inflammatory agent, and therefore helpful with conditions such as arthritis; it is found in the herb frankincense.

Capsaicin   Abundant in hot peppers, it helps protect DNA from damage.

Carotenoids   As the name implies, carotenoids – one type of which is betacarotene – are rich in carrots. They are also rich in other fruit and vegetables including sweet potato, watercress and peas. They act as important anti-ageing antioxidants.

Chlorophyll   This is the substance that makes green plants green. Chlorophyll-rich foods like wheat grass, algae, seaweeds and green vegetables help to 'build' the blood. Vitamins C, B12, B6, A, K and folic acid are among the nutrients needed to keep blood healthy. Research has shown that components of chlorophyll found in foods, when fed in very small, purified amounts, may stimulate the production of red blood cells in the bone marrow. Chlorophyll has been shown to help protect against cancer and certain forms of radiation, to kill germs and to act as a powerful wound-healer. Cereal grasses have the nutrient profile of a dark green vegetable rather than that of a grain, so they are gluten-free and safe for those who have coeliac disease (due to allergy to gluten).

Coumarins and chlorogenic acid   These substances prevent the formation of cancer-causing nitrosamines and are found in a wide variety of fruit and vegetables, including tomatoes, green peppers, pineapple, strawberries and carrots.

Curcumin   A powerful antioxidant found in mustard, turmeric, corn and yellow peppers.

Ellagic acid   Present in strawberries, grapes and raspberries, ellagic acid neutralises carcinogens before they can damage DNA. A common cancer-producing chemical found in some meat, called nitrosamine, is put out of action by strawberries. In fact, research has shown that strawberries are second only to garlic for their anti-cancer properties against nitrosamines.[67] One of the reasons, apart from their high antioxidant levels, that strawberries and raspberries come out top is that they are very high in another anti-cancer nutrient, called ellagic acid. According to research at the Indiana University School of Medicine in the US, ellagic acid in strawberries and raspberries protects healthy cells from developing into cancer cells.[68] Ellagic acid also protects you from another common carcinogen, aflatoxin.[69] This is found in low levels in a number of foods, including peanuts.

Genistein   Abundant in soya beans, this substance, a type of phyto-estrogen (see below), prevents breast, prostate and other lumps from growing and spreading. Research is beginning to focus on two isoflavonoids – genistein and daidzein. Japanese women, who generally have a lower risk of breast cancer than women in other industrialised societies, have been found to have higher levels of these in their bodies. They may protect against the harmful effects of unopposed oestrogen. In fact, a recent study from Singapore, which monitored a group of women for early signs of breast cancer, found that the more soya a woman ate, the less chance there was of her having pre-cancer changes in her breast cells.

A likely ideal intake for cancer prevention is around 5mg a day of genistein and daidzein, which you can get from a 12oz serving of soya milk or a serving of tofu. Soya milk can be used in drinks and on cereal like cow's milk, while tofu is excellent in stir-fries. Tofu is the richest source of isoflavones, while very processed soya products are the poorest source. However, I don't advise having much more than this. Even plant oestrogens could, theoretically, be oestrogenic in excess, and you can develop allergies to soya if you eat too much of it.

Glucosinolates   These are one of the most important anti-cancer and liver-friendly nutrients found in food. According to the World Cancer Research Fund there's convincing evidence that foods high in glucosinolates reduce risk for lung cancer, stomach cancer, colo-rectal cancer and probably breast cancer. That's why broccoli is considered so good for you. Tenderstem is the richest source by far discovered, followed by broccoli and Brussels sprouts and other cruciferous vegetables. Glucosinolates have this profound anti-cancer effect by helping the liver detoxify.

In an ingenious study volunteers were given Brussels sprouts that had their glucosinolates removed, versus regular Brussels sprouts. Those eating the regular Brussels sprouts had 30 per cent more active liver enzyme function, showing just how powerful glucosinolates are for boosting your ability to detoxify.

Isothiocyanates (ITCs) and indoles   These are plentiful in cruciferous vegetables, which include broccoli, Brussels sprouts, cabbage, cauliflower, cress, horseradish, kale, kohlrabi, mustard, radishes and turnips. One of the highest food sources is tenderstem, which is a cross between kale and broccoli. Strawberries and raspberries are another rich source.

Eating fruit or vegetables rich in ITCs is now linked to a lower incidence of cancer, particularly of the colon. Research has shown that if you eat cabbage more than once a week, you are only one-third as likely to develop colon cancer as someone who never eats cabbage. This means that one serving of cabbage a week could cut your chances of colon cancer by 60 per cent. Both broccoli and Brussels sprouts also show a dose-dependent protective response against cancer. Isiothiocyanates don't just help prevent cancer; they reverse it by killing cancer cells. Strawberries and raspberries, for example, have been shown to inhibit cancer development in cervical,[70] oesophageal[71] and oral cancer, [72] and probably prostate cancer.

Lentinan   Two species of mushrooms, shiitake and reishi, are rich sources of this powerful anti-cancer agent. In animal studies it has shown anti-tumour properties. Lentinan is widely used in Japanese hospitals to treat cancer. It also induces the production of interferon, the body's own anti-viral chemical used to fight off infection. Other research suggests that lentinan may have potential in the fight against AIDS. It has demonstrated anti-HIV activity and in one US study, 30 per cent of patients taking lentinan who were HIV+ showed an increase in their T-cell counts after twelve weeks.

Lignans   These are part of the group of compounds known as phytoestrogens, plant substances that can induce biological responses in the body. They do this by mimicking the actions of endogenous oestrogens, usually by binding to the oestrogen receptors. They are ingested as inactive compounds and then activated by the gut microflora. The main source of lignans is linseeds (flax seeds) and they are also found in beans, nuts, fruit and cereals in smaller quantities.

Lutein   This is a powerful antioxidant found in many fruits and vegetables. It is remarkably heat-stable and can survive cooking. A recent study by the Florida International University found that people whose eyes contained higher amounts of lutein were up to 80 per cent less likely to be suffering from age-related macular degeneration (ARMD), a condition that includes cataracts. Lutein protects the eye by forming pigments in the macula – the part of the eye right behind the lens in the centre of the retina. These pigments help with vision by filtering out harmful blue light wavelengths that can damage the eye. The more pigments your eye contains, the less likely it is to fall prey to ARMD.

As the body does not naturally generate lutein, you need to make sure you are getting enough from other sources. The best are green leafy vegetables such as cabbage, spinach, broccoli, cauliflower and kale. A study in the *American Journal of Clinical Nutrition* found that eating a teaspoon of green leafy vegetables (with a small amount of fat) raised blood lutein levels by nearly 90 per cent.

Lycopene   This is a powerful antioxidant with anti-cancer properties, found in tomatoes.[73] Tomatoes also contain many other antioxidants. Lycopene in tomatoes becomes considerably more bioavailable when you juice, mash or cook the tomatoes. Lycopene is also found in other red foods, including watermelon. It's worth eating something red most days.

Phenols   These are potent antioxidants particularly rich in green tea. These substances have been investigated for their cancer-protective effects, which have been found to be even more powerful than those in vitamins C and E. It's believed that green tea consumption in Japan, which averages about three cups a day, is partly responsible for the low levels of cancer found in that country.

Phytoestrogens   These substances play a protective role by binding excess oestrogens made in the body, or taken in from the environment via pesticides, plastics and other sources of oestrogen-like chemicals, to a protein made in the blood. This action reduces the amount of oestrogens available to oestrogen-sensitive tissues. Foods rich in phytoestrogens include soya, particularly in the forms tofu and miso, other pulses, citrus fruits, wheat, liquorice, alfalfa, fennel and celery. A high intake of phytoestrogens is associated with a low risk for breast and prostate cancer, menopausal symptoms, fibroids and other hormone-related diseases. For a complete list of the phytoestrogen content of different foods please see my website www.patrickholford.com.

Phytosterols The term 'phytosterols' covers plant sterols and plant stanols. These are naturally occurring substances present in the diet, principally in vegetable oils, and are effective in lowering plasma total and low-density lipoprotein (LDL) cholesterol. They do this by inhibiting the absorption of cholesterol from the small intestine. In order to achieve a cholesterol-lowering benefit, approximately 1g a day of plant sterols or plant stanols needs to be consumed. In comparison, the normal dietary intake is between 200 and 400mg a day. The best food sources are seeds, beans and lentils, plus seed oils. Some margarine is now being enriched with phytosterols.

Piperine This is found in black pepper and actually helps you absorb more nutrients from your food. So effective is piperine at improving the uptake of nutrients that you might literally double the nutrients you take in from food simply by going heavy on the pepper. Piperine is particularly high in black pepper, not white, and it's not present in the other so-called peppers, such as chilli, paprika and cayenne; these are all fruits from the capsicum family with their own interesting properties. Chillies, for example, are one of the richest known sources of vitamin C. Some people are allergic to these 'capsicum' peppers, but allergy to black pepper is rare. (It can, however, make you sneeze.)

Quercetin Nature usually provides a solution to cope with ailments – and in the case of hay fever it's strawberries. Why? Because strawberries, as well as other berries, are especially high in a quirky bioflavonoid call quercetin. Quercetin, along with other bioflavonoids in berries, can also improve the health of capillaries and connective tissues. Because of this, the many benefits of quercetin include alleviating bruising, oedema, varicose veins and fragile capillaries.

A major benefit of quercetin is its ability to inhibit the release of histamine. As such, it is said to help mitigate conditions brought on by some types of allergen (e.g. eczema, asthma, hay fever, etc.) and has been ascribed anti-inflammatory properties, which means that berries could be good for arthritis sufferers as well.

At the prestigious Mayo Clinic in the US, research has been conducted into quercetin to help treat and prevent prostate cancer, the fastest-rising cancer, now affecting one in six men at some point in their life. In the words of the Mayo Clinic researcher Dr Nianzeng Xing, 'Our laboratory results showed quercetin blocks the androgen activity in androgen-responsive human prostate cancer cells. By blocking the androgen activity,' he continued, 'the growth of prostate cancer cells can be prevented or stopped.'

Sulforaphane   Sulforaphane is another of nature's great healers found in brassicas – broccoli, cauliflower, Brussels sprouts, turnips, kale and especially tenderstem. Originally it was discovered to reduce risk of stomach cancer and stomach ulcers, but now we know this is mainly because sulforaphane is one of nature's best anti-bacterial compounds. As many as half of all stomach ulcers are triggered by infection with the *Helicobacter pylori* bacterium. Sulforaphane kills off this unpleasant bacterium, helping to keep your digestive tract healthy. Sulforaphane also lessens the incidence of breast cancer in animals.

Zeanxanthin   This is an antioxidant that gives corn its yellow colour. It is also found in spinach, cabbage, broccoli and peas.

When you realise just how many active compounds there are in natural foods, the idea of separating and concentrating each nutrient and supplementing it on its own seems ridiculous. That is why the foundation of optimum nutrition is to eat as much whole, unadulterated natural food as possible and then supplement on top. Natural foods also contain enzymes that help you derive the most benefit from these foods.

Enzymes – the keys of life

We are what we eat, runs the familiar saying. Well, not quite – we are what we can digest and absorb. The food we eat cannot nourish us unless it is first prepared for absorption into the body. This is done by enzymes, chemical compounds that digest and break down large food particles into smaller units. Protein is broken down into amino acids; complex carbohydrate into simple sugars; and fat into fatty acids and glycerol. Every day 10 litres of digestive juices, mainly produced by the pancreas, liver, stomach and intestinal wall, pour into the digestive tract.

For the body to make these enzymes it needs nutrients. If you become nutrient-deficient, enzyme deficiency soon follows (which means your body will be less able to make use of the nutrients it does take in, which makes you become even more enzyme-deficient – and so the cycle continues). For example, zinc is needed to make both stomach acid and protein-splitting enzymes called proteases. A zinc-deficient person soon stops breaking down protein efficiently. This makes large food molecules end up where they should not, in the small intestine. If the intestinal wall is not 100 per cent intact – a common defect in zinc deficiency – these undigested food particles can get inside the body where they are seen as invaders and attacked. This is the basis of most food allergies.

Once a food becomes the subject of an allergy, every time it is eaten the reaction in the gut leads to inflammation. This reaction disturbs the normal balance of beneficial bacteria and other micro-organisms in the gut. Food allergy triggered by digestive enzyme deficiency is always a possible cause if you are suffering from indigestion, bloating, flatulence, digestive pain, colitis, irritable bowel syndrome, Crohn's disease or candidiasis.

The main families of digestive enzymes are amylases, which digest carbohydrate; proteases, which digest protein; and lipases, which digest fat. As an aid to digestion, many nutritional supplements contain these enzymes. Freeze-dried plant enzymes are often used for this purpose. The most common of them are bromelain from pineapples and papain from papaya, which is chemically similar to pepsin, a powerful protein-digesting enzyme capable of digesting between 35 and 100 times its own weight in protein.

Enzymes from raw food

A good way of boosting your enzyme potential is to eat foods raw, because in this state they contain significant amounts of enzymes. The cooking process tends to destroy enzymes. Professor Artturi Virtanen, Helsinki biochemist and Nobel prize winner, showed that enzymes are released in the mouth when raw vegetables are chewed: they come into contact with the food and start the act of digestion. These food enzymes are not denatured by stomach acid, as some researchers have suggested, but remain active throughout the digestive tract.

Extensive tests by Kaspar Tropp in Würzburg, Germany, have shown that the human body has a way of protecting enzymes that pass through the gut so that more than half reach the colon intact. There they alter the intestinal flora by binding free oxygen, reducing the potential for fermentation and putrefaction in the intestines, a factor linked to cancer of the colon. In so doing they also help to create conditions in which lactic acid-forming beneficial bacteria can grow.

Some foods unfortunately contain enzyme blockers. For example, lentils, beans and chickpeas contain trypsin inhibitors, preventing protein from being completely digested. However, this anti-enzyme factor is destroyed either by sprouting these pulses or by cooking them. So bean sprouts or cooked beans are OK. The same is true for grains rich in phytates, which can bind to beneficial minerals.

The two main digestive enzymes, amylase and protease, are found in many foods. For centuries humans have put these food enzymes to work by pre-digesting foods before eating them. Fermented and aged foods are examples of this. However, raw foods too contain these enzymes, which become active when we chew them. These foods need to be chewed properly, which helps to liberate and activate the enzymes they contain. Some foods, like apples, grapes and mangoes, also contain the antioxidant enzymes peroxidase and catalase, which help to disarm free radicals. The chart below shows those foods that have so far been found to contain significant levels of health-promoting enzymes; many foods have still not been investigated.

▪ Enzymes naturally present in raw foods

	Amylase (digests sugars)	Protease (digests protein)	Lipase (digests fat)	Peroxidase and catalase (disarm free radicals)
Apples				*
Bananas	*			
Cabbage	*			
Eggs (uncooked)	*	*	*	*
Grapes				*
Honey (raw/unpasteurised)	*			*
Kidney beans	*	*		*
Mangoes				*
Milk (raw/unpasteurised)	*			*
Mushrooms	*	*		*
Pineapple	*	*		
Rice	*			
Soya beans		*		
Sweet corn	*			*
Sweet potatoes		*		
Wheat	*	*		

Probiotics – the inside story

Inside our bodies are twenty times as many bacteria as living cells, and the role they play in keeping you healthy is no less important. Having the right bacteria is vital for healthy digestion, keeping your immune system strong and consequently for fighting infections.

However, not all bacteria are good for you. There are harmful or pathogenic bacteria that can either cause infection directly, or produce toxic substances that contribute to inflammation or cancer, particularly of the digestive tract. The good guys, principally two families of bacteria called the *Lactobacillus* and *Bifodobacteria*, to a large extent keep the bad guys under control.

What you eat and supplement makes a big difference to the balance of bacteria inside you and consequently your health. The ingesting of beneficial bacteria, known as probiotics, has a number of proven benefits.

■ The proven benefits of probiotics

- Improving your digestion
- Producing vitamins
- Lowering cholesterol levels
- Regulating hormones
- Boosting your immunity
- Increasing resistance to infections
- Relieving symptoms of irritable bowel syndrome (IBS)
- Relieving symptoms of thrush
- Reducing risk for certain cancers

The value of probiotics was first brought to light in 1907 by Metchnikoff, a Nobel laureate working at the Pasteur Institute in Paris, who was impressed by the robust health and longevity of Bulgarian peasants who were in the habit of drinking fermented milk. In the 1930s Dr Minoru in Japan isolated a strain of *Lactobacillus* bacteria now used in the yoghurt drink Yakult, and by the 1990s an estimated twenty million people in Asia were consuming probiotics. In the UK about a million people consume probiotic supplements or food. Interestingly, the addition of probiotics into animal feed has increased fivefold in the last ten years because this has proven to increase the animals' growth and reduce signs of stress. This potential benefit has yet to be studied in humans.

When you need probiotics

There is a good case for recommending probiotics, either in fermented foods or as supplements, every single day to promote health and prevent disease. It certainly worked for the Bulgarians. The case is even stronger for the elderly since the amount of colonic bacteria decreases with age. The same is probably true for those under continuous stress. In animal studies probiotics have been shown to help reduce the symptoms of stress when animals are transported – so if you're a stressed-out commuter they may help you too! Probiotics may help:

- Infections, especially sore throats, candida or bladder infections
- Food poisoning, traveller's diarrhoea or irritable bowel syndrome
- Inflammatory bowel problems such as Crohn's disease or colitis
- Cancer, especially of the stomach or bowel
- Constipation or any digestive disturbance including indigestion
- After a course of antibiotics
- After surgery
- At times of prolonged stress.

Choosing the best probiotic foods and supplements

Many cultures have observed the health-promoting effects of fermented foods and include them as a regular part of their diet. These foods include:

- Yoghurt, cottage cheese, kefir (from dairy produce)
- Sauerkraut, pickles (from vegetables)
- Miso, tofu, natto, tempeh, tamari, shoyu, soya yoghurt (from soya)
- Wine (from grapes)
- Sourdough bread (from wheat or rye)

However, most of these foods don't contain strains of *Lactobacillus* or *Bifidobacteria* that can colonise in the digestive tract. Yoghurt and other fermented dairy products often contain *Lactobacillus thermophilus* or *L. bulgaricus*. These bacteria will hang around for a week or so doing good work. They, like the other beneficial bacteria, can make vitamins as well as turning lactose, the main sugar in milk, into lactic acid. This makes the digestive tract slightly more acidic, which inhibits disease-causing microbes. Including these foods in your diet is a good way to promote healthy intestinal flora, although it is not as powerful as supplementing the strains of bacteria that can easily colonise the digestive tract. These resident strains are shown below. The most effective probiotic supplements provide these strains, often in combination.

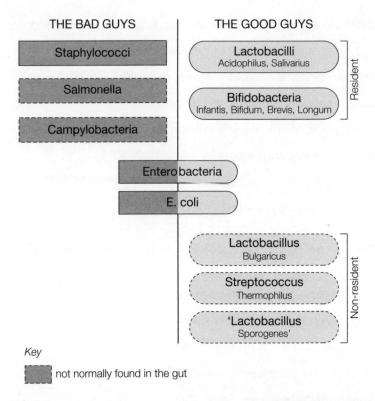

THE BAD GUYS | THE GOOD GUYS

Staphylococci

Salmonella

Campylobacteria

Lactobacilli
Acidophilus, Salivarius

Bifidobacteria
Infantis, Bifidum, Brevis, Longum

Resident

Enterobacteria

E. coli

Lactobacillus
Bulgaricus

Streptococcus
Thermophilus

'Lactobacillus
Sporogenes'

Non-resident

Key

not normally found in the gut

'Good' and 'bad' bacteria. Not all the 'good' bacteria shown on the right take up residence in you. The 'non-residents' do good work on their way through, but the best bacteria are Lactobacillus acidophilus and Bifidobacteria (think of A and B). Some bacteria, such as E. coli, are often present in the gut in tiny amounts. If they proliferate they become bad news. Other bacteria, such as salmonella, shouldn't be there at all and cause disease such as food-poisoning.

■ Resident and transient bacteria strains in adults

RESIDENT	L. acidophilus
	L. salivarius
	B. infantis
	B. bifidum
	B. brevis
	B. longum
PASSING THROUGH	L. bulgaricus
	L. casei
	L. sporogenes
	S. thermophilus

Key   B. = Bifidus   L. = Lactobacillus   S. = Streptococcus

Another way to boost the healthy bacteria inside you is to eat foods that feed them. The best food for your health-promoting bacteria are something called fructo-oligosaccharides, or FOS for short, sometimes known as a prebiotic. Bananas are especially rich in these, as are other fruit, barley, garlic, Jerusalem artichoke, onions, soya beans and wheat. One study found that eating banana powder thickened the stomach lining, as opposed to aspirin, which thins the stomach lining.[74]

The best probiotic supplements also contain FOS for the bacteria to feed off, promoting their rapid multiplication. FOS can also be supplemented alone and have been shown to help promote more of the good guys and less of the bad guys, as well as relieving constipation.[75]

Overall, eating a plant-based diet, high in fruit and vegetables, which are naturally high in fibre and FOS, is much more likely to encourage healthy bacteria than a diet that does not include many of these ingredients. On the other hand, a diet high in meat is – apart from being the primary source of gastrointestinal infections – more likely to introduce toxic breakdown products as well as slowing down gastrointestinal transit time.

Are your probiotics getting through?

Even if you supplement the right probiotics, in food, powders or capsules, the next question is to what extent they make it through your stomach to the small and large intestines. The vast majority of gut bacteria reside in the colon – about 100 trillion in one individual, to be precise, which is more than the total number of people on this planet. Stomach acid kills off a lot of bacteria, but certainly not all. There are four ways you can help more get through:

- Supplement at least 100 million viable organisms.

- Supplement with FOS.

- Supplement away from food.

- Use enteric-coated supplements.

- Use spore-form *Lactobacillus* supplements.

Supplementing enough bacteria is the starting point. You probably need 100 million to a billion viable bacteria to start with. Supplements are made by culturing bacteria, then freeze-drying them. If this is done properly probiotic supplements are stable for many months, if not years, and do not need to be kept in the fridge. When you swallow them and they come into contact with moisture, they come back to life.

A supplement containing FOS will promote rapid multiplication, so you may not need so many as is suggested above. The same is true for micro-encapsulated or enterically coated supplements, which should be taken with food; otherwise take supplements away from meals to minimise their destruction from gastric acid in the stomach (stomach acid will normally destroy a percentage of the bacteria you ingest – good and bad). *Lactobacilli* and *Bacillus coagulans* (formerly known as *Lactobacillus sporogenes*) are particularly resistant to stomach acid and are therefore a good choice as a supplement. *Bacillus coagulans* is especially effective at producing lactic acid, which is the primary way in which probiotics fight infection. Although not resident, *Bacillus coagulans* hangs around for a week or so doing good work.

If you are taking probiotics therapeutically, for example to reinoculate the digestive tract after antibiotics or as part of an anti-infection strategy, for instance to kill off candidiasis, you may need three times the amount needed for general health promotion. Higher levels of probiotics and pre-biotics such as FOS do sometimes result in increased flatulence, at least in the short term. This is not necessarily a bad sign – as less desirable organisms die off, symptoms sometimes get worse before they get better.

Living food in action

Every time you eat a combination of fresh, living foods, such as fruit and vegetables, you are giving yourself a cocktail of essential vitamins, minerals, amino acids, antioxidants, enzymes, probiotics and phytochemicals that work together synergistically to promote your health. The idea of separating out each ingredient and then treating it like a drug to cure a specific illness is not just impractical but nonsensical. The moral of this story is to eat foods that you can pick out of the ground or pluck from a tree.

Here is a simple checklist of good habits to develop to ensure that living foods, and the nutrients they contain, form a regular part of your diet:

- Eat at least three pieces of fresh fruit a day.

- Have a salad as a major part of one meal each day.

- Eat frequently the many foods rich in antioxidants and phytochemicals such as sweet potatoes, broccoli, watercress, peas, carrots and berries.

- Eat a multicoloured variety of foods, as each natural colour contains different health-promoting phytochemicals.

- Eat whole foods, rather than refined or processed foods full of artificial chemicals.

- Eat as much raw food as possible. Steam food where you can, and fry as little as possible.

- Wherever possible, buy organic food. If this is not possible, peel or throw away outer leaves and wash to reduce pesticide residues.

- Buy fresh foods when you need them, rather than buying ahead and storing them. The longer you keep them, the more their nutrients are destroyed.

- Eat fermented foods such as yoghurt, cottage cheese, miso, shoyu, sauerkraut and sourdough bread, especially those cultured with *Lactobacillus* or *Bifodobacteria*.

- Take a probiotic supplement containing beneficial strains of bacteria as well as FOS.

- Supplement your diet with a synergistic collection of vitamins, minerals, antioxidants and other phytochemicals (see Part 6).

18.

Your Body Is 66 per cent Water

It is an astonishing fact that the human body is basically two-thirds water. Without it most people are dead in four days. In normal circumstances in twenty-four hours we lose 1.5 litres of water in urine, 750ml through the skin, 400ml in the breath and 150ml in faeces. That's a total of 2.8 litres a day.[76] A simple equation would suggest that this is what you need to drink.

It isn't quite that simple, however. Firstly, the body makes water by metabolising food, normally around 300ml a day. Then there is the water in food itself, which normally provides around 1 litre a day. This totals 1.3 litres, leaving the average person 1.5 litres short on an average day. That's the equivalent of six glasses of water.

Why eight glasses is better

Drinking a total of 1.5 litres of water a day is really a minimum since if it is hot or if you exercise you will need more because you will sweat more. Also, drinking more is generally helpful for the kidneys. This is because many toxins, both those generated by the body and the ones that are consumed, are eliminated via the kidneys. By diluting the concentration of these toxins in the blood you give your kidneys an easier time, up to a point.

In fact, it's essential to ensure that enough fluid is available for the excretion of soluble minerals in the blood and nitrogenous waste material, especially from protein metabolism. The maximum intake from oral liquids should be that which the kidneys can reasonably excrete in twenty-four hours, and in adults this is around 2 litres per day (30–35 ml/kg body weight), according to research by S. M. Kleiner at the University of Washington, published in the *Journal of the American Dietetics Association* in 1999.[77]

Contrary to popular opinion, drinking more water doesn't leach minerals from the body according to mineral expert Dr Neil Ward of the University of Surrey, who has never found any evidence of this or reason why it would happen.

Why more than eight glasses is worse

Drinking more than you need, which is around 1.5 to 2 litres a day in normal circumstances, isn't better for you, and may be worse. This is because too much water taxes the kidneys and can lead to overhydration. Taken to the extreme this can kill you. A man died recently after drinking 10 litres in a few hours, while almost every year somebody dies from drinking too much water while on Ecstasy, for fear of drinking too little. This drug, and others, disturbs the normal thirst reflex. Far more people die as a consequence of drinking too little.

What happens if you don't get enough?

Water has many roles throughout the body other than flushing the kidneys, including dissolving minerals, and acting as a delivery system, a lubricant and a temperature regulator.

Even very mild dehydration can lead to constipation, headaches, lethargy and mental confusion, while increasing the risk of urinary tract infections and kidney stones. When just 1 per cent of body fluids is lost, body temperature goes up and concentration becomes more difficult.

The thirst mechanism kicks in when we've lost between 1 and 2 per cent of body water. However, the thirst reflex is often mistaken for hunger. If we ignore it or mistake it for hunger, dehydration can continue to around 3 per cent, where it seriously affects both mental and physical performance. Sports nutritionists have found that a 3 per cent loss of body water results in an 8 per cent loss in muscle strength.

Dr Batmanghelidj, author of *Your Body's Many Cries for Water*, cites many other health problems resulting from chronic low-level dehydration, including gastric ulcers (water is needed for the mucosal lining of your stomach and digestive system to protect it from your digestive juices), joint pain (the discs and cartilage cushioning joints are dependent on their water content for proper functioning), asthma and allergies (concentrated blood reaching the lungs results in increased production of histamine) and many more conditions. After more than a decade of research he confirms that we need a minimum of six to eight 250ml glasses of water per day.[78]

How to tell how much water you need

At first glance you'd think that thirst indicates only that you need more water. While this is obviously true in most circumstances, there are other factors that can trigger the thirst reflex. So if you're constantly thirsty it can mean that you don't drink enough, but it could mean something else. The two most common reasons other than water deficiency are blood sugar problems and essential fat deficiency.

People with diabetes, or borderline diabetes, are often thirsty. This is because their blood sugar levels are too high – in these cases, the body wants to dilute glucose in the blood, which can be toxic to cells, by drinking more. This is why very sweet drinks make you drink more. It wouldn't surprise me if the sugared-drink industry hadn't worked out the perfect balance here to keep you drinking all day long!

The other reason for thirst is essential fat deficiency. Many people, especially children, are deficient in essential fats from fish and seeds and their oils. Without the right fats cells can't maintain their right water balance, and excessive thirst can result. The solution, of course, is to eat more fish, seeds and cold-pressed seed oils, or to supplement the essential fats.

Any combination of the symptoms below might help you become more in tune with your body's cries for water.

- Are you prone to constipation?

- Are you often thirsty?

- Do you have joint problems?

- Do you feel tired?

- Are you having difficulty concentrating?

- Are you overheating?

- Do you have dry skin, mouth or lips?

- Do you get frequent infections?

- Do you have dry, brittle hair?

The other way to tell whether you need to drink more is by checking the colour of your urine. If your urine is very strongly coloured, then you're not drinking enough. This simple gauge is, however, complicated by the fact that riboflavin (vitamin B2) makes the urine a fluorescent kind of yellow. This is different from dark yellow, once you get used to it. Ideally, your urine should be a light, straw-coloured yellow. If, however, your urine is often clear, like water, you may be drinking too much and not taking in enough nutrients.

Do tea and coffee count?

Water-consumption advice almost always specifically discounts caffeinated beverages, but this is now being questioned, and may need revising. Caffeine does cause a loss of water, but only a fraction of what you're adding by drinking the beverage. In people who don't regularly consume caffeine, for example, researchers say that a cup of coffee actually adds about two-thirds the amount of hydrating fluid that's in a cup of water.

Regular coffee- and tea-drinkers become accustomed to caffeine and lose little, if any, fluid. In a study published in the *Journal of the American College of Nutrition*, researchers at the Center for Human Nutrition in Omaha, Nebraska, measured how different combinations of water, coffee and caffeinated sodas affected the hydration status of eighteen healthy adults who drank caffeinated beverages routinely.[79] 'We found no significant differences at all,' said nutritionist Ann Grandjean, the study's leading author. 'The purpose of the study was to find out if caffeine is dehydrating in healthy people who are drinking normal amounts of it. It is not.'

The same goes for tea, juice, milk and caffeinated sodas: one glass provides about the same amount of hydrating fluid as a glass of water. The only common drinks that produce a net loss of fluids are those containing alcohol – and usually it takes more than one of those to cause noticeable dehydration, doctors say.

I would still advise the consumption of pure filtered or bottled water in preference to tea, coffee, sugary drinks and juice because these drinks have effects other than just hydrating you. They all disrupt your blood sugar balance; tea, coffee and cola rob the body of minerals; and sugary drinks (including some juice drinks) provide calories but few nutrients, hindering an optimal nutrient intake, as well as potentially causing too-high concentrations of glucose in the blood.

If you want hydration, go for water. If you don't like water, try flavouring it with lemon, lime, ginger, mint or herbal teas.

What's the best water?

The best water to drink is natural mineral water, which contains significant amounts of minerals – for example 60 to 100mg of calcium in 2 litres of water. This can be still or sparkling. Carbonation makes no difference to calcium absorption. However, fizzy drinks containing phosphorus can inhibit calcium absorption, as can drinks containing caffeine. A cola drink that contains both is therefore bad news. If you drink only pure water or distilled water, ensure that you are getting all the minerals you need from your diet and supplements. The majority of water filters cannot help but remove some of the good minerals along with the bad, so the same applies. Most important of all, whatever kind of water you drink, make sure you drink enough.

In summary:

- Drink the equivalent of eight glasses of water a day, as water, diluted juices or caffeine-free drinks.

- Choose natural mineral water, pure water or filtered tap water.

chapter 19.

Food Combining – Facts and Fallacies

Many people find that certain types or combinations of food do not suit them. Based on this observation and on his research into health and nutrition, in the 1930s Dr Howard Hay devised a diet plan popularly known as 'food combining', which has helped millions of people towards better health. He recommended eating a healthy diet consistent with the optimum nutrition approach, and formulated rules about which foods you can eat together. The key elements in Dr Hay's original theory were to eat 'alkaline-forming foods', to avoid refined and heavily processed foods, to eat fruit on its own, and not to mix protein-rich and carbohydrate-rich foods.

Protein and carbohydrate are digested differently. That is a fact. Carbohydrate digestion starts in the mouth when the digestive enzyme amylase, which is present in saliva, starts to act on the food you chew. Once you swallow food and it enters the relatively acid environment of the stomach, amylase stops working. Only when the food leaves the stomach, where the digestive environment becomes more alkaline, can the next wave of amylase enzymes, this time secreted into the small intestine from the pancreas, continue and complete the digestion of carbohydrate.

Protein, on the other hand, is not digested in the mouth at all. It needs the acid environment of the stomach and may hang out there for three hours until all the complex proteins are broken down into smaller collections of amino acids known as peptides. This happens in the stomach only because it contains the high levels of hydrochloric acid needed to activate the protein-digesting enzyme pepsin. Once peptides leave the stomach they meet peptidase enzymes, again from the pancreas, which break them down into individual amino acids, ready for absorption.

The myth of the bean

The simplistic view of food combining is that carbohydrate and protein foods should be separated because they are digested differently. The fact that eating certain kinds of beans produces flatulence is often quoted as a negative effect, because beans contain both protein and carbohydrate. However, it is now known that this is not the reason for beans' boisterous reputation.

Some beans contain proteins such as lectin, which cannot be digested by the enzymes in our digestive system, even when eaten alone. These proteins can, however, be digested by the bacteria that live in the large intestine. So when you eat beans you feed not only yourself but also these bacteria. After a good meal of lectin, these bacteria produce gas, hence the flatulence. It has got nothing to do with food combining. Many healthy cultures throughout the world have evolved to eat a diet in which beans or lentils are a staple food – but they suffer no digestive problems.

Protein and carbohydrate – foods that fight?

Of course, since items of food do not consist exclusively of either carbohydrate or protein, in practical terms separating them means not combining concentrated protein foods with concentrated starch foods. Meat is 50 per cent protein and 0 per cent carbohydrate. Potatoes are 8 per cent protein and 90 per cent carbohydrate. In between are beans, lentils, rice, wheat and quinoa. So where exactly do you draw the line, if a line should be drawn at all?

A brief excursion into our primitive past may solve the puzzle. The general consensus is that the human race has been eating a predominantly vegetarian diet for millions of years, with the occasional meal of meat or fish. Monkeys or apes can be divided into two types: those that have a ruminant-like digestive tract and slowly digest even the most indigestible fibrous foods, much like a cow; and those that have a much speedier and technologically advanced digestive system that produces a whole series of different enzyme secretions. We fit into the second category. The system is more efficient but can handle only foods that are easier to digest – fruit, young leaves, certain vegetables. No stalks for us! Evolutionary theorists believe that this digestive system did two things: firstly, it gave us the motive to improve our mental and sensory processing so that we would know when and where to find the food we needed, and secondly, it gave us the nutrients to develop a more advanced brain and nervous system.

Did monkeys eat meat and two vegetables?

I believe the human body has three basic programmes for digestion. The first is for digesting concentrated protein, which means meat, fish and eggs. To digest these foods we have to produce vast amounts of stomach acid and protein-digesting enzymes. After all, when our early ancestors had hunted down and killed an animal, do you think they then went off to hand-pick a few tasty morsels of vegetation to create that 'balanced meal'? I doubt it. I imagine they ate their catch, organs and all, as fast as possible before it went off and other predators moved in. They might have spent a couple of days living on nothing but concentrated animal protein. Fresh, raw, organic meat is, after all, highly nutritious.

Fruit – the Lone Ranger

At certain times of the year, early humans would have had access to certain fruit. No doubt we were not the only fruit-eating creatures. Since fruit is the best fuel for instant energy, requiring very little digestion, our second programme produces the enzymes and hormones necessary to process the simple carbohydrates in fruit. Again, my guess is that we mainly ate fruit on its own. After all, once you had chomped three bananas there would be little reason to go digging up a few roots.

Many kinds of soft fruit ferment rapidly once ripe. They will do the same if you put them in a warm, acidic environment, which is what the stomach is. That is what happens if you eat a slice of melon followed by a steak. So Dr Hay's advice to eat fruit separately makes a lot of sense. Since fruit takes around thirty minutes to pass through the stomach, whereas whole concentrated protein takes two to three hours, the best time to eat fruit is as a snack more than thirty minutes before a meal, or not less than two hours after a meal – possibly more if you eat a lot of concentrated protein. The only exception to this advice is combining fruits that do not readily ferment, like bananas, apples or coconut, with complex carbohydrate-rich foods such as oats or millet. So a chopped apple on your porridge or a whole-rye banana sandwich would be fine.

However, for most of the time our ancestors seem to have eaten a varied vegan diet. That means leaf vegetables, root vegetables, nuts, seeds, pulses and sprouts. This, I propose, is the third and most common digestive programme – for a mixture of foods containing a mixture of carbohydrate and protein, but never as protein-dense as meat. I see no problem in combining rice, lentils, beans, vegetables, nuts and seeds.

80 per cent alkaline

One of Dr Hay's greatest observations was that people with more acidic blood were more likely to be ill. He identified a range of acidity, a pH of 7.4 to 7.5, which is slightly alkaline and associated with good health. A pH of 7 or below is increasingly acid, while a pH above 7 is increasingly alkaline.

Many factors affect the acid–alkaline balance of the blood.

When foods are metabolised, acids are produced which are neutralised by the alkaline salts (carbonates) of calcium, magnesium, potassium and sodium. So our intake of these mineral salts affects our acid–alkaline balance, as does the type of food we eat. Foods containing large amounts of chlorine, phosphorus, sulphur and nitrogen, for example most animal products, tend to be acid-forming. Those rich in calcium, potassium, magnesium and sodium, for example most vegetables, tend to be alkaline-forming. Exercise too has an effect – it makes the blood more acidic. Deep breathing makes the blood more alkaline.

In her book *The Wright Diet*, Celia Wright describes the over-acidic person as being grouchy, sensitive and exhausted, inclined to aches and pains, headaches, problems with sleeping and acidity of the stomach. Smokers have been found to have a high acid level in their urine. Cravings appear to decrease on a more alkaline diet.

Nearly all fresh fruit, vegetables and pulses are alkaline-forming. Exceptions include butter beans and broad beans, asparagus, olives and mustard and cress. Meat, fish, eggs and butter are acid-forming, while skimmed milk and whole milk are mildly alkaline-forming. A few grains are acidic, including oatmeal, wholemeal flour, sago and tapioca. Walnuts and hazelnuts are acidic, but other nuts are alkaline. (For a comprehensive list of acid and alkaline foods see the chart on page 516.)

No doubt part of the success of Dr Hay's approach was his emphasis on alkaline-forming foods. This, as you can see, means eating plenty of fruit and vegetables that are naturally high in many vital nutrients.

Refined carbohydrates are out

Refining food, or cooking it, Dr Hay did not recommend either. As explained earlier, the more refined, processed or cooked a food is, the less nutrition it will provide. The obvious advice is to eat raw or lightly cooked whole foods instead of overcooked and over-processed junk foods. Refined high-sugar foods are a new invention as far as your digestive system is concerned. Very few naturally occurring foods contain the kinds of concentrations of fast-releasing sugars that modern food can provide. The body is simply not adapted to deal with a flood of fast-releasing sugars which not only make your blood sugar levels rocket, requiring all sorts of hormones to swing into emergency action to restore the balance, but also feed potentially undesirable micro-organisms that can occur in the gut.

Improve your digestion

In a nutshell, food combining can be condensed into five simple steps, as shown in the illustration below. If you still have problems digesting these food combinations you may have a digestive enzyme deficiency, a food intolerance or a gut infestation of candida or unfriendly bacteria, and should see a nutritionist. Vegans have only one rule to follow, which is to eat certain fruit separately. Easy, isn't it?

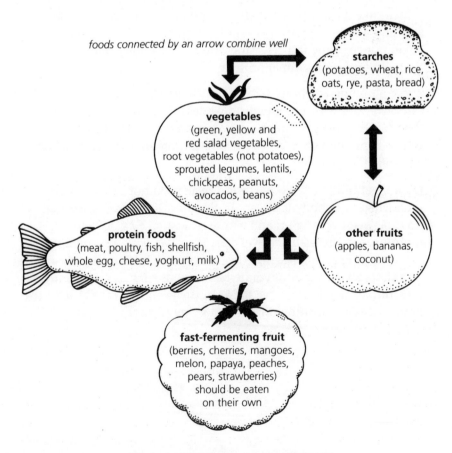

foods connected by an arrow combine well

starches
(potatoes, wheat, rice, oats, rye, pasta, bread)

vegetables
(green, yellow and red salad vegetables, root vegetables (not potatoes), sprouted legumes, lentils, chickpeas, peanuts, avocados, beans)

protein foods
(meat, poultry, fish, shellfish, whole egg, cheese, yoghurt, milk)

other fruits
(apples, bananas, coconut)

fast-fermenting fruit
(berries, cherries, mangoes, melon, papaya, peaches, pears, strawberries) should be eaten on their own

Food combinations – do's and don'ts

Here are five quick guidelines to help improve your digestion:

- Eat 80 per cent alkaline-forming foods, 20 per cent acid-forming foods. This means eating large quantities of vegetables and fruit, and less-concentrated protein foods like beans, lentils and whole grains instead of meat, fish, cheese and eggs.

- Eat fast-fermenting and acid fruit on their own as snacks. Most soft fruits, including peaches, plums, mangoes, papayas, strawberries and melons, ferment quickly. High-acid fruit (although alkaline-forming) may also inhibit digestion of carbohydrate; they include oranges, lemons, grapefruit and pineapple. All these fruits require little digestion, releasing their natural fructose content quickly. Eat them on their own as a snack when you need an energy boost.

- Eat animal protein on its own or with vegetables. Concentrated protein like meat, fish, hard cheese and eggs requires lots of stomach acid and a stay of about three hours in the stomach to be digested. So do not combine fast-releasing or refined carbohydrates or food that ferments with animal protein.

- Avoid all refined carbohydrates. Eat unrefined, fast-releasing carbohydrates with unrefined slow-releasing carbohydrates. Fruits that do not readily ferment, such as bananas, apples and coconut, can be combined with slow-releasing carbohydrate cereals like oats and millet.

- Do not eat until your body is wide awake. Do not expect to digest food when your body is asleep. In the morning, leave at least an hour between waking up and eating. If you take exercise in the morning, eat afterwards. Never start your day with a stimulant (tea, coffee or a cigarette), because the 'stress' state inhibits digestion. For breakfast, eat only carbohydrate-based foods such as cereal and fruit, just fruit, or whole grain rye toast. In the evening, leave at least two hours between finishing dinner and going to sleep.

chapter 20

Eat Right for Your Blood Type

E ach of us is unique, and each of us has a unique set of inherited genes, which determine our own individual 'perfect diet'. Some of us are programmed to function better on more protein, others do well on more carbohydrate. Some of us need more folic acid than others. In the future it will be possible to determine your 'ideal' diet and nutrient intake by testing your pattern of genes, as well as taking into account your diet, lifestyle and environment.

One example of your inherited genetic uniqueness is provided by your blood type. There are four blood types and, owing to the pioneering research of naturopath Peter D'Adamo, some nutritionists consider that each of them may be best suited to a specific type of diet. Why? Because blood types have evolved, from O to A to B to AB, as humanity has evolved, with each phase representing a different pattern of diet and environmental challenges. Knowing your blood type may therefore be a key to knowing how your immune system will react to certain foods and to certain diseases, and to what you need to eat to maximise your potential for health and vitality.

The story begins about 50,000 years ago with the emergence of our early humanoid ancestors, first Neanderthal man then Cro-Magnon man, who through cunning became the most dangerous predators on earth, the kings of the food chain. Their diet was high in animal protein, and the blood group O – the predominant blood type today – was born. These were the original hunters and every culture still has many type Os. With no natural predators other than themselves, the population of our ancestors exploded. As a consequence, their hunting grounds became exhausted. Cro-Magnon man migrated further afield from his African roots, exhausting big game along the way. By 20,000 BC Cro-Magnon man was in what is now Europe and Asia, and eventually migrated to Australasia and the Americas. The failing food supply probably led to rivalry, migration and wars, and may have propelled our early ancestors towards a more omnivorous diet of berries, nuts, grubs, roots and small animals.

Then, somewhere between 20,000 and 15,000 BC, a new blood type gained dominance in Western Europe – type A. A is for 'agrarian' and reflects the emergence of peasant farmers who grow their own grain and domesticated animals. Type A reflected a whole new digestive and immune programme – for much better-adapted individuals, who are more resistant to contagious diseases such as cholera, plague and smallpox, able to digest grain and able to co-operate; who are less the hunter and more the cultivator, working in network communities. Very rapidly, type A took over from type O, particularly in Western Europe, where it is still most concentrated. Even today, type Os are more susceptible to death from infections than are type As.

Another mutation took took place in the Himalayan highlands somewhere between 15,000 and 10,000 BC and blood type B emerged. It was the hallmark of the great tribes of the steppe dwellers – the Caucasian and Mongolian tribes. These tribes were herdsmen. Their diet was more nomadic than that of people living in Western Europe, and included meat and cultured dairy products. Soon type B spread throughout Asia and into Eastern Europe. B stands for 'balance' – a mixture of the vegetarian and meat-eating diets of the As and Os.

AB blood type is thoroughly modern. Emerging only in the last ten or twelve centuries, it is a very recent evolution of blood type and accounts for less than 5 per cent of the world's population. It probably started as the nomad warriors (type Bs) moved in on the collapsing civilisation of the Roman Empire and other European cultures. The result was a multi-faceted blood type, complex and unsettled – a perfect metaphor for modern life.

Blood type – the blueprint for immunity

Your blood type is your blueprint for immunity. Your cells are tagged with an antigen (a marker), which tells the immune system which cells belong to you. The immune system produces weapons – antibodies – to anything that isn't you, for example a virus. It also produces antibodies to other blood types, so that a type A will have antibodies to type O or type B cells.

That's why a type A will react to type B or O blood – the blood cells don't have the right marker so the immune system goes ballistic.

Those with blood type AB carry no antibodies to O, A or B and can receive blood from any group. On the other hand, they cannot donate blood to those having any of the other types of blood. Their cells are tagged with both A and B antigens, so type A reacts to the B antigen, type B reacts to the A antigen and type O reacts to both!

Food is the major invader of the body. The need for the immune system to react appropriately to digested material is of paramount importance to survival. That's why there are more immune cells and activity in the gastrointestinal tract than anywhere else in the body.

Not unexpectedly, different blood types programme the immune system to tolerate different kinds of foods. It really doesn't matter what you or your immediate ancestors have got used to eating. Your immune system is programmed to accept the kinds of foods that were the major part of your ancestors' diet thousands of years ago. That's why a type A (the grain-growing vegetarian) is more likely to react badly to dairy products, the staple of nomadic type Bs, or to a high-meat diet, the staple food of type Os.

The key to how this works is lectins, which are proteins found in most foods. These proteins have sticking or 'agglutinating' properties that help them to attach to other molecules, and other molecules to attach to them. Germs and immune cells use lectins to their own benefit. Cells in the liver's bile ducts have lectins on their surfaces that snatch up bacteria and parasites. Microbes and bacteria use lectins to stick to slippery surfaces such as the gastrointestinal wall. These lectins are often blood-type specific, as are those found in some foods. The lectins in milk have B-like qualities, so type As are more likely to react to them.

This, in a nutshell, is the basis behind Peter D'Adamo's work identifying which foods are most suited to which blood type. However, his work isn't based just on this logic. It's also based on testing thousands of foods and people and noting which foods raised toxic by-products of these lectin reactions. His research led him to produce certain dietary guidelines for each blood type (see page 177).

Blood types and disease risk

Knowing your blood type does more than help identify which foods are likely to suit you best. It reflects your unique metabolism and even possibly gives clues to your personality, although the latter is more plausible conjecture than scientific fact. However, what is becoming clear is that your risk of getting certain diseases, and your chances of recovery, may depend on your blood type. D'Adamo's book explains the connection between blood types and many common diseases, and outlines the best strategies for different blood types.

Perhaps the most interesting story emerging from the ongoing research into disease and blood types is the link to cancer. There is undeniable evidence, says D'Adamo, that people with type A or AB blood have an overall higher rate of cancer and poorer odds of survival than those with type O or B. The high risk of cancer among type ABs was reported as early as the 1940s by the American Medical Association, although the scientific community didn't pick up on this important discovery.

This is the first of many discoveries that will unfold, now that the link between blood types, immunity, diet and disease has been uncovered. In my view we owe an enormous debt to Dr Peter D'Adamo and his father, who first developed the blood-type theory and published it in 1980. Dr D'Adamo's book *Eat Right for Your Type* is the place to start for those wanting to unravel the mysteries of the evolutionary code hidden in your blood type and what it means for you in terms of your ideal diet and lifestyle.

Be aware, however, that you are even more unique than your blood type. The best way to find out which foods suit you and which foods don't is to have an allergy test (see Resources, page 527) that literally measures whether or not you produce specific antigens to specific foods. The dietary guidelines below, applicable to specific blood types, are just that – guidelines. By all means try them out. See how you feel. Many people find this way of eating works well for them. Others find that it makes little difference to them.

Also bear in mind that times and food have changed. If you were a type O back in the Stone Age, all that was available for you to eat was fit, organic meat, and you were not exposed to hormone-disrupting chemicals. Today, in the twenty-first century, most meat is from unfit animals, so it is fatty and contains undesirable chemical residues that over-stimulate cell growth. Beans, on the other hand, were not an available food source back in the Stone Age, but do have protective effects against cancer. So, even if a 'blood-type' diet has to be altered to fit the age we live in, it is one piece of the jigsaw of finding out your optimum nutrition.

STRENGTHS	WEAKNESSES	MEDICAL RISKS	DIET PROFILE	
Type O THE HUNTER strong, self-reliant, leader				
Hardy digestive tract Strong immune system Natural defences against infections System designed for efficient metabolism and preservation of nutrients	Intolerant to new dietary, environment conditions Immune system can be overactive and attack itself	Blood-clotting disorders Inflammatory diseases, arthritis, low thyroid function, ulcers, allergies	High protein: meat, fish, vegetables, fruit Limited: grains, beans, legumes	Avoid: wheat, corn, kidney beans, navy beans, lentils, cabbage, Brussels sprouts, cauliflower, mustard grains Aids: kelp, seafood, salt, liver, red meat, kale, spinach, broccoli
Type A THE CULTIVATOR settled, co-operative, orderly				
Adapts well to dietary and environmental changes Immune system preserves and metabolises nutrients more easily	Sensitive digestive tract Vulnerable immune system, open to microbial invasion, while resistant to contagious infections	Heart disease Cancer Anaemia Liver and gallbladder disorders Type 1 diabetes	Vegetarian: vegetables, tofu, seafood, grains, beans, legumes, fruit	Avoid: meat, dairy, kidney beans, lima beans, wheat Aids: vegetable oil, soy foods, vegetables, pineapple
Type B THE NOMAD balanced, flexible, creative				
Strong immune system Versatile adaptation to dietary and environmental changes Balanced nervous system	No natural weaknesses, but imbalance causes tendency toward auto-immune breakdowns and rare viruses	Type 1 diabetes Chronic fatigue syndrome Auto-immune disorders – Lou Gehrig's disease, lupus, multiple sclerosis	Balanced omnivore: meat (no chicken), dairy, grains, beans, legumes, vegetables, fruit	Avoid: corn, lentils, peanuts, sesame seeds, buckwheat, wheat Aids: greens, eggs, venison, liver, licorice, tea
Type AB THE ENIGMA rare, charasmatic, mysterious				
Designed for modern conditions Highly tolerant immune system Combines benefits of Types A and B	Sensitive digestive tract Tendency for over-tolerant immune system, allowing microbial invasion Reacts negatively to A-like and B-like conditions	Heart disease Cancer Anaemia	Mixed diet in moderation: meat, seafood, dairy, tofu, beans, legumes, grains, vegetables, fruit	Avoid: red meat, kidney beans, lima beans, seeds, corn, buckwheat Aids: tofu, seafood, dairy, greens, kelp, pineapple

Eat right for your blood type

Part 3

The Wonderful World Within

chapter 21.

You Are What You Eat

Nothing created by man compares to the magnificent design of the human body. As you read this book 2.5 million red blood cells are being made every second within your bone marrow in order to keep your body cells supplied with oxygen. Meanwhile, today you will produce 10 litres of digestive juices to break down the food you eat and enable it to pass through your 'inside skin', the gastrointestinal wall, a 30-foot-long tract with a surface area the size of a small football pitch which effectively replaces itself every four days.

The health of your gastrointestinal tract is maintained by a team of some 300 different strains of bacteria and other micro-organisms, as unique to you as your fingerprint, which exceed the total number of cells in your entire body. Meanwhile, your immune system replaces its entire army every week and, when under viral attack, has the capacity to produce 200,000 new immune cells every minute. Even your outside skin is effectively replaced every month, while most of your body is renewed over a seven-year period. Your brain, a mere 3lb/1.4kg of mainly fat and water, is processing information of immense complexity through its trillion nerve cells, each connected to 10,000 others in a network whose connections are formed as our life, and the meaning we attach to it, unfolds. In fact, by the time you finish this chapter you will have hard-wired thirty new connections between your brain cells.

The energy produced from a small amount of food powers all these unseen processes, with plenty left over to keep us warm and allow us to undertake a wide range of physical activities. The by-products are water and carbon dioxide, both of which are essential for plants, which in turn produce carbohydrate, our fuel, and oxygen, the spark that lights our cellular fires. It is estimated that we use only a quarter of a per cent of our brain's capacity and, in many cases, half the potential lifespan of our bodies. The design, the capacity and the resilience of the human body is truly awesome.

Yet, unlike a new car, we arrive without a maintenance manual and rely on instructions developed by those who have made their livelihood from a study of the human body – usually sick bodies at that. These instructions are in their infancy, a fact that is obvious when you consider how much of medicine is based on giving drugs that poison the body, radiation that burns it and surgery that removes defective parts. Most of us only begin to think about body maintenance when something goes wrong. Yet, because of the body's incredible resilience, most serious diseases like cancer and cardiovascular disease take twenty to thirty years to develop. By the time we notice the symptoms it may already be too late.

Learning from experience

Once you realise that your body is a collection of highly organised cells, designed by the forces of nature, adapting to the changing environment over millions of years, it becomes natural to give that body what it needs, with the tangible benefit of health. Experience is, of course, the greatest motivator. If something you eat makes you feel good you are likely to continue eating it, while if something makes you feel bad you are likely to stop – unless you have become addicted. But in order to learn from experience we must first understand something called the general adaptation syndrome. It was first described in 1956 by Professor Hans Selye, who proposed three basic stages of reaction to any event. This can be applied to a cigarette, a food, a stress or a physical activity. Let's see these stages, using your reaction to a stimulant such as caffeinated drinks or cigarettes as an example.

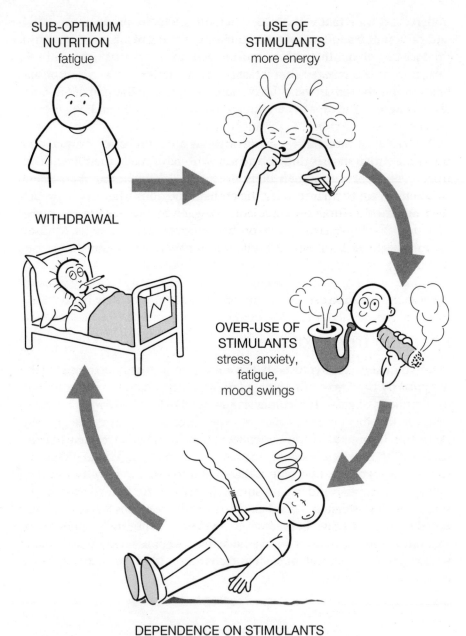

SUB-OPTIMUM
NUTRITION
fatigue

USE OF
STIMULANTS
more energy

WITHDRAWAL

OVER-USE OF
STIMULANTS
stress, anxiety,
fatigue,
mood swings

DEPENDENCE ON STIMULANTS
exhaustion, depression,
chronic fatigue, can't cope with stress

The general adaptation syndrome

Stage 1: the initial response   Your first response to any event or substance is the best indicator of whether or not it suits you. Remember your first cigarette, your first alcoholic drink or your first cup of coffee? You are unlikely to remember your first taste of sugar, meat or milk or other foods introduced when you were very young.

Stage 2: adaptation   Very quickly your body learns to adapt. Gone is the pounding heart after a cup of coffee, or coughing after a cigarette. An example of this stage is the rise and subsequent fall to normal levels of the blood pressure of country dwellers, not normally exposed to air pollution, who move to a city. The cells in the lungs of a smoker change form to protect themselves from smoke. Plaque develops in the arteries to repair damaged tissue. What is going on behind the scenes in all these cases? The body is trying to protect itself, and in so doing is in an unseen state of stress.

Stage 3: exhaustion   Continue the insult for long enough and one day you are sick. Your energy is gone, your digestive system is not functioning properly, your blood pressure is raised, and you develop anything from chest infections to cancer. The body cannot cope, it cannot adapt any more. This is the stage at which most people seek help from a health practitioner.

We could add two further stages to this process.

Stage 4: recovery   To enable the body to recover, it is usually necessary to avoid or greatly restrict the initial insult and other undesirable substances. This means being as puritanical as possible for a period during which you may have to wean yourself off all sorts of things to which you have become addicted or allergic. Generally these are the substances of which you would say, 'I can give up anything but not my . . .' This is the nature of addiction. To help the body recover, much larger amounts of vitamins and minerals are needed than would normally be required just to maintain good health.

Stage 5: hypersensitivity   Once you have recovered and your body is basically healthy, which can take years, you are effectively back to stage one. But this time, because your diet and lifestyle are much improved, you may seem to be hypersensitive and react to all sorts of things that you never reacted to before: certain wines that contain additives, ordinary foods like wheat or milk, fumes and so on. This is healthy because, just as in an initial reaction, your body is telling you what suits you. The more you follow this guidance the healthier you will become. In due course, as your reserve strength builds up, you can tolerate the odd insult without such hypersensitivity, but by then it is to be hoped that you will have learnt (or suffered) enough not to indulge those old bad habits!

Once you understand this cycle and why it is that you can sometimes apparently abuse the body without noticeable ill-effects, and at other times react strongly to small insults, it is easier to interpret what happens to you, and alter your diet or lifestyle accordingly. Think about the substances that you have suspected may not suit you. What do they have in common? Perhaps there are subtle signs that you have chosen to ignore. Here is a list of the most common suspects that my clients have found they react to.

■ Chemicals that commonly cause reactions

Wheat and other grains	Yeast-based alcohols (beer and
Milk and dairy produce	wine, but not champagne)
Chocolate	Additives in alcohol
Sugar	Cigarettes
Coffee, including decaffeinated	Fumes
Tea	Vehicle exhaust
Food additives	Gas fires
Alcohol	Grass pollens
Yeast in bread and processed foods	

It is interesting that our ancestors, who until relatively recently in evolutionary terms were not cultivating grains or milking animals, were not exposed to any of these substances.

The delayed effect

Another noteworthy phenomenon is the delayed effect. The general adaptation syndrome describes a long-term delayed effect, but with many foods there is a short-term delay of up to twenty-four hours before you notice their effect on you. For example, if you eat something very sweet you may feel fine as your blood sugar level rises. But when it plummets four hours later you may fall asleep. And alcohol has its worst effects many hours later. This is largely because, once the liver's ability to detoxify alcohol is exceeded, the remaining alcohol is changed into a toxic by-product, which is what induces headaches and nausea. Many substances that are not good for you show an initial reaction within twenty-four hours.

A hairy bag of salty soup

Scientists believe that we, like all other mammals, evolved from the sea. We carry our 'sea' around inside us: we have many of the same constituents as the oceans from which we came. We are 66 per cent water, 25 per cent protein and 8 per cent fat, the rest being carbohydrate plus minerals and vitamins. Saddam Hussein, Tony Blair, Posh and Becks, you and I are all just 66 per cent water. 'Hairy bags of salty soup,' said Dr Michael Colgan, a British-born scientist who has pioneered the optimum nutrition approach. Yet if you were to throw all these compounds together you would not end up with a human being. So what is it that makes life happen?

The answer, as explained in Chapter 22, is enzymes. They turn the food we eat into fuel for every single cell, be it a muscle cell, a brain cell, an immune cell or a blood cell. Further enzymes within these cells turn the fuel into usable energy that makes our heart beat, our nerves fire and all other bodily functions take place.

Everything in this universe is part of a vast ongoing chemical reaction. Our part, as temporary living organisms, is to provide ourselves and others with the best possible components to allow this process to continue in such a way that we all have a good, long, enjoyable life. And what makes our life-giving enzymes function at their peak? The answer is vitamins and minerals. Nearly all the thousands of enzymes in the body depend directly or indirectly on the presence of vitamins and minerals. Once you understand that the body, and health itself, depend on this vast and complex interacting network you will appreciate that there is little point in taking extra quantities of a single vitamin. That would be like replacing only one dirty spark plug and expecting your car to run smoothly. Yet most medical research into nutrition has done just that, by taking one nutrient and measuring its effect on one aspect of health.

As you will see, the research that has produced the most astonishing results in improving energy, mental performance, longevity, fertility and resistance to disease has involved a multi-nutrient approach that recognises the fact that nutrients interact. Parts 4 and 5 of this book explain the kinds of results that can be achieved and the conditions helped by applying the optimum nutrition approach.

chapter 22

Improving Your Digestion

Like all other animals, we spend our physical lives processing organic matter for waste. How good we are at it determines our energy level, longevity and state of body and mind. A lack of nutrients and the wrong kind of food can result in faulty digestion, faulty absorption, abnormal gut reactions including bloating and inflammation, gut infections and poor elimination. The knock-on effects disrupt every body system – immunity, the brain and nervous system, hormonal balance and our ability to detoxify.

Stomach acid – the right balance

Digestion starts in the senses. The sight and smell of food initiate chemical reactions that get us ready to assimilate and digest food. Chewing is particularly important because messages are sent to the digestive tract to prepare different enzyme secretions according to what is in the mouth.

Food then passes into the stomach, where large proteins are broken down into smaller groups of amino acids. The first step in protein digestion is carried out by hydrochloric acid released from the stomach wall, which is dependent on zinc. Hydrochloric acid production often declines in old age, as do zinc levels. The consequence is indigestion, particularly noticeable after high-protein meals, and the likelihood of developing food allergies because undigested large food molecules are more likely to stimulate allergic reactions in the small intestine.

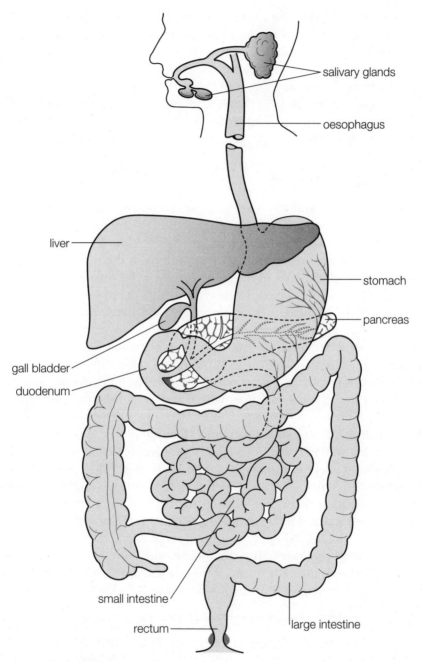

The digestive system

The nutritional solution for too little stomach acid is to take a digestive supplement containing betaine hydrochloride, plus at least 15mg of zinc in an easily absorbable form such as zinc citrate. Some people, however, produce too much stomach acid, a possible cause of 'acid stomach', experienced as indigestion and a burning sensation. This is usually rectified by avoiding acid-forming and irritating foods and drinks; alcohol, coffee, tea and aspirin all irritate the gut wall. Meat, fish, eggs and other concentrated proteins stimulate acid production and can aggravate over-acidity. The minerals calcium and magnesium are particularly alkaline and tend to have a calming effect on people suffering from excess acidity.

Digestive enzymes

The stomach also produces a range of enzymes, collectively called proteases, to break down protein. Protein digestion continues in the first part of the small intestine, the duodenum, into which flow digestive enzymes produced in the pancreas and liver. The pancreas is the primary organ of digestion, and special cells in it produce enzymes for breaking down carbohydrates, fats and proteins. These enzymes are called amylases, lipases and, once again, proteases. Again, there are many different kinds.

The production of digestive enzymes depends on many micronutrients, especially vitamin B6. Sub-optimum nutrition often results in sub-optimum digestion, which in turn creates sub-optimum absorption so that nutritional intake gets worse and worse. The consequence is undigested food in the small intestine, which encourages the proliferation of the wrong kind of bacteria and other micro-organisms; symptoms can include flatulence, abdominal pain and bloating.

The easiest way to correct this kind of problem is to take a broad-spectrum digestive enzyme supplement with each meal. This can make an immediate difference. You can test the effects of these enzyme supplements by crushing them and stirring them into a thick porridge made from oats and water. If the product is good, the porridge will become liquid in thirty minutes. While there is no harm in taking digestive enzymes on an ongoing basis, correcting their levels with supplements paves the way for increasing nutrient levels in the body. Once this is achieved the digestion often improves of its own accord and the supplements may no longer be necessary.

Before being digested, fat has to be specially prepared. This is achieved by a substance called bile, produced by the liver and stored in the gall bladder. Bile contains lecithin, which helps to emulsify large fat particles and turn them into tiny particles with a greater surface area for the fat-splitting lipase enzyme to work on. Supplementing lecithin as granules or capsules improves emulsification and can help people with poor tolerance of fat – for instance, anyone who has had their gall bladder removed and therefore cannot store bile.

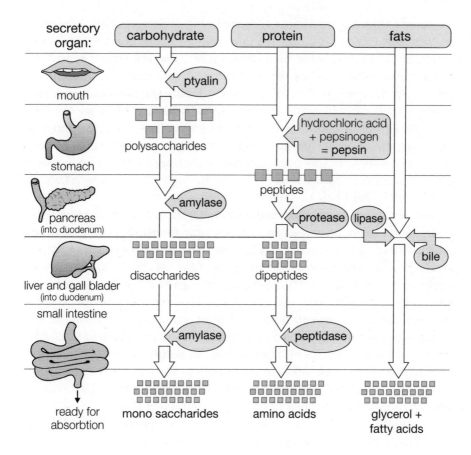

Digestive enzymes. *Digestive enzymes, such as amylase, protease or lipase, help turn large food molecules into tiny molecules that your digestive tract then allows to pass into the bloodstream.*

Probiotics

Probiotics are your digestive tract's best friend for a number of reasons. First, they help to digest your food. Both proteins and fats can be broken down into amino acids and fatty acids by *Lactobacilli* bacteria. The sugar in milk, lactose, is also broken down, into glucose and galactose. This is especially helpful for those who are lactose-intolerant, lacking the digestive enzyme lactase which would normally do this. They also improve the absorption of calcium and other minerals, manufacture vitamins, primarily the vitamins K, B12 and folic acid, relieve constipation and are important healers in a wide variety of digestive disorders.

Among these disorders are Crohn's disease, ulcerative colitis, diarrhoea and irritable bowel syndrome. In one study in Poland on irritable bowel syndrome 100 people were given *Lactobacilli*, a placebo or anti-spasmodic drugs.[1] Three-quarters of those taking *Lactobacilli* had significant improvement, compared with 27 per cent taking the drug and 0 per cent taking the placebo. Twenty-two patients who had no relief on the drug were then given probiotics plus the drug. Seventy-seven per cent reported improvement. Clearly probiotics were much more effective than anti-spasmodic drugs. It has been estimated that about half of all people diagnosed with irritable bowel syndrome have abnormal bacteria balance and therefore are likely to benefit from probiotics.[2]

Inflammatory bowel disorders such as Crohn's disease and ulcerative colitis have also been proven to respond favourably to probiotics. *Lactobacillus salivarius*, a particular strain of *Lactobacilli*, has proven particularly effective for colitis sufferers. One of the ways in which probiotics may help is by promoting healing and repair of the digestive tract. When the digestive tract is inflamed, perhaps owing due to these diseases, infection or irritation by alcohol, painkillers or antibiotics, it can become abnormally permeable, which is a major cause of the development of food allergies and detoxification problems. This sequence of events can also cause other inflammatory diseases such as arthritis, which has also been shown to benefit from probiotics.[3] The digestive tract can be restored to health by short-chain fatty acids (SCFAs) which are naturally produced by *Lactobacilli*, *Bifidobacteria* and *Eubacteria*. (*Eubacteria* are generally not used as probiotics because supplementation makes little difference to their numbers in the gut.)

The most proven benefit of probiotics is in cases of diarrhoea, especially those brought on by bacterial infections. In most cases, provided the right strain of bacteria at the right strength is used, probiotics can halve recovery time from a bout of diarrhoea. Hence, probiotics are an exotic traveller's best friend.

If you suffer from food allergies the chances are probiotics will help you too. Many food reactions may not be solely due to food allergy but also due to the feeding of unfriendly bacteria which then produce substances that activate the immune system in the gut.[4] Probiotics have been shown to help reduce inflammatory reactions in food allergies by lessening the response in the gut to allergenic foods.[5] (There's more on probiotics in Chapter 17.)

Gut reactions

While indigestion can be caused by a lack or excess of stomach acid, a lack of digestive enzymes or a lack of probiotics, these are not the only possibilities. Many of the foods we eat irritate and damage our very sensitive and vitally important interface with the inside world. One such food is wheat, in which a protein called gluten contains gliadin, a known intestinal irritant. A small amount may be tolerated, but most people in Britain consume wheat in the form of biscuits, toast, bread, cereals, cakes, pastry and pasta at least three times a day. Modern wheat is very high in gluten, and baking increases its ability to react with the gut wall. In cases of severe gluten sensitivity the villi, the tiny protrusions that make up the small intestine, get completely worn away. For those with gluten sensitivity, all foods containing gluten must be avoided. Rice, corn, quinoa and buckwheat are fine, as all are gluten-free.

Gut infections

The best way to get a gut infection is to eat plenty of sugar, suffer from indigestion and have regular courses of antibiotics. There are around 300 different strains of bacteria in the gut, most of which are essential. They protect us from harmful bacteria, viruses and other dangerous organisms.

Antibiotics wipe out all the bacteria in the body, good as well as bad, and are best not taken unless absolutely necessary. If the gut contains the wrong kind of bacteria, or perhaps an overgrowth of a yeast-like organism called *Candida albicans*, a high-sugar diet, including fruit, can exacerbate the problem. Feelings of intoxication, drowsiness and bloating after consuming sugar are good indicators of a potential imbalance. In the same way that yeast ferments sugar to produce alcohol, it is possible to check for the presence of yeast-like organisms by testing the blood, eating sugar and then testing the blood again for the presence of alcohol.

A number of powerful natural remedies have been proven to help with gut infections. Caprylic acid, extracted from coconuts, and olive leaf extract are both powerful anti-fungal agents. Grapefruit seed extract, taken as drops in water, is anti-fungal, anti-viral and anti-bacterial, but does not destroy all the essential strains of bacteria. Even so, it is best not taken with meals. Another remedy, probiotics (see page 155), aims to improve the strength of the beneficial bacteria in the gut. This is easily achieved by short (one-month) courses of supplements. Since bacteria are fragile it is best to choose a high-quality product containing *Acidophilus* and *Bifidus* bacteria.

Preventing wind and constipation

Indigestion is a cause of wind, as is eating foods that contain indigestible carbohydrates. These carbohydrates are found particularly in beans and vegetables. The enzyme alpha-galactosidase (sometimes called glucoamylase) breaks down these indigestible carbohydrates and reduces flatulence, and is found in better digestive enzyme supplements.

Constipation has many causes, the most common of which is hard faecal matter. Natural foods stay soft in the digestive tract because they contain fibres that absorb water and expand. Fruit and vegetables naturally contain a lot of water. Provided they are prepared properly, whole grains such as oats and rice absorb water and provide soft, moist bulk for the digestive tract. Meats, cheese, eggs, refined grains and wheat (because of its gluten content) are all constipating. While it should not be necessary to add fibre to the diet, oat fibre has particular benefits in that it has been shown to help eliminate excess cholesterol and slow down carbohydrate uptake, as well as preventing constipation. It is naturally present in oats, which are best soaked and eaten cold.

Some foods and nutrients exert a mild laxative effect. These include flaxseeds, which can be ground and sprinkled on food, prunes, and vitamin C in doses of several grams. But most laxatives, even natural ones, are gastrointestinal irritants and, while they work, they do not solve the underlying issue. A new kind of laxative, fructo-oligosaccharides, supplied in powder form, is a complex carbohydrate that helps keep moisture in the gut and stimulates production of healthy lactic acid bacteria. While the results are not quite so rapid, this is a far preferable way of dealing with constipation. Eating plenty of fruit, vegetables and whole grains, plus drinking lots of water, is essential as well.

For some people long-term constipation can result in physical blockages and distension of the bowel. Dietary changes help but are not always enough to clean out the intestinal tract. A combination of particular fibres, such as psyllium husks, beet fibre, oat fibre and herbs, will assist in loosening up old faecal material. These are available via colon-cleansing formulas consisting of powders and capsules to be taken over a one- to three-month period. Another helpful treatment is colonic therapy: water is passed into the bowel by enema under pressure and this, together with abdominal massage, helps to release and remove old faecal material. Exercise that stimulates the abdominal area also helps to improve digestion, as do breathing exercises that relax the abdomen. It is a natural reflex of the body to stop digesting in times of stress.

Improving digestion is the cornerstone to good health. Energy levels improve, the skin becomes softer and clearer, body odour is reduced and the immune system is strengthened. The trick is to work from the top down, first ensuring good digestion, then good absorption and finally good elimination. If you have any specific digestive difficulties the best person to see is a nutrition consultant. With current testing methods and recent advances in natural treatments most digestive problems can be solved with relative ease, little expense and no need for invasive tests or treatment.

Dig deeper by reading my book *Improve your Digestion*.

chapter 23

Secrets for a Healthy Heart

You have a 50 per cent chance of dying from heart or artery disease. That is the bad news. The good news is that heart disease is, in most cases, completely preventable. Yet so widespread is this epidemic that we almost take it for granted. We fail to protect ourselves from a disease more life-threatening than AIDS, a condition whose cause for the most part is known and whose cure is already proven.

There is nothing natural about dying from heart disease. Many cultures do not experience a high incidence of strokes or heart attacks. For example, by middle age British people in general have nine times as much heart disease as the Japanese, although the Japanese are now showing signs of catching up. Autopsies performed on the mummified remains of Egyptians who died around 3000 BC showed signs of deposits in the arteries but no actual blockages that would result in strokes or heart attacks.

Despite the obvious signs of a heart attack (severe chest pain, cold sweats, nausea, fall in blood pressure and weak pulse), in the 1930s it was so rare that it took a specialist to make the diagnosis. According to American health records, the incidence of heart attacks per 100,000 people was none in 1890 and had risen to 340 by 1970. Although deaths did occur from other forms of heart disease, including calcified valves, rheumatic heart and other congenital defects, the incidence of actual blockages in the arteries causing a stroke or heart attack used to be minimal.

Even more worrying is the fact that heart disease is occurring earlier and earlier. Autopsies performed in Vietnam showed that one in two soldiers killed in action, with an average age of twenty-two, already had arterial blockages (atherosclerosis). Nowadays most teenagers can be expected to show signs of atherosclerosis, heralding the beginning of heart disease. Obviously something about our lifestyle, diet or environment has changed radically in the last sixty years to bring on this modern epidemic.

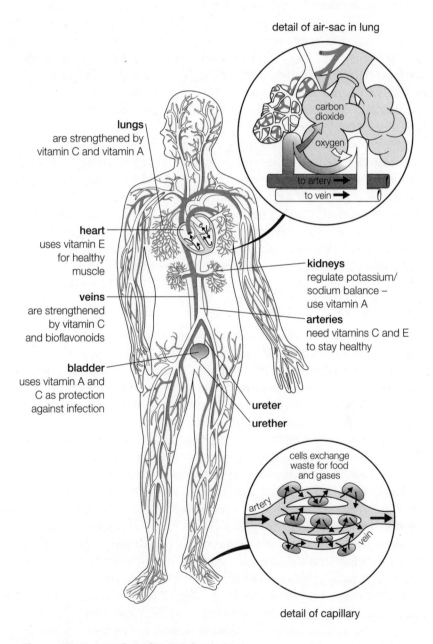

detail of air-sac in lung

carbon dioxide

oxygen

to artery →
to vein →

lungs
are strengthened by
vitamin C and vitamin A

heart
uses vitamin E
for healthy
muscle

veins
are strengthened
by vitamin C
and bioflavonoids

bladder
uses vitamin A and
C as protection
against infection

kidneys
regulate potassium/
sodium balance –
use vitamin A

arteries
need vitamins C and E
to stay healthy

ureter

urether

cells exchange
waste for food
and gases

artery

vein

detail of capillary

The respiratory and cardiovascular system

What is heart disease?

The cardiovascular system consists of blood vessels that carry oxygen, fuel (glucose), building materials (amino acids), vitamins and minerals to every single cell in your body. The blood is oxygenated when tiny blood vessels, called capillaries, absorb oxygen from the lungs and in turn discharge carbon dioxide, which we then exhale. These blood vessels feed into the heart, which pumps the oxygenated blood to all cells. At the cells the blood vessels once more become a network of extremely thin capillaries, which give off oxygen plus other nutrients and in return receive waste products. Oxygen plus glucose is needed to make energy within every cell of the body; the waste products are carbon dioxide and water.

The blood vessels that supply cells with nutrients and oxygen are called arteries, while the blood vessels that carry away waste products and carbon dioxide are called veins. Arterial blood is a brighter red than venous blood because oxygen is carried on a complex called haemoglobin, which contains iron. The pressure in the arteries is also greater than in the veins. As well as returning to the heart after it has visited the cells, all blood passes through the kidneys. Here, waste products are removed, and formed into urine that is stored in the bladder.

Diseases of the arteries

Heart disease is wrongly named. The main life-threatening diseases are diseases of the arteries. Over a number of years a deposit can start to form in the artery wall. This is called arterial plaque or atheroma, from the Greek word for porridge, because of the porridge-like consistency of these deposits. The presence of arterial deposits is called atherosclerosis, and it occurs only in certain parts of the body.

Atherosclerosis, coupled with thicker than normal blood containing clots, can lead to a blockage in the artery, which stops the flow of blood. If this occurs in the arteries feeding the heart, the part of the heart fed by these blood vessels will die from lack of oxygen. This is called a myocardial infarction or heart attack. Before this occurs many people are diagnosed as having angina, a condition in which there is a limited supply of oxygen to the heart owing to partial blockage of coronary arteries which feed oxygen plus glucose to the heart muscle, causing chest pain, most classically on exertion or when under stress.

If a blockage occurs in the brain, part of the brain may die. This is called a stroke. The arteries in the brain are especially fragile and sometimes a stroke occurs not as a result of a blockage but because an artery ruptures. This is called a cerebral haemorrhage. If a blockage occurs in the legs it can result in leg pain, which is a form of thrombosis (a thrombus is a blood clot). When peripheral arteries get blocked this can result in poor peripheral circulation, for example in the hands and feet.

Reversing high blood pressure

So two main factors are responsible for so-called heart disease: atherosclerosis (the formation of deposits) and the presence of blood clots (thick blood). However, there is a third problem that can and usually does occur along with atherosclerosis. That is arteriosclerosis, the hardening of the arteries. Arteries are elastic and, whether or not atherosclerosis is present, tend to lose their elasticity and harden with age. One reason for this is a lack of vitamin C, which is needed to make collagen, the intercellular 'glue' that keeps skin and arteries supple. Arteriosclerosis, atherosclerosis and thick blood can all raise blood pressure, putting you at greater risk of thrombosis, angina, a heart attack or a stroke.

In the same way that the pressure in a hosepipe increases and decreases as the tap is turned on and off, the pressure in the arteries increases when the heart beats and decreases in the lull before the next beat. These are called your systolic and diastolic blood pressure respectively, and a normal reading should be 120/80 irrespective of age. However, if the arteries are blocked, or if the blood is too thick, the pressure increases. Given that blood pressure increases with age in most people, conventional medical wisdom is that a systolic blood pressure of 100 plus your age (say 150 for a fifty-year-old) means that you are in 'normal' health. Yet, these are the very same normal people who drop dead unexpectedly from heart attacks. These guidelines are certainly not ideal.

Strategies for lowering blood pressure

There are four ways to lower blood pressure:

Taking extra minerals and avoiding salt
The arteries are surrounded by a layer of muscle, and an excess of sodium, or a lack of calcium, magnesium or potassium, can increase the muscular pressure. Increasing your intake of these minerals, while avoiding added salt (sodium chloride), can make a substantial difference to blood pressure in just a month. Of these, magnesium is the most important. There is a strong association between magnesium deficiency and heart-attack risk. A pronounced magnesium deficiency can cause a heart attack by cramping a coronary artery even in the absence of an atherosclerotic blockage. So checking your magnesium level is essential.

Vitamin E protects your arteries

Another way to change blood pressure is to thin the blood. Conventionally aspirin is used, and reduces the risk of a heart attack by 20 per cent. Vitamin E, however, was four times as effective, according to Professor Morris Brown, whose double-blind controlled trial of vitamin E at Cambridge University Medical School showed a 75 per cent reduction in heart-attack risk.[6]

These results are consistent with many studies that show a reduced risk of heart attack, especially if vitamin E is given before a problem develops. In one study, whose findings were published in the *New England Journal of Medicine*, 87,200 nurses were given 67mg of vitamin E daily for more than two years. A 40 per cent drop in fatal and non-fatal heart attacks was reported compared with the rate among those not taking vitamin E supplements.[7] In another study 39,000 male health professionals were given 67mg of vitamin E for the same length of time and achieved a 39 per cent reduction in heart attacks.[8]

While these results confirm the first reports of vitamin E's protective effect, made in the 1950s by Drs Wilfred and Evan Shute who treated 30,000 patients with heart disease with an 80 per cent success rate, not all trials have been positive. A trial at Oxford University, giving people who had had a heart attack 600mg of vitamin E, plus 250mg of vitamin C and betacarotene, failed to find a reduction in mortality.[9] I would suggest that if a person has had a heart attack much better results could be achieved by making dietary changes, plus taking more substantial supplementation, including Omega 3 fats.

The benefits of fish oils

The Omega 3 fish oils, which contain EPA and DHA, have also been shown to reduce risk of heart disease. So too has eating fish. If you've had a heart attack and start eating Omega 3-rich fish three times a week you could halve your risk of a further heart attack. Other trials giving people Omega 3 fish oils have found that they do indeed confer protection from heart disease.[10] Exactly how they work is still under investigation. Omega 3 fats are anti-inflammatory, and artery damage involves inflammation. They also thin the blood and, in combination with vitamin E, are much more effective and considerably safer than aspirin.

Nutritional solutions for narrowing arteries

However, the major risk associated with high blood pressure is the narrowing of arteries caused by atherosclerosis. A number of nutritional strategies have been shown to stop and even reverse this process. The main results have been produced by supplements of antioxidants, fish oil, and a combination of vitamin C and lysine. Vitamin C also helps to stop arterial tissue from hardening, another cause of high blood pressure. Supplementing a combination of these nutrients is more effective in the long term than taking drugs designed to lower blood pressure – they deal with the cause of the problem, rather than the symptom. The results of a survey in Sweden showed that people who took supplements had a much lower risk of having a heart attack, with women reducing their risk by 34 per cent and men by 21 per cent.[11]

At the Institute for Optimum Nutrition we conducted a three-month trial on people with high blood pressure and achieved an average eight-point drop in systolic and diastolic blood pressure, with the greatest decreases in those with the highest initial blood pressure.[12] Dr Michael Colgan found that, irrespective of age, people placed on comprehensive nutritional supplement programmes showed gradual decreases in blood pressure from an average of slightly above 140/90 to below 120/80. The optimal range is a systolic blood pressure no higher than 125 and a diastolic blood pressure no higher than 85, irrespective of age. Certainly blood pressure above 140/90 is cause for concern.

Dr Colgan also found that pulse rate, which is more a measure of heart strength and is therefore lower in fitter people, decreased from 76 to an average of 65 over a period of five years among those on nutritional supplements. Again, an ideal pulse rate is probably below 65 beats per minute.

What causes heart disease?

To understand how nutritional supplementation, as well as dietary changes, make all the difference we need to examine the underlying cause of arterial disease. Back in 1913 a Russian scientist, Dr Anitschkov, thought he had got the answer. He found that feeding cholesterol (an animal fat) to rabbits induced heart disease. What he failed to realise was that rabbits, being vegetarians, have no means of dealing with this animal fat. Since the fatty deposits in the arteries of people with heart disease had also been found to be high in cholesterol, it was soon thought that these deposits were the result of excess cholesterol in the blood, possibly caused by excess cholesterol in the diet. Such a simple theory had its attractions, and many doctors still advocate a low-cholesterol diet as the answer to heart disease – despite a consistent lack of results.

The cholesterol myth

In 1975 a research team headed by Dr Alfin-Slater from the University of California decided to test the cholesterol theory.[13] They selected fifty healthy people with normal blood cholesterol levels. Half of them were given two eggs per day (in addition to the other cholesterol-rich foods they were already eating as part of their normal diet) for eight weeks. The other half were given one extra egg per day for four weeks, then two extra eggs per day for the next four weeks. The results showed no change in blood cholesterol. Later Dr Alfin-Slater commented, 'Our findings surprised us as much as ever.'

Many other studies have also found no rise in blood cholesterol levels caused by eating eggs. In fact, as long ago as 1974 a British advisory panel set up by the government to look at 'medical aspects of food policy on diet related to cardiovascular disease' issued this statement: 'Most of the dietary cholesterol in Western communities is derived from eggs, but we have found no evidence that relates the number of eggs consumed to heart disease.'

A review in 2000 of all studies that had investigated cholesterol and egg intake and heart disease published in the *Journal of the American College of Nutrition* concluded that no association was seen between consumption of more than one egg per day and the risk of heart disease'.[14] The bottom line is that there's no evidence that eating up to seven eggs a week makes any difference to your cardiovascular risk.

Since high blood cholesterol levels are associated with a high risk of coronary artery disease, it is assumed that having a low cholesterol level is good news. Not so, according to three independent research groups. One, in Japan, found that while high levels are associated with cardiovascular disease, which is low in Japan, low levels are associated with strokes. As cholesterol levels dropped below 190mg/dl in the blood in this group of 6,500 Japanese men, incidence of strokes increased. Meanwhile, a Finnish researcher, Jykri Penttinen, has found low levels to be associated with a higher rate of depression, suicide and death from violent causes.[15]

These findings were confirmed by David Freedman of the Centers for Disease Control in Atlanta – he found that people with anti-social personality disorders had lower cholesterol levels. Freedman believes that very low levels of cholesterol lead to aggression.

While there is no doubt that high blood cholesterol represents a risk factor for arterial disease, eating a diet containing moderate amounts of cholesterol, for example in eggs, is not associated with an increased risk of heart disease. So what is ideal? According to a survey carried out by medical researcher Dr Cheraskin, comparing overall health with cholesterol levels, there is a very narrow band that represents a 'healthy' cholesterol level in the blood.[16] This is between 190 and 210mg/dl or 4.9 and 5.4 mmol/l. (Some countries, including the UK, measure cholesterol in mmol/l (millimoles per litre), while others, including the US, use mg/dl (milligrams per decilitre).) Variations either side correlate with increasing rates of disease. The UK National Heart Forum recommends a cholesterol level below 5mmol/l, while the UK average is more like 5.5mmol/l. They, however, set no minimum level, implying that the lower one's cholesterol the better. This denies the fact that cholesterol is a vital precursor of hormones and much needed by the body and brain.

■ Ideal test scores for cardiovascular health

	High Risk	Medium Risk	Healthy
Cholesterol (US)	<120–>330mg/dl	>240mg/dl	190–210mg/dl
(UK)	<3.1–>8.5 mmol/l	>6.2mmol/l	4.9–5.4 mmol/l
Cholesterol/HDL	>8:1	>5:1	<3.5:1
Blood pressure	>140/90	>130/85	<125/80
Pulse	>85	<85	<70

> = more than   < = less than

Good cholesterol

Of course, the nail in the coffin of the dietary cholesterol hypothesis was hammered in by the Inuit (Eskimos). Although they have one of the highest-cholesterol diets in the world they also have one of the lowest incidences of cardiovascular disease. We now know that there is 'good' and 'bad' cholesterol.

When cholesterol, which is a component of bile, is reabsorbed into the bloodstream it is carried to the arteries by a lipoprotein (fat/protein complex) called LDL (short for low-density lipoprotein). If a large proportion of a person's cholesterol is combined with LDL it is more likely to be deposited in the artery walls. Another lipoprotein called HDL (short for high-density lipoprotein) can take cholesterol out of the arteries and back to the liver. Not surprisingly, it has been popularised as 'good' cholesterol – the higher a person's HDL cholesterol compared with their LDL cholesterol, the lower the risk. The ideal ratio is one part HDL cholesterol to three parts total cholesterol.

Once again, multivitamin and mineral programmes are highly effective at achieving this ideal cholesterol balance. Dr Michael Colgan has demonstrated that by putting people on a supplement programme for six months, then taking them off for three months, and doing this repeatedly over two years, he could consistently lower blood cholesterol and increase the ratio of HDL to LDL.[17] Vitamin B3 (niacin) is also highly effective at increasing HDL levels, although you need to supplement 500–1,000mg a day. Because niacin can produce an unfortunate blushing effect, many people take niacin inositolate or 'no-flush niacin'.

Another effective way to raise HDL and lower LDL and total cholesterol is by consuming significant quantities of Omega 3 oils.[18] In practical terms this means taking an EPA fish oil supplement or eating a lot of oily fish. This is what is understood to have protected the Inuit.

Another important point about cholesterol is that, like any fat, it can be damaged by oxidation. Cigarette-smoking, for instance, increases the oxidation of fats. Once damaged, cholesterol becomes more difficult to clear from the arteries. Oxidation can also injure the cells that line the artery wall, causing them to get clogged up. Antioxidant nutrients are protective, while low dietary and blood levels of betacarotene and vitamins A, C and E have repeatedly been shown to increase the risk of heart disease. By increasing intake of antioxidants and decreasing your exposure to free radicals (see Chapter 15) you can reduce your risk.

The combination of the right diet plus supplements is likely to be far quicker and more effective than the current main medical treatment – statin drugs. While these do lower the risks of both heart attack and stroke in the long term (there is usually no risk reduction in the first year) by blocking the enzyme that makes cholesterol, this enzyme also makes an important heart nutrient, Co-enzyme Q10, so blocking it potentially increases risk for heart failure since CoQ10 is vital for the proper functioning of the heart itself. If you are on a statin drug make sure you supplement at least 30mg of CoQ10.

New theory on heart disease – lipoprotein A

According to Dr Linus Pauling and Matthias Rath, even these factors may be but a small part of the underlying cause of atherosclerosis.[19] On the understanding that our ancestors lost the ability to make vitamin C when living in a tropical environment, Pauling and Rath wondered how we survived through repeated Ice Ages without dying from scurvy, a disease that once used to decimate ships' crews. The first sign of scurvy is vascular bleeding, as blood vessels start to leak – nowhere else in the body is membrane under such pressure.

According to Pauling and Rath, we may have developed the ability to deposit lipoproteins (fat-protein complexes) along the artery wall in order to increase our chances of surviving during vitamin C-deficient times. Two groups of proteins that normally accumulate at injury sites to carry out repairs are fibrinogen and apoprotein. Apoproteins have a natural affinity with fat (lipids) and become lipoprotein A (LpA), which can repair damaged or leaky blood vessels. However, it also increases the risk of heart disease by building up deposits on the artery wall. In fact, of all the factors that can be measured, a person's level of lipoprotein A is the best indicator of risk.

Genetic research is now strongly suggesting that the development of lipoprotein A was most likely a genetic response to a threat of extinction through leaky blood vessels. Could this have been nature's way of dealing with life-threatening scurvy? The estimated dates for the development of lipoprotein A in monkeys correlate with the period in which primates are thought to have lost the ability to produce vitamin C.

How well does the theory of vitamin C deficiency as a root cause for cardiovascular disease fit with the facts? Vitamin C deficiency raises cholesterol, triglycerides (fats in the blood), bad LDLs, apoprotein and lipoprotein A, and lowers the beneficial HDLs. Conversely, increasing vitamin C intake lowers a high cholesterol, triglyceride, LDL or LpA level and raises HDLs.

The significance of all these beneficial effects for our ancestors could have been that during the summer, when they could take in enough vitamin C, the increased HDL production would remove excess cholesterol. Vitamin C also inhibits excessive cholesterol production and helps convert cholesterol to bile. All this would lead to a decrease in unnecessary atherosclerotic deposits. In one study it was shown that a daily 500mg of vitamin C can lead to a reduction in atherosclerotic deposits within two to six months. 'This concept also explains why heart attacks and strokes occur today with a much higher frequency in winter than during spring and summer, the seasons with increased ascorbate intake,' said Pauling.

If vitamin C deficiency does prove to be the common cause of human cardiovascular disease, then vitamin C supplementation is destined to become the universal treatment for this disease. Pauling and Rath recommend somewhere between 3 and 10 grams a day and, for those with cardiovascular disease, the addition of the amino acid lysine at around 3 grams a day. The combination of these two nutrients appears to reverse atherosclerosis.

Homocysteine – the heart attacker

While a lack of vitamin C may weaken arteries, what actually causes the damage? One answer is a dangerous protein called homocysteine. If you've had a heart attack or stroke, there's a more than 50 per cent chance you have a high homocysteine level.

The homocysteine theory was first proposed by Dr Kilmer McCully, a pathologist at the VA Medical Center in Providence, Rhode Island, USA, in 1969. It wasn't until the 1990s that the evidence for the homocysteine theory started to become very convincing.[20] In 1992 a study of 14,000 male doctors found that those with homocysteine levels in the top 5 per cent had three times the heart-attack risk, compared with those in the bottom 5 per cent. This increased risk was confirmed by the Massachusetts-based

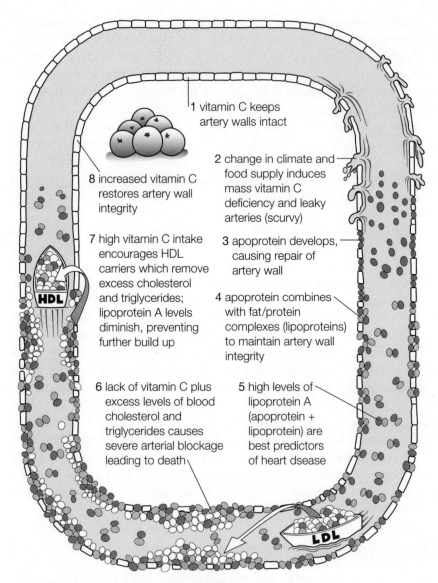

1 vitamin C keeps artery walls intact

2 change in climate and food supply induces mass vitamin C deficiency and leaky arteries (scurvy)

8 increased vitamin C restores artery wall integrity

7 high vitamin C intake encourages HDL carriers which remove excess cholesterol and triglycerides; lipoprotein A levels diminish, preventing further build up

3 apoprotein develops, causing repair of artery wall

4 apoprotein combines with fat/protein complexes (lipoproteins) to maintain artery wall integrity

6 lack of vitamin C plus excess levels of blood cholesterol and triglycerides causes severe arterial blockage leading to death

5 high levels of lipoprotein A (apoprotein + lipoprotein) are best predictors of heart dsease

HDL

LDL

How lipoprotein A causes heart disease

Framingham Heart Study in 1995 which found that having more than 11.4 units of homocysteine in the blood increased the risk.[21] Another study at the University of Washington found that having high homocysteine doubles the risk of heart attack in young women.

The real clincher was a study carried out by the European Concerted Action Group, a consortium of doctors and researchers from nineteen medical centres in nine European countries.[22] They studied 750 people

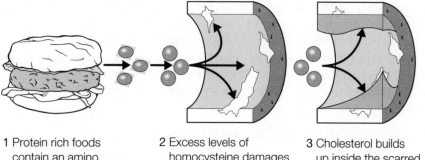

1 Protein rich foods contain an amino acid, methionine, that converts to homocysteine

2 Excess levels of homocysteine damages the lining of arteries

3 Cholesterol builds up inside the scarred arteries, which can lead to fatal blockages

How homocysteine causes heart disease

under the age of 60 with atherosclerosis, compared with 800 people without such cardiovascular disease. They found that having a high level of homocysteine in the blood was as great a risk factor for cardiovascular disease as smoking or having a high blood cholesterol level.

To put this in perspective, every 12 per cent increase in your homocysteine score triples your risk of a heart attack, if you are a man. If you have both a high homocysteine score and a family history of heart disease, this increases your personal risk of heart attack, regardless of sex, a whopping thirteen to fourteen times! Those with a homocysteine level above 14 units have an 82 per cent increased risk of total stroke, compared with those below 9.2 units. Since this study, in 1998, more than a thousand studies have confirmed the incredibly strong link between homocysteine and heart disease – much stronger and more important than cholesterol, yet hardly ever tested.

While much of the spotlight on heart-disease diagnosis has been on cholesterol, the fact is that your homocysteine level is roughly forty times more predictive of a heart attack than your cholesterol level. Time and time again I encounter heart-attack patients who don't have high cholesterol levels, haven't been checked for homocysteine and are still put on cholesterol-lowering drugs such as statins. While these drugs do decrease the rate of death from heart attacks, they don't have as great an effect on overall mortality, adding, on average, a mere eighteen months to life. Lowering your homocysteine score, on the other hand, dramatically reduces death from all causes, not just heart attacks.

So the question is: how do you lower your homocysteine level? The answer is with B vitamins, not drugs. Specifically, folic acid, B12 and B6. The ideal amount to supplement depends on your homocysteine level, but suffice it to say that anyone at any risk should be supplementing at least 400mcg of folic acid, 12mcg of vitamin B12 and 50mg of B6. Much larger amounts are needed to lower very raised homocysteine scores. Since homocysteine not only damages arteries but also damages cholesterol, making it accumulate in arteries, lowering your homocysteine can be expected to lower your cholesterol too. Homocysteine is discussed in full in Chapter 16, together with details on how to lower it.

Supernutrition for a healthy heart

Much is known about the causes of cardiovascular disease and how to prevent it, and no doubt more is yet to be discovered. However, few if any general practitioners are applying what is already known to prevent and reverse heart disease.

The following guidelines apply to us all as a means of eliminating risk and adding at least ten healthy years to our lifespan:

- Avoid fried food and limit your intake of meat and foods high in saturated fat. Oily fish such as mackerel, herring, salmon and tuna are better.

- Eat plenty of fresh fruit and vegetables, which are high in calcium, magnesium and potassium, especially green leafy vegetables and beans, which are high in folate.

- Eat seeds, high in vitamin E, essential fats and minerals.

- Do not add salt when cooking, or to your plate, and restrict your consumption of foods with added salt. If you do use salt, use Solo salt.

- Keep fit, not fat.

- No smoking.

- Avoid prolonged stress.

- Know your blood pressure and have your blood lipid level checked every five years.

- Take a supplement of antioxidant nutrients, including at least 400mg of vitamin E and 2 grams of vitamin C, plus the Omega 3 fats EPA and DHA and a multivitamin containing B6, B12 and folic acid.

If you have cardiovascular disease or high blood pressure the following also apply:

- See a nutritionist and have your blood lipid levels and homocysteine measured.

- If you have low HDL, take 1 gram of 'no flush' niacin a day.

- If you have high cholesterol or triglycerides, take an EPA fish oil supplement giving you 1,000mg of EPA.

- If you have high lipoprotein, A, take a supplement of at least 5 grams of vitamin C and 3 grams of lysine.

- If you have high homocysteine, increase your intake of vitamins B6, B12 and folic acid (see Chapter 16 for amounts).

- If you have high blood pressure, take a magnesium supplement.

- Do all you can to improve your diet and lifestyle.

Dig deeper by reading my book *Say No to Heart Disease*.

chapter 24

Boosting Your Immune System

Louis Pasteur, who discovered in the nineteenth century that microorganisms were responsible for infections, realised late in his life that strengthening the body, rather than conquering the invading organism, might prove a more effective strategy. Yet for the last hundred years medicine has focused on drugs designed to destroy the invader – antibiotics, anti-viral agents, chemotherapy. By their very nature these drugs are poison to the body. AZT, the first prescribable anti-HIV drug, is potentially harmful and proving less effective than vitamin C.[23] Although initially antibiotics fight bacterial infection, in the long term they may do more harm than good as they encourage the evolution of new drug-resistant strains of bacteria.[24] Chemotherapy depletes the immune system and, even in the best situations, wins a victory at a cost.

Only recently, with the seemingly endless onslaught of new infectious agents, has attention turned within – towards strengthening our immunity. The immune system is one of the most remarkable and complex systems within the human body. When you realise that it has the ability to produce a million specific 'straitjackets' (called antibodies) within a minute and to recognise and disarm a billion different invaders (called antigens), the strategy of boosting immune power makes a lot of sense. The ability to react rapidly to a new invader makes all the difference between a minor twenty-four-hour cold or stomach bug and a week in bed with flu or food-poisoning. It may also be the difference between a non-malignant lump and breast cancer, or symptom-free HIV infection and full-blown AIDS.

Immune power

How do you boost your immune power? Exercise, your state of mind and your diet all play a part. Overtraining or vigorous exercise actually suppresses the immune system, while the Chinese art of t'ai chi has been shown to increase the count of T-cells (one of the body's types of immune cell) by 40 per cent. Calming rather than stressful forms of exercise are probably best for immunity. This may be because corticosteroids, substances produced by the adrenal glands as a response to stress (and also taken as the drug cortisone), suppress the immune system. This too may be a key explanation for numerous studies which have found that low psychological states such as stress, depression and grief depress the immune system. Learning how to cope with stress, deal with psychological issues and relax is an important part of boosting the immune system. Meditation, for example, has been shown to increase T-cell counts and improve the T-helper/suppressor ratio (see page 211).[25]

Understanding immunity

The purpose of the immune system is to identify the body's enemies and destroy them. These enemies include defective body cells as well as foreign agents such as bacteria and viruses. The main 'gates' into the body are the digestive tract, which lets in food, and the lungs, which let in air. Within the digestive tract is the 'gut-associated immune system', which is programmed to allow completely digested food particles, such as amino acids, fatty acids and simple sugars, to pass unhindered through the gut wall into the body. Incompletely digested food can result in immune reactions and eventually allergies, especially if large food molecules pass into the bloodstream. The nasal passages help to prevent unwanted agents from entering the lungs. Healthy, strong mucous membranes in the respiratory and digestive tract are the first line of defence against invaders.

The immune army

Inside the body, the immune system has an army of special cells to deal with invaders. These defenders differ in their function and territory. For example, some cells operate in the blood, keeping an eye out for invaders, and whistling up other troops that can destroy specific invaders. The three main types of immune cell found in the blood, collectively called white cells, are B-cells, T-cells and macrophages.

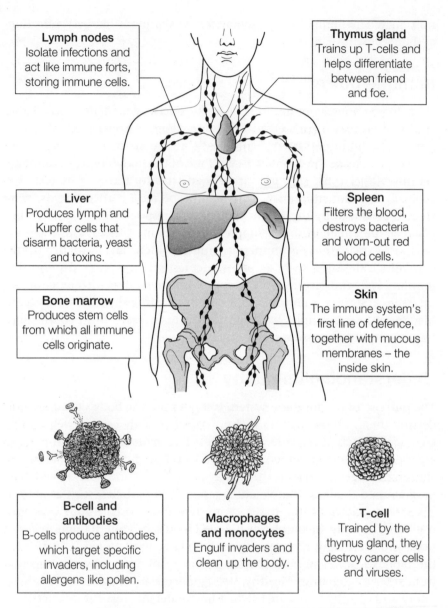

Lymph nodes
Isolate infections and act like immune forts, storing immune cells.

Thymus gland
Trains up T-cells and helps differentiate between friend and foe.

Liver
Produces lymph and Kupffer cells that disarm bacteria, yeast and toxins.

Spleen
Filters the blood, destroys bacteria and worn-out red blood cells.

Bone marrow
Produces stem cells from which all immune cells originate.

Skin
The immune system's first line of defence, together with mucous membranes – the inside skin.

B-cell and antibodies
B-cells produce antibodies, which target specific invaders, including allergens like pollen.

Macrophages and monocytes
Engulf invaders and clean up the body.

T-cell
Trained by the thymus gland, they destroy cancer cells and viruses.

The immune army and battleground. The immune system trains up specialised cells, such as B or T lymphocytes, from 'stem cells' made in bone marrow. These travel around the body, especially in the lymph, protecting you from invaders, be it a virus or a food you are allergic to, or even a misbehaving cancer cell.

B-cells, or B-lymphocytes, are produced in an antibody for each specific invader or antigen. When a B-cell comes into contact with an antigen it grows larger and divides into several cells which secrete specific antibodies that latch on to the invader. Antibodies cannot destroy bacteria and viruses, but they do give them a hard time. They stop bacteria producing toxins, and they prevent viruses from entering body cells. Since a virus cannot reproduce unless it enters a body cell and takes over the cell's control centre, reprogramming it to produce more viruses, antibodies are a major nuisance for viruses. Antibodies also whistle up other, more belligerent members of the immune army, such as T-cells.

T-cells, or T-lymphocytes, are derived from the thymus gland at the top of the chest. There are three kinds: T-helpers, T-suppressors and NK (natural killers). NK cells produce toxins that can destroy the invader. T-helpers help to activate B-cells to product antigens, while T-suppressors turn off the reactions once the battle is won. Normally, there are roughly twice as many T-helpers as T-suppressors. In AIDS the HIV virus selectively destroys T-helpers, resulting in too many T-suppressors, which depress the immune system, leaving the sufferer susceptible to other infections.

Macrophages finish off the battle by completely engulfing and digesting the invader that has been identified by B- and T-cells. This action is called phagocytosis. Phagocytic cells that operate in the blood are called monocytes, while those that operate in other tissues are called macrophages.

The immune battleground

At any time there are a small number of immune cells roaming the body. Many of them have only a short life: T-cells, for example, live for about four days. When an invader is identified, new troops are produced in the bone marrow and thymus and posted to forts such as lymph nodes, the tonsils, appendix, spleen and Peyer's patches in the digestive tract which concentrate lymphocytes. Lymphatic vessels drain into these forts, bringing in invaders to be destroyed. That is why lymph nodes, for example in the neck, armpits and groin, become inflamed during an infection. This means they are doing their job. Since the lymphatic system doesn't have a pump, lymphatic fluid is moved along by muscle movement, so physical exercise is important for lymphatic drainage.

Immune-boosting nutrients

Your immune strength is totally dependent on an optimal intake of vitamins and minerals. Deficiency of vitamins A, B1, B2, B6, B12, folic acid, C and E suppresses immunity, as does deficiency of iron, zinc, magnesium and selenium. Vitamins B1, B2 and B5 have mild immune-boosting effects compared with B6. The production of antibodies, so critical in any infection, depends upon B6, as does T-cell function. The ideal daily intake is probably 50–100mg. B12 and folic acid also both appear essential for proper B-cell and T-cell function. B6, zinc and folic acid are all needed for the rapid production of new immune cells to engage an enemy.

Since no nutrients work in isolation, it is a good idea to take a good high-strength multivitamin and mineral supplement. The combination of nutrients at even modest levels can boost immunity very effectively. Dr Ranjit Chandra, from the Memorial University of Newfoundland, and colleagues, in a research study published in the *Lancet*, took a group of ninety-six healthy elderly people and gave some a supplement of this kind, and others a placebo.[26] Those on the supplement suffered fewer infections, had a stronger immune system as measured by blood-test determination of immune factors, and were generally healthier than those given the placebo.

Antioxidant power

The nutrients worth adding in larger amounts to fight off infection are the antioxidants and particularly vitamin C. Most invaders produce the dangerous oxidising chemicals known as free radicals to fight off the troops of your immune system. Antioxidant nutrients such as vitamins A, C and E, zinc and selenium disarm these free radicals, weakening the invader. Vitamin A also helps to maintain the integrity of the digestive tract, lungs and all cell membranes, preventing foreign agents from enter- ing the body and viruses from entering cells. In addition, vitamin A and betacarotene are potent antioxidants. Many foreign agents produce oxi- dising free radicals as part of their defence system. Even our own immune cells produce free radicals to destroy invaders. Therefore a high intake of antioxidant nutrients helps to protect your immune cells from these harmful weapons of war.The ideal intake of betacarotene is 3,300mcgRE to 16,000mcgRE per day.

Vitamin E, another important all-rounder, improves B- and T-cell func- tion. Its immune-boosting properties increase when it is given in conjunction with selenium. The ideal daily intake is between 100 and 600mg. Selenium, iron, manganese, copper and zinc are all involved in anti-oxidation and have been shown to affect immune power positively. Of these, selenium and zinc are probably the most important. While zinc is critical for immune cell production and proper functioning of B- and T- cells, excess zinc can suppress the ability of macrophages to destroy bacteria. The ideal daily intake is 15–25mg. While zinc may be a beneficial supplement during a viral infection, it may not be a good idea to supple- ment it during a bacterial infection. The same is true for iron. While iron deficiency suppresses immune function, too much iron interferes with the ability of macrophages to destroy bacteria. When an infection is pres- ent, the body initiates a series of defence mechanisms designed to stop the invader absorbing iron, so supplementing iron is not recommended during a bacterial infection.

How much C?

Vitamin C is unquestionably the master immune-boosting nutrient. To date more than a dozen roles in this capacity have been identified for it. It helps immune cells to mature, improves the performance of antibodies and macrophages and is itself anti-viral and anti-bacterial, as well as being able to destroy toxins produced by bacteria. In addition, it is a natural anti-histamine, calming down inflammation, and stimulates another part of the immune-defence system to produce interferon that boosts immunity. Excessive levels of the stress hormone cortisol, a potent immuno suppressant, are controlled by sufficient vitamin C. However, the dosage of vitamin C is crucial. Professor Harry Hemilia from the Department of Health at the University of Helsinki examined all studies that tested the effects of vitamin C or a placebo on the common cold, selecting only those that gave 1 gram daily or more. Thirty-seven out of thirty-eight concluded that supplementing 1 gram, twenty times the RDA, had a protective effect. Studies using less than this amount tend not to be conclusive.

Probiotics – nature's antibiotics

Infectious agents are all around us. Whether or not you succumb to them is determined not only by your exposure, but also by your balance of bacteria. The reason for this is that beneficial bacteria both consume the nutrients that would otherwise feed the bad guys and also block receptor sites that harmful bacteria have to latch on to to cause an infection, for example by entering the bloodstream. However, the main reason that probiotics protect you is that they produce substances such as lactic acid and hydrogen peroxide, which stop harmful bacteria from growing. These are nature's antibiotics. They not only keep less desirable residents, such as *E. coli* or *Enterobacteria*, at bay, but also make it very hard for bugs such as *Staphylococci* (responsible for many sore throats), *Salmonella* and *Campylobacter*, which cause most cases of food poisoning, to survive. Worldwide, more than a million people die from food-poisoning each year.[27] In the UK alone there are around 60,000 reported cases of food poisoning a year, although the real numbers are probably ten times this.

Probiotics don't just give pathogenic bacteria a hard time, they positively boost your immune system. Six research studies have specifically found that different strains of beneficial bacteria improve the fighting power of the immune system. This means that probiotics are also important in the treatment of cancer and allergies, as well as infections caused by viruses, parasites and yeasts such as *Candida albicans*, which is responsible for thrush.

One research study published in the *Annals of Internal Medicine* in 1992 gave women prone to thrush either a live yoghurt containing *Lactobacilli* for six months or no yoghurt.[28] After six months those on yoghurt were asked to switch to no yoghurt, and vice versa. Most of the women on no yoghurt dropped out of the study, while those on daily yoghurt refused to switch after six months. They had experienced a substantial reduction in the number and severity of yeast infections. Even more effective is the use of suppositories to deliver probiotics directly into the vagina.

Probiotics have also proven helpful in treating recurrent bladder infections, sinusitis and tonsillitis.

The immune power diet

The ideal immune-boosting diet is, in essence, no different from the ideal diet for anyone. Since immune cells are produced rapidly during an infection, sufficient protein is essential. However, too much suppresses immunity, probably by using up available vitamin B6. Diets high in saturated or hydrogenated fat suppress immunity and clog up the lymphatic vessels; but essential fats, found in cold-pressed seed oils, boost immunity. Therefore a well-balanced protein, low-fat diet, with fats obtained from essential sources such as seeds and nuts, together with plenty of fresh fruit and vegetables rich in vitamins and minerals, is best for maximum immunity.

During a viral infection that increases mucus production, it is best to avoid meat, dairy produce and eggs, and also any foods that you suspect you might be allergic to. Great foods are all vegetables, especially carrots, beetroots and their tops, sweet potatoes, tomatoes and beansprouts. Fruit is particularly beneficial, especially watermelon and berries, plus ground seeds, lentils, beans, whole grains such as brown rice, and fish. All foods should be eaten as raw as possible, avoiding frying, which introduces free radicals.

Foods for a power diet

Here are some typical items in an immune power diet:

Watermelon juice Blend the flesh and the seeds in an electric blender. The husks will sink to the bottom, leaving the seeds, which are rich in protein, zinc, selenium, vitamin E and essential fats, in the juice. Drink a pint for breakfast and another pint during the day.

Carrot soup Blend three organic carrots, two tomatoes, a bunch of watercress, a third of a packet of tofu, half a cup of rice milk or soya milk, a teaspoon of vegetable stock (bouillon or Vecon), and (optional) some ground almonds or seeds. Eat cold or heat to serve, accompanied by oat-cakes or rice cakes. Alternatively, boil carrots, sweet potato or butternut squash and make a soup adding vegetable stock, loads of ginger and some coconut milk.

A large salad Include a selection of 'seed' vegetables like broad beans, broccoli, grated carrot, beetroot, courgettes, watercress, lettuce, tomatoes and avocados, adding seeds or marinated tofu pieces – organic if possible. Serve with a dressing of cold-pressed oil containing some crushed garlic.

Berries as a snack Strawberries have more vitamin C than oranges. Blueberries have the highest antioxidant power 'ORAC' score of all. Raspberries and strawberries are also excellent. Berries contain many phytonutrients that boost your immune system. So, when you are under attack, snack on berries – the more the merrier.

Useful supplements

These supplements help to fight infections naturally:

- A good, high-strength multivitamin and mineral
- A good, high-strength antioxidant formula giving at least 2,000mcg of vitamin A, 300mg of vitamin E, 100mg of B6, 20mg of zinc and 100mcg of selenium
- Vitamin C, 3 grams every four hours including last thing at night and immediately on rising (it may have a laxative effect – if it does, reduce the dose accordingly); choose a supplement that contains berry extracts, especially elderberry
- Cat's-claw tea with ginger four times a day
- Echinacea, ten drops three times a day
- Grapefruit seed extract, ten drops three times a day

For maintenance have 1 to 2 grams of vitamin C a day. Some supplements also contain other antioxidants and immune-friendly nutrients such as berry extracts, zinc or cat's claw.

25.

Balancing Hormones Naturally

S ome of the most powerful chemicals in the body are hormones. These are biochemicals produced in special glands and, when present in the bloodstream, they give instructions to body cells. Insulin, for example, tells the cells to take up glucose from the blood. Thyroxine, from the thyroid gland, speeds up the metabolism of cells, generating energy and burning fat. Oestrogen and progesterone, from the ovaries, control a sequence of changes that maintain fertility and the menstrual cycle. Hormone imbalances can wreak havoc on your health.

Hormones are either fat-like, called steroid hormones, or protein-like, such as insulin. They are made from components of your food, and diet can play a crucial part in keeping your hormone levels in balance. Most hormones work on feedback loops, with the pituitary gland as the conductor of the orchestra. For example, the pituitary releases thyroid-stimulating hormone (TSH), which tells the thyroid gland to release thyroxine, which speeds up the metabolism of the cells in the body. When the blood level of thyroxine reaches a certain point, the pituitary stops producing TSH.

The thyroid gland and metabolism

The thyroid hormone thyroxine is made from the amino acid tyrosine. The enzyme that converts one into the other is dependent on iodine, zinc and selenium. A lack either of tyrosine or of iodine, zinc or sele-

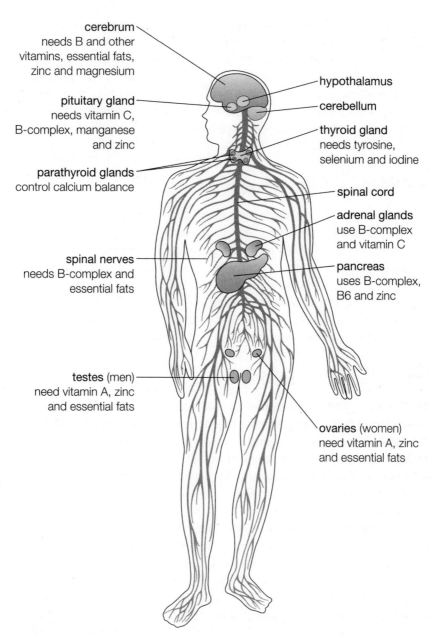

cerebrum
needs B and other
vitamins, essential fats,
zinc and magnesium

hypothalamus

pituitary gland
needs vitamin C,
B-complex, manganese
and zinc

cerebellum

thyroid gland
needs tyrosine,
selenium and iodine

parathyroid glands
control calcium balance

spinal cord

adrenal glands
use B-complex
and vitamin C

spinal nerves
needs B-complex and
essential fats

pancreas
uses B-complex,
B6 and zinc

testes (men)
need vitamin A, zinc
and essential fats

ovaries (women)
need vitamin A, zinc
and essential fats

The endocrine glands and hormones

nium can reduce thyroxine levels. However, an underactive thyroid, which can cause symptoms such as weight gain, mental and physical lethargy, constipation and thickening skin, is quite common. Many people suspected of having thyroid problems have borderline 'normal' thyroxine levels on being tested, but experience amazing health transformations after taking a low dose of thyroxine. Some people develop underactive thyroids because their body is destroying their thyroxine. These people test positive to 'anti-thyroid antibodies'. This is often due to gluten allergy. The immune system, it seems, becomes hypersensitive to a food and attacks thyroid tissue by mistake. Therefore, if you have an underactive thyroid it's worth testing yourself for allergies, as well as anti-thyroid antibodies.

Maintaining calcium balance

The thyroid gland also produces a hormone responsible for maintaining calcium balance in the body. Calcitonin from the thyroid works in balance with parathormone (PTH) from the parathyroid glands, four tiny glands attached to the thyroid. PTH converts vitamin D into an active hormone that helps to increase available calcium. While most of the body's calcium is in the bones, a small amount is in the blood and cells because every single nerve and muscle reaction uses calcium. PTH stimulates the bones to give up calcium, while calcitonin puts calcium back into the bones.

Stress and the adrenals

The adrenal glands sit on top of the kidneys and produce hormones that, among other things, help us adapt to stress. The hormones adrenalin, cortisol and DHEA help us respond to emergencies by channelling the body's energy towards being able to 'fight or take flight', improving oxygen and glucose supply to the muscles, and generating mental and physical energy. It is a design that helped our remote ancestors cope with truly life-threatening situations.

During a stress reaction the blood thickens to help wounds to heal. In modern life all this happens when you open your bank statement to find you are overdrawn, get stuck in a traffic jam or have a row with your partner. Tea, coffee, chocolate and cigarettes have the same effect as they contain caffeine, theobromine, theophylline or nicotine, which stimulate the release of adrenalin. This instant energy has a downside. The body slows down digestion, repair and maintenance to channel energy into dealing with stress, As a consequence, prolonged stress is associated with speeding up the ageing process, with a number of the diseases of the digestion and with hormone balance.

By living off stimulants such as coffee and cigarettes, high-sugar diets or stress itself, you increase your risk of upsetting your thyroid balance (which means your metabolism will slow down and you will gain weight) or calcium balance (resulting in arthritis), or of getting problems associated with sex-hormone imbalances and excessive cortisol. These are the long-term side effects of prolonged stress, because any body system that is over-stimulated will eventually under-function.

After only two weeks of the raised cortisol levels of stress, the dendrite 'arms' of brain cells that reach out to connect with other brain cells start to shrivel up, according to research carried out at Stanford University in California by Robert Sapolsky, professor of neuroscience.[29] The good news is that such damage isn't permanent. Stop the stress and the dendrites grow back. One way to reduce your stress levels is to reduce you intake of sugar and stimulants. The more dependent on stimulants you are, the more your blood sugar levels fluctuate, with more 'rebound' low blood sugar levels triggering the release of adrenal hormones. Your adrenals think you're starving and go into 'fight/flight' mode, when in truth you are just having a blood sugar dip as the body overcompensates after one more high-sugar food.

Nutrients for the stress hormones

The stress hormones rely on certain nutrients for their production. For adrenalin you need enough of vitamins B3 (niacin), B12 and C. Cortisol, which is also a natural anti-inflammatory substance, cannot be produced without enough vitamin B5 (pantothenic acid). Your need for all these nutrients, along with those needed for energy production such as vitamins B and C, goes up with prolonged stress.

Supplementing DHEA

Levels of DHEA, a vital adrenal hormone, fall as a result of prolonged stress. This hormone, which can be bought over the counter in the US, can be supplemented in small amounts to restore stress resistance.

A new kind of test can tell you where you are on the stress cycle. Saliva taken at five specific times of the day is analysed to determine its levels of cortisol and DHEA. DHEA can also be used to make the sex hormones testosterone and oestrogen, and is considered 'anti-ageing'. However, too much can also over-stimulate the adrenal glands and, for example, induce insomnia. So it is best not to take it unless you need it, as revealed by an adrenal stress test (see Resources on page 527).

Sex hormones

In women the balance between progesterone and oestrogen is critical. A relative excess of oestrogen, called oestrogen dominance, is associated with an increased risk of breast cancer, fibroids, ovarian cysts,

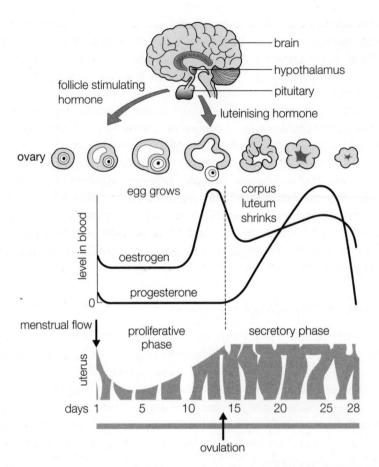

Hormones in the menstrual cycle. In the first half of the menstrual cycle a woman's body produces oestrogen, which makes the lining of the womb grow, ready to receive a fertilised egg. If the egg is released, the remaining sac then produces progesterone, which rises in the second half of the cycle, keeping the womb healthy. If no fertilised egg is implanted the sac (the corpus luteum) shrivels up and progesterone levels plummet. This triggers menstruation.

endometriosis and PMS. The early warning symptoms of oestrogen dominance include PMS, depression, loss of sex drive, sweet cravings, heavy periods, weight gain, breast swelling and water retention.

Oestrogen dominance can be due to excess exposure to oestrogenic substances, or a lack of progesterone, or a combination of both. Oestrogenic compounds are found in meat, much of which is hormone-fed, in dairy products, in many pesticides and in soft plastics, some of which leach into food when used for wrapping. Oestrogen is also contained in most birth-control pills and HRT.

If a woman does not ovulate, which ironically can be because of a slight lack of oestrogen, no progesterone is produced. This is because progesterone is produced in the sac that contains the ovum, once the ovum is released. If no progesterone is produced, there is a relative oestrogen dominance.

Stress raises levels of the adrenal hormone cortisol, which competes with progesterone and lowers levels of DHEA, the precursor of progesterone. DHEA is also a precursor of testosterone, and evidence is accumulating to suggest that men too can suffer from oestrogen dominance and testosterone deficiency. While men produce very little oestrogen, they are exposed to this hormone in their diet and in the environment. Some substances, such as breakdown products of the pesticide DDT, and Vincloxaline, used to spray lettuces, are known to interfere with the body's testosterone, creating a deficiency. This may explain the increase in the incidence of genital defects and undescended testes in male infants, and the rise in infertility as well as prostate and testicular cancer (see page 282). In later life some men have the equivalent of a 'male menopause'. The symptoms, according to male-hormone expert Dr Malcolm Carruthers, include fatigue, depression, decreased sexual performance, redistribution and gain in weight, including growth of excessive breast tissue.

Prostaglandins, made from essential fatty acids, sensitise cells to hormones. There is considerable interaction between prostaglandins and hormones, especially sex hormones. Deficiency in essential fats, which is endemic in the Western world, or deficiency in the nutrients needed to convert essential fats into prostaglandins (vitamins B3, B6 and C, biotin, magnesium and zinc), can also create the equivalent of hormonal imbalances.

These nutrients, plus essential fats, have proved very helpful in relieving PMS and menopausal symptoms. So too have the herbs agnus castus, dong quai, black cohosh and St John's wort. Vitamin E is also helpful for menopausal symptoms. One possible explanation is that vitamin E protects essential fats and prostaglandins from oxidation.

Balancing your hormones

The following guidelines will help you keep your hormones in balance. However, if you are suffering from a major hormone imbalance such as oestrogen dominance it may be necessary also to take small amounts of natural progesterone. This is very different from synthetic progestins, which are included in some birth-control pills and HRT, often in massive amounts in comparison to what the body naturally produces. Natural progesterone (and, for men, testosterone) is available only on prescription.

To keep your hormones in balance:

- Keep animal fats very low in your diet.

- Choose organic vegetables and meat wherever possible to reduce pesticide and hormone exposure.

- Don't eat fatty foods wrapped in non-PVC cling film.

- Use stimulants such as coffee, tea, chocolate, sugar and cigarette infrequently, if at all. If you are addicted to any of these, break the habit.

- Do not let stress become a habit in your life. Identify sources of stress and make some positive changes to your circumstances and the way you react to them.

- Make sure you are getting enough essential fats from seeds, their oils or supplements of evening primrose or borage oil (Omega 6) or flax oil (Omega 3).

- Make sure your supplement programme includes optimal levels of vitamins B3 and B6, biotin, magnesium and zinc.

- If you have PMS or menopausal symptoms, consider supplementing a hormone-friendly supplement containing extra vitamins B3, B6 and C, biotin, magnesium and zinc and/or the herbs agnus castus, dong quai, black cohosh and St John's wort (see Supplement resources, page 533).

Dig deeper by reading my book *Balancing Hormones Naturally* co-authored with Kate Neil.

26.

Bone Health – a Skeleton in the Cupboard

Not many people think about nourishing their skeleton. There is almost a belief that once your bones are formed they are there for good – until they start to break down, as in arthritis or osteoporosis. Yet the bones, like every other part of the body, are continually being rebuilt. They are a structure of protein and collagen (a kind of intercellular glue) that collects mainly calcium, plus phosphorus and magnesium. We even store heavy metals like lead in our bones when our body cannot get rid of them.

There are two kinds of bone cells: osteoblasts build new bone, while osteoclasts break down and get rid of old bone. The bone ends are made of cartilage, which is softer so that joints can work smoothly. While bones use calcium, phosphorus and magnesium as building materials, the ability to absorb calcium into bones depends on vitamin D and is assisted by the trace mineral boron. Vitamin C makes collagen, and zinc helps make new bone cells. This orchestra of nutrients is often found in 'bone-friendly' supplements.

Osteoporosis

The epidemic of osteoporosis has made many women think seriously about the health of their bones. It is the silent thief that robs up to 25 per cent of your skeleton by the time you reach the age of fifty. Particularly prevalent in women after the menopause, it increases the risk of bone fractures which occur in one in three women and one in twelve men by the age of seventy.

The conventional explanation is that once a woman stops menstruating she produces little of the oestrogen that helps keep calcium in her bones, hence the recommendation for women to have hormone replacement therapy (HRT). But this is far from the truth. Firstly, analyses of skeletal remains of our ancestors, and across cultures, show that post-menopausal women do not routinely suffer decreased bone density. It is a more recent phenomenon, particularly in Western society. Secondly, oestrogen, which stimulates osteoclast cells, does not help build new bone but only stops the loss of old bone. Progesterone, on the other hand, stimulates osteoblasts, which do build new bone. Taking natural progesterone increases bone density four times more effectively than oestrogen.

In the time leading up to the menopause, and afterwards, a woman stops ovulating. If no ovum is released no progesterone is produced, even though the body continues to produce small amounts of oestrogen. Scientists are now coming round to thinking that it is the relative excess of oestrogen to progesterone, which is in effect progesterone deficiency, that is precipitating osteoporosis, not deficiency in oestrogen.

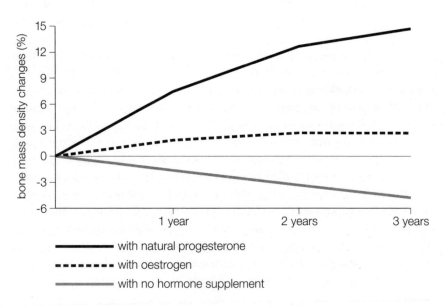

Typical bone mass density changes in menopausal women

Of course, this is not the only factor. Changes in diet are strongly related to increased risk of osteoporosis and may explain why many cultural groups have no osteoporosis at all. But while people with very low calcium intakes may benefit from taking more, there is no strong association between osteoporosis and calcium levels. The Bantu tribes of Africa, for example, have an average calcium intake of 400mg a day, well below the recommended intake for post-menopausal women, yet virtually no osteoporosis. And the Inuit (Eskimos), who consume vast amounts of calcium, have an exceptionally high incidence of osteoporosis. Why? And what have countries and cultures with a *high* incidence of osteoporosis got in common? The answer certainly isn't a lack of calcium, since milk consumption is exceedingly high in both the US and the UK, where osteoporosis is endemic. It may be too much dietary protein.

Protein-rich foods are acid-forming. The body cannot tolerate substantial changes in acid level in the blood and neutralises this effect through two main alkaline agents – sodium and calcium. When the body's reserves of sodium are used up, calcium is taken from the bones. Therefore the more protein you eat, the more calcium you need. One big difference between the Bantus and the Inuit is their level of protein consumption.

The idea that high-protein diets lead to calcium deficiency is nothing new. Numerous studies have demonstrated that a high protein intake increases urinary calcium excretion and that, on average, 1mg of calcium is lost in urine for every 1g rise in dietary protein. This effect is primarily attributable to metabolism of sulphur-containing amino acids present in all animal and some vegetable proteins, resulting in a greater acid load and buffering response by the skeleton – your body uses calcium to neutralise the acid.[30] And research is beginning to show that if you eat a high-protein diet no amount of calcium will correct the imbalance.

In one piece of research published in the *American Journal of Clinical Nutrition*, the group of people studied were given either a moderately high-protein diet (80g protein a day) or a very high-protein diet (240g protein) plus 1400mg of calcium. The overall loss of calcium was 37mg per day on the 80g-protein diet and 137mg per day on the 240g-protein diet. The author concluded that 'high-calcium diets are unlikely to prevent probable bone loss induced by high-protein diets'. In another study a protein intake of 95g a day (bacon and eggs for breakfast supplies 55g) resulted in an average calcium loss of 58mg per day, which means a loss of 2 per cent of total skeletal calcium per year, or 20 per cent each decade. The negative effects of too much protein have been clearly demonstrated in patients with osteoporosis. Some medical scientists now believe that a lifelong consumption of a high-protein, acid-forming diet may be a primary cause of osteoporosis.

Say no to arthritis

According to Dr Robert Bingham, a specialist in the treatment of arthritis, 'No person who is in good nutritional health develops rheumatoid or osteoarthritis.' Yet by the age of sixty, nine in every ten people have it. For some it is a living hell that can even be life-threatening. For all of them, arthritis means living with pain and stiffness. Arthritis is not, however, an inevitable consequence of ageing and can be prevented, provided the underlying causes are eliminated.

In the search for the cause of arthritis many things have been considered, including diet, physical exercise, posture, climate, hormones, infections, genetics, old age and stress. Most of these factors have proved relevant to some arthritis sufferers. I believe the occurrence of the symptoms of arthritis, or any type of arthritic disease, is the result of an accumulation of stresses that eventually causes joint, bone and muscle degeneration.

1 A healthy joint consists of strong bones, which are essentially minerals in a collagen (protein) matrix. Cartilage on the edge of bones is protected from the opposing bone and cartilage by a sac containing synovial fluid, which effectively lubricates the joint.

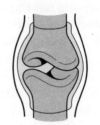

2 Overuse and dietary imbalances can lead to a breakdown of cartilage. Synovial fluid becomes less lubricating. Loss of cartilage components in both cartilage and bone. Bone ends become uneven and osteophytes (large bone spurs) form. Inflammation restricts movement.

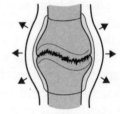

3 Loss of calcium balance can lead to calcium being dumped in soft tissues, causing muscle pain. In rheumatoid arthritis (ringed) bone ends can become fused together.

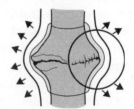

How arthritis develops

Why arthritis develops

The likely factors that lead to the development of this painful condition are:

Poor lubrication of the joints In between joints is a substance called synovial fluid. Good nutrition is needed to make sure that the synovial fluid stays fluid and able to lubricate. Cartilage and synovial fluid contain mucopolysaccharides, which can be provided by certain foods.

Hormonal imbalance Hormones control the calcium balance in the body. If the calcium balance is out of control the bones and joints can become porous and subject to wear and tear, and calcium can be deposited in the wrong place, resulting in arthritic 'spurs'. The fault is not so much calcium intake, but the loss of calcium balance in the body. A lack of exercise, too much tea, coffee, alcohol or chocolate, exposure to toxic metals like lead, excessive stress or underlying blood sugar or thyroid imbalances can all upset calcium control. While calcium control can be worse after the menopause, probably owing to the loss of oestrogen, too much oestrogen also makes arthritis worse. It is all a question of balance. Another hormone, insulin, stimulates the synthesis of the mucopolysaccharides, from which cartilage is made. People with underactive thyroid glands are particularly susceptible to arthritis.

Allergies and sensitivities Almost everyone who suffers from rheumatoid arthritis and many people who have osteoarthritis have food and chemical allergies or sensitivities that make their symptoms flare up. The most common food allergies are to wheat and dairy produce. Chemical and environmental sensitivities can include gas and exhaust fumes. These are well worth strictly avoiding for one month so you can see whether they contribute to the problem.

Free radicals In all inflamed joints a battle is taking place, with the body trying to deal with the damage. One of the key weapons of war in the body are free radicals (see page 128). If the immune system is not working properly, as in rheumatoid arthritis, it will produce too many free radicals, which can damage tissue around the joint. A low intake of antioxidant nutrients can make arthritis worse.

Infections Any infection, be it viral or bacterial, weakens the immune system which controls inflammation. But some viruses and bacteria particularly affect the joints by lodging in them and recurring when immune defences are low. Often the immune system can harm surrounding tissue in an attempt to fight an infection, like an army that obliterates its own country in trying to get rid of an invader. Building up your immune defences through optimum nutrition is the natural solution.

High homocysteine Several studies have found a link between high homocysteine levels and both osteoporosis and arthritis. It's well worth checking your level and lowering it by supplementing specific nutrients (see Chapter 16).

Bone strain and deformities   Any damage or strain, so often caused by bad posture, increases the risk of developing arthritis. A yearly check-up with an osteopath or chiropractor, plus regular exercise that helps to increase joint suppleness and strength, is the best prevention. Once arthritis has set in, special exercises help to reduce pain and stiffness.

State of mind   Research at the Arthritis and Rheumatism Foundation and at the University of Southern California Medical School has shown a link between arthritis and emotional stress. 'Hidden anger, fear or worry often accompanies the beginning of arthritis,' says Dr Austin from USC.

Poor diet   Most arthritics have a history of poor diet, which paves the way for many of the above risk factors. Too much refined sugar, too many stimulants, too much fat and too much protein are all strongly associated with arthritic problems. A lack of any of a large number of vital vitamins, minerals and essential fatty acids could, in itself, precipitate joint problems.

Nature's painkillers

Whatever the cause, once arthritis develops there is usually inflammation, causing pain, redness and swelling. Anti-inflammatory drugs fall into two main categories – cortisone-based and non-steroidal anti-inflammatory drugs (NSAIDs). NSAIDs account for more adverse drug reactions and deaths than any other class of drug.

The good news is that there are highly effective alternatives.

Omega 3 fish oils

One of the most popular is fish oils, which can be converted in the body to anti-inflammatory prostaglandins called PG3s. These counteract the inflammatory PG2s. Research has conclusively shown that fish-oil supplementation can reduce the inflammation of arthritis.[31] An effective amount is the equivalent of 1,000mg of EPA and DHA a day, which means two or three capsules. Cod liver oil, the richest source of omega 3 fats, has also been shown to reduce the pain and inflammation of arthritis.

A recent study giving osteoarthritis patients scheduled for knee-replacement surgery cod liver oil is a case in point. Half of the thirty-one patients were given two daily capsules of 1,000mg extra-high-strength cod liver oil, rich in Omega 3 fats (DHA and EPA), and the other half were given placebo oil capsules containing no Omega 3 fats for ten to twelve weeks. A total of 86 per cent of pre-operative patients with arthritis who took the cod liver oil capsules had absent or markedly reduced levels of enzymes that cause cartilage damage, as opposed to 26 per cent of those given a control oil. Results also showed a reduction in the inflammatory markers that cause joint pain among those who took the cod liver oil.[32]

Natural painkillers

Turmeric, boswellia, ashwagandha, hop extract and ginger all help reduce the over-production of leukotrienes that cause pain and inflammation.

The bright yellow pigment of the spice turmeric contains the active compound curcumin, which has a variety of powerful anti-inflammatory actions – trials in which it was given to arthritic patients showed it to be similarly effective to the anti-inflammatory drugs, without the side effects. You need about 500mg, one to three times a day.

Frankincense may be the ultimate gift for an arthritic friend. Its botanical name is *Boswellia serrata*, and it is also known as Indian frankincense; it is proving to be a very powerful natural anti-inflammatory agent, without the side effects of current drugs. In one study where patients initially received boswellic acid, the active ingredient within the plant, and then later a placebo, arthritic symptoms were significantly reduced, but then returned with a vengeance when the treatment was switched over to placebo.[33] Boswellic acid appears to reduce joint swelling, restores and improves blood supply to inflamed joints, provides pain relief, increases mobility, improves morning stiffness and prevents or slows the breakdown of the components of cartilage. Preparations are available in tablet and cream form – the ideal dose is 200 to 400mg, one to three times a day; the creams are especially useful in the treatment of localised inflammation.

Ashwagandha is a promising natural remedy that has been used for hundreds of years as part of Ayurvedic medicine in India. The active ingredient of this powerful natural anti-inflammatory herb are 'withanolides'. In animal studies ashwagandha has proven highly effective against arthritis. In one study animals with arthritis were given ashwagandha, hydrocortisone or placebo. While hydrocortisone produced a 44 per cent reduction in symptoms, ashwagandha produced an 89 per cent reduction, making it substantially more effective than cortisone.[34] Try 1,000mg a day of the root, providing 1.5 per cent withanolides.

One of the most effective natural painkillers of all is an extract from hops called IsoOxygene. It works just as well as painkilling drugs but without the associated gut problems. You need about 1,500mg a day.

Ginger is also anti-inflammatory, as well as being rich in antioxidants. In one study, supplementing ginger (500–2000mg a day) reduced pain and swelling in three-quarters of those with arthritis. Alternatively, eat a 1cm (½ inch) slice of fresh ginger each day.[35]

Inflammation reducers

Antioxidant nutrients help reduce inflammation, so keep eating those berries and supplementing an antioxidant formula. However, there are some exciting plant extracts that have very powerful antioxidant and anti-inflammatory effects. One of these is an extract from olives called hydroxytyrosol. This is what is called a polyphenol. Other plant foods containing polyphenols include green tea, grape skins and onions, both of which contain quercetin, but none is as powerful as this extract of olives. Compared with that of vitamin C its ORAC rating, a measure of antioxidant power, is more than ten times higher. Try 400mg a day.

Glucosamine and MSM: the joint-builders

Glucosamine is an essential part of the building material for joints and the cellular 'glue' that holds the entire body together, although joint cartilage contains the highest concentration of glucosamine.[36] The mechanism by which glucosamine appears to stop or reverse joint degeneration is by providing the body with the materials needed to build and repair cartilage.

Scientists originally thought glucosamine just helped reduce the pain of arthritis, but recent research in Belgium has proven that it actually helps rebuild cartilage, thereby reversing joint damage. So if you do have any joint problems from injury or arthritis, glucosamine could well help you repair the damage as well as relieving the pain. Usual dosage for glucosamine is 500mg, three times daily. Glucosamine hydrochloride works better than glucosamine sulphate. Glucosamine is a major component of joint tissue, and as a supplement works to stimulate joint function and repair. It is most effective in battling osteoarthritis, the most prevalent type of arthritis. A number of studies over the last twenty years have shown this. For example, a 1982 clinical study compared usage of the NSAID ibuprofen with that of glucosamine sulfate, for osteoarthritis of the knee. During the first two weeks, the ibuprofen decreased pain faster, but by the fourth week the glucosamine group was well ahead in pain relief. The overall results showed that 44 per cent of people in the glucosamine group had pain relief, compared with 15 per cent of those taking ibuprofen. Because glucosamine is not an anti-inflammatory drug, it takes longer to start working, but it works equally well. Some researchers now feel that glucosamine hydrochloride may be the best form because it has a slightly higher concentration of glucosamine in the molecule (83 per cent versus 80 per cent for glucosamine sulfate) and has better stability.[37]

MSM, which stands for methyl sulfonyl methane, is a source of the essential mineral sulphur. Sulphur is involved in a multitude of key body functions, including pain control, regulation of inflammation, detoxification and tissue-building. Extraordinary results are starting to be reported in terms of pain relief and relief from arthritis, from supplementing around 3 grams of MSM daily. One possibility is that sulphur deficiency is far more common than has been realised.

Some pain is due to pressure changes in cells, which in turn affect the nerves that sense pain. If cells inflate as a result of excess build-up of fluid or a drop in the pressure surrounding them, the nerves register the pain. MSM may also help improve cell-membrane fluidity, thereby improving the exchange of fluids in and out of cells, and reducing pressure build-up. One study at UCLA School of Medicine found that on 2,250mg of MSM a day, patients with arthritis had an 80 per cent improvement in pain within six weeks compared with a 20 per cent improvement among those who had taken dummy pills. The therapeutic dose appears to be around 1,500mg to 3,000mg.

My favourite natural anti-inflammatory regime is a combination of Omega 3 fats, boswellia, hop extract, hydroxytyrosol from olives, plus glucosamine and MSM. Look out for combinations of these nutrients and herbal extracts (see Supplement resources, page 533).

In summary, if you want to keep your bones and joints in good health:

- Keep fit and supple and see an osteopath or chiropractor once a year. Reduce your meat consumption to avoid excessive protein.

- Get out of the 'stress cycle' and keep stimulants to a minimum.

- Make sure your diet is rich in minerals from seeds, nuts and root vegetables.

- If you have arthritis, check out possible food allergies.

- If you have osteoporosis, consider natural progesterone (as a cream, not as HRT).

- If you have joint inflammation, take a daily supplement of 1,000mg of EPA/DHA fish oil or cod liver oil and a natural anti-inflammatory formula containing ashwagandha, turmeric, boswellia or hop extracts, as well as glucosamine hydrochloride and MSM.

Dig deeper by reading my book *Say No to Arthritis.*

chapter 27

Skin Health – Eat Yourself Beautiful

S kin. Where would we be without it? Not only does it keep our insides in, but also it protects us from infection, radiation and dehydration, keeps us warm and makes us look good. While we are most aware of our 'outside skin', the 'inside skin' of the lungs and digestive tract covers a much larger area. This entire surface is replaced every twenty days, and the degree to which the condition of your skin is influenced by what you eat and drink, as well as other factors such as your environment and, more obviously, cosmetics, is quite remarkable.

Skin is, after all, the largest organ in the body: in an adult it weighs around 11lb (5kg), and has a surface area of 22 square feet (2m²), about the size of a double bed. No other organ in the body is so exposed to damage or disease from the outside such as from injury, sunlight, smoking, environmental pollution and germs, so it really can have a rough time. At the same time, skin reflects many conditions and emotions that come from within, for example when it blushes or sweats.

Similarly, some skin disorders, such as warts, are confined just to the skin, while others – indeed most of them – tell a story of what is going on inside. Cold sores and chicken pox show that there is some sort of internal infection which the immune system is fighting off, a rash may be the result of an allergic reaction to a food that has been eaten, and a yellowish skin tone may indicate that there is a problem with the liver. So you can see that the condition of your skin is sensitive to a number of factors including your age, genes, hygiene, circulation, digestion, detoxification, immune system, the environment, your psychology and, of course, what you eat.

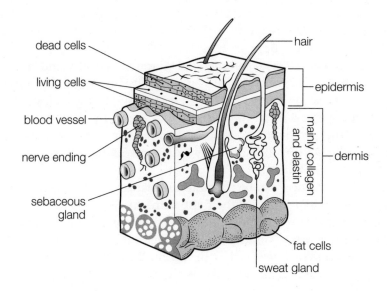

A cross-section of the skin

Nutrition is fundamentally involved at every stage of skin development. Starting with the inner layer of the skin, the dermis, collagen is made when vitamin C converts the amino acid proline into hydroxyproline. No vitamin C, no collagen. The flexibility of collagen and elastin fibres declines in time owing to damage caused by free radicals. This damage is limited by antioxidants such as vitamins A, C and E, selenium and many others.

Vitamin A helps to control the rate of keratin accumulation in the skin. A lack of this vitamin can therefore result in dry, rough skin. Both eating a diet rich in vitamin A and taking supplements of vitamin A can help to maintain healthy skin, but even more effective is to apply vitamin A-rich skin cream (see Resources, page 526). The membranes of skin cells are made from essential fats. A lack of essential fats makes these cells dry out too quickly, resulting in dry skin and excessive need of moisturisers. The health of skin cells depends on sufficient zinc, which is needed for accurate production of new generations of skin cells. Lack of zinc leads to stretch marks and poor healing, and is associated with a wide variety of skin problems from acne to eczema. Skin cells also produce a chemical that, in the presence of sunlight, is converted into vitamin D, which is needed to maintain the calcium balance of the body. So in many ways what you eat today you wear tomorrow.

The following good dietary guidelines are especially important for people with skin problems. Limit alcohol, coffee, tea, sugar and saturated fat (as in meat and dairy products), and increase your intake of fresh fruit, vegetables, water, herb teas and diluted juices. It is also well worth taking a good all-round multivitamin and mineral supplement, plus at least 1,000mg of vitamin C a day.

Your skin is a remarkable barometer of your body's health and, as such, is very much affected by how well you are internally. We've all looked a bit pale after a few too many parties – all sorts of signs of what is going on inside the body show up in the skin, such as a red face when we are hot and sweaty after strenuous exercise, or a rash in response to something we've eaten. So getting all your body systems working well is crucial to addressing skin problems.

Many skin disorders can be traced to imbalances in the digestive tract. While an insufficient intake of the right nutrients can affect the health of your skin, so can poor digestion and absorption. Some people eat healthy food but, for one reason or another, don't digest it properly and therefore don't get the nutrients they need. Other factors linked to digestion can contribute to skin problems, such as insufficient 'good' bacteria, or an overgrowth of the candida yeast. Once too many toxins and large molecules start 'gate-crashing' through the digestive tract, the body's ability to detoxify starts to weaken. This results in compromised liver function. By this stage even the slightest increase in toxins results in a whole host of symptoms such as fatigue, headaches and inflammation, as well as poor skin condition.

Dry skin

Slapping on moisturising cream certainly goes some way to relieving or preventing dry skin – but only some way. Without enough water each one of the cells in your body becomes dehydrated, losing its plumpness and structure, so the first step in keeping your skin well hydrated is to do just that – hydrate it by drinking at least 1.5 litres of water a day. You can keep your skin well 'oiled' from the inside by eating essential fatty acids from fish, nuts and seeds (see below). If you have particularly dry skin, it's best to supplement them too, as either fish, linseed or evening primrose oil or as a special blend such as Udo's Choice or Essential Balance.

Another, more subtle, factor that can contribute to dry skin is poor metabolism of the mineral calcium in the body – if you are not processing calcium well it will get dumped in certain tissues, including the skin. Calcium is a drying mineral – think chalk – so excess in the skin will dry it out. (A hair mineral analysis, available through nutritional therapists, can show how well you are metabolising calcium.)

Skin's enemies

Various outside factors as well as processes inside our bodies bring on the signs of ageing. The culprit is oxidative damage, caused by oxidants (free radicals).[38] They come from pollution, cigarette smoke, fried and burnt foods, processed cooking oils, sunlight, combustion and, ironically, even the body's own burning of oxygen to produce energy. Just as oxygen can damage iron to form rust, so it can damage molecules in our bodies. The oxidants are overall very destructive as they damage fats, proteins, connective tissue and nucleic acids (DNA and RNA). Parts of the body that are particularly vulnerable to such attack are the membranes of our cells and the DNA within them – obviously affecting the condition of the skin and its ability to generate new cells.

The good guys

Diet

A good diet consisting of fresh, untreated foods is crucial for the health of your entire body, not just your skin. It reduces the speed at which the skin ages or degenerates in any way. Eating plenty of antioxidant-rich foods every day is therefore a key dietary essential. These foods include red, orange and yellow vegetables and fruits such as sweet potatoes, carrots, apricots and watermelon, purple foods such as berries and grapes, green foods such as watercress, kale, alfalfa sprouts and broccoli, 'seed' foods such as peas and whole grains, fresh nuts, seeds and their oils, and onions and garlic.

Another important component of a good skin diet is the Omega 3 and 6 essential fats. Each cell membrane – in effect the skin of each cell – is composed partly of essential fats, and in turn your skin is made up of countless cells. So the fatty-acid content of your cell membranes is vital. Not only do the essential fats keep cell membranes smooth and soft, but also they help the membranes to do a better job of controlling what goes in and out of cells. Without enough fats in the cell membranes, they are not able to retain water and they lose their plumpness. So for soft skin, include plenty of essential-fat-rich foods in your diet such as fish, nuts, and seeds and their oils. Have seeds in salads, as snacks or ground up, and on cereals, yoghurt or soups.

Given the importance of keeping your digestive tract and liver in good working order for healthy skin, it is important to have a diet that includes unprocessed foods naturally high in fibre, such as whole grains, root vegetables, lentils and beans. These should be well chewed, and eaten when you are relaxed. The above recommendations are in addition to a wholesome, fresh diet.

Water – nature's moisturiser

One of the most important nutrients is water. Imagine a balloon filled with water – taut and firm to the touch. Allow some of the water out and the balloon will shrink, and the rubber may even become a little shrivelled. Deprive a cell of water and it will produce a similar result – in addition to the change in structure, the way it works will also be diminished. The process of removing water , or dehydration, leaves all the cells in our body gasping for replenishment, not least those in the skin, which are exposed to the harsh elements of the outside world – sun, cold, heating, air-conditioning, pollution. Without an adequate supply of water, your cells cannot rebuild your body, and waste products that stack up in the cells and your blood cannot be cleared. This turns into a vicious cycle whereby the cells cannot receive enough oxygen or nutrients to work or cleanse properly. Deep in your skin water is a crucial component, providing a basis for the healthy, soft, taut look of youthful skin.

Skin supplements

Following on from the recommendations above, a standard good multivitamin can be supplemented with extra antioxidants and some EFAs (linseed, fish oils or GLA). In addition to this, individual conditions will require specific supplementation.

One other nutrient that deserves a mention is sulphur. This essential mineral is a constituent of keratin and collagen – substances in skin, nails and hair, so it's no surprise that they improve when people take supplements in the form of MSM (methyl sulfonyl methane). Rather than taking collagen, or using expensive creams that contain it, you will be better off supplying your body with the raw materials it needs to make collagen, such as MSM (along with vitamin C). Sulphur is needed for new cell formation (remember your skin is constantly renewing itself), keeping the bonds between cells pliable, and it's also a great detoxifier. MSM has been shown not only to enhance the beauty of skin, nails and hair, but also to help skin healing (for instance after burns or wounds), acne, allergies, arthritis and much more. Start by taking 1,000mg three times a day. The recommendations above are in addition to a good diet and a multivitamin/mineral supplement.

A to Z of skin problems and nutritional solutions

Acne

Factors to consider   Excess fat blocks the skin pores. High-histamine types (see page 337) produce more sebum, an oily secretion in the skin. Vitamin A deficiency produces skin congestion through over-keratinisation of skin cells. Vitamin A and zinc deficiency lead to lowered ability to fight infection, as does lack of beneficial bacteria (often through over-use of antibiotics).

Diet   Low in fat, low in sugar, plenty of water, fresh fruit, vegetables (high-water-content foods) and regular cleansing diets/fasts.

Supplements   Vitamin A, zinc, vitamin C, all antioxidants, niacin to combat skin-flushing, vitamin E for wound-healing.

Skin treatments   Use a cream containing significant amounts of vitamins A, C and E in forms that can penetrate the epidermis (such as retinyl palmitate, ascorbyl palmitate and vitamin E acetate – see Resources, page 526).

Cellulite

Factors to consider   Excess saturated fat or fat-based toxins render fat cells immobile. If you strictly avoid dietary sources of saturated fat and eat only sources of essential oils, fat cells decongest and become softer. The body takes in many toxins, for example pesticide residues, which are hard to get rid of. These are dumped in fat cells to keep them away from vital organs. Hard fat and fat-based toxins can be eliminated by improving the circulation. Circulation to and from fat cells is stimulated by high water content while lymphatic drainage is achieved by massage, movement, exercise and skin-brushing.

Diet   A strict no-saturated-fat diet, which means no meat or dairy products. Essential fatty acids can be acquired from seeds. Drink lots of water and eat plenty of high-water-content foods such as fruit and vegetables, all organic. Apples are particularly good at eliminating cellulite. The pectin found in apples, carrots and other fruit and vegetables is an important phytochemical, which strengthens the immune and detoxification systems of the body. Consider a three-day apple-only fast or eat only organic apples one day a week.

Supplements   Lecithin granules, hydroxycitric acid, high-dose vitamin C and niacin.

Dermatitis

Factors to consider   Dermatitis literally means skin inflammation, and is similar to eczema. The term is used when the primary cause appears to be a contact allergy. Consider all possibilities, such as metals in jewellery, watches, etc., perfumes or cosmetics, detergents in washing-up liquid, soaps, shampoos or washing powders. Where there is a contact allergy there is often a food allergy too: common culprits are dairy products and wheat. Sometimes a combination of eating an allergy-provoking food and contact with an external allergen is needed for symptoms to develop. Another factor that makes dermatitis more likely is a lack of essential fatty acids from seeds and their oils, which turn into anti-inflammatory prostaglandins in the body. Their formation is blocked if you eat too much saturated fat or fried food, or lack certain key vitamins and minerals. The skin is also a route that the body can use to get rid of toxins. One kind of dermatitis, called acrodermatitis, is primarily caused by zinc deficiency and responds exceptionally well to zinc supplementation.

Diet   Keep it low in saturated fat, eat sufficient essential fats and very little meat or dairy produce – stay mainly vegan, although fish is all right. Test for dairy or wheat allergy, if suspected, by avoiding these foods for a couple of weeks and seeing if there is any improvement. Consider a cleansing diet.

Supplements   Essential oils such as flax, evening primrose and borage oil; vitamin B6, biotin, zinc and magnesium, plus antioxidant vitamins A, C and E.

Skin treatments   Use a cream containing significant amounts of vitamins A, C and E in forms that can penetrate the epidermis (such as retinyl palmitate, ascorbyl palmitate and vitamin E acetate – see Resources, page 526).

Dry skin

Factors to consider   Possible disturbed water balance due to essential-fatty-acid deficiency, poor intake of water or lack of vitamin A.

Diet   Should be low in saturated fat, high in essential fatty acids (from seeds and their oils). Drink at least 1 litre of water a day and eat plenty of water-rich foods (fruit and vegetables). Alcohol and stimulants such as coffee and tea should be limited.

Supplements   Essential oils such as flax, borage and evening primrose oil, vitamin A, vitamin E.

Skin treatments   Use a cream containing significant amounts of vitamins A and E in forms that can penetrate the epidermis (such as retinyl palmitate and vitamin E acetate – see Resources, page 526).

Eczema

Factors to consider   As for dermatitis. Most common contributory factors are the combination of a food allergy (most often wheat or dairy) and a lack of essential fatty acids from seeds and their cold-pressed oils, which have powerful anti-inflammatory effects.

Diet   Should be low in saturated fat, but with sufficient essential fats from seeds and their cold-pressed oils, low in meat and dairy produce, mainly vegan. Fish is all right. Test for dairy and wheat allergy, if suspected, by avoiding these foods for a set period. Consider a cleansing diet.

Supplements   Essential oils such as flax, evening primrose and borage oil; vitamin B6, biotin, zinc and magnesium, plus antioxidant vitamins A, C and E.

Skin treatments   Use a cream containing significant amounts of vitamins A, C and E in forms that can penetrate the epidermis (such as retinyl palmitate, ascorbyl palmitate and vitamin E acetate – see Resources, page 526).

Facial puffiness and water retention

Factors to consider   Food allergy, lack of essential fatty acids, hormonal imbalance such as progesterone deficiency or oestrogen dominance.

Diet   Test for food allergy (wheat and dairy the most common). Ensure a high intake of seeds and their oils, plenty of water and water-rich foods (fruit and vegetables).

Supplements   Essential oils such as flax, evening primrose and borage oil; vitamin B6, biotin, zinc and magnesium.

Oily skin

Factors to consider   Excess fat in the diet, high-histamine type (see page 337) and excessive adrenal stimulation resulting from stress, all of which increase sebum production.

Diet   Low in fat; ensure sufficient essential oils from seeds and their cold-pressed oils; low in alcohol, sugar and stimulants.

Supplements   Vitamin C, pantothenic acid (if you are stressed).

Skin treatments   Use a cream containing significant amounts of vitamin A in forms that can penetrate the epidermis (such as retinyl palmitate – see Resources, page 526). This helps to control excessive sebum production.

Psoriasis

Factors to consider   Psoriasis is a completely different kind of skin condition from eczema or dermatitis and does not generally respond as well to nutritional intervention. It can occur when the body is 'toxic' – perhaps owing to an overgrowth of the organism *Candida albicans*, to digestive problems leading to intoxication, or to poor liver detoxification. Otherwise consider the same factors as for eczema and dermatitis.

Diet   Start with a cleansing diet followed by one low in saturated fat but with sufficient essential fats, low in meat and dairy produce, and with a high vegan content. Fish is all right. Test for dairy and wheat allergy, if suspected, by avoiding these foods for a certain time.

Supplements   Essential oils such as flax, evening primrose and borage oil, vitamin B6, biotin, zinc and magnesium, plus antioxidant vitamins A, C and E.

Skin treatments   Use a cream containing significant amounts of vitamins A, C and E in forms that can penetrate the epidermis (such as retinyl palmitate, ascorbyl palmitate and vitamin E acetate – see Resources, page 526).

Rashes

Factors to consider   Possible over-inflammation due to lack of essential fatty acids, or food or contact allergy, or a stress reaction due to adrenal overload, or (for example in shingles) a viral, fungal or bacterial infection.

Diet   Low in saturated fat but with sufficient essential fats, low in meat and dairy produce, high vegan content. Fish is all right. Test for dairy and wheat allergy, if suspected, by avoiding these foods for a certain time.

Supplements   Essential oils such as flax, evening primrose and borage oil, vitamin B6, biotin, zinc and magnesium, plus antioxidant vitamins A, C and E.

Skin treatments   Use a cream containing significant amounts of vitamins A, C and E in forms that can penetrate the epidermis (such as retinyl palmitate, ascorbyl palmitate and vitamin E acetate – see Resources, page 526).

Rough skin

Factors to consider   Lack of vitamin A, dehydration, lack of essential fatty acids.

Diet   Should be high in fruit and vegetables (especially yellow, orange and red ones, which are high in betacarotene), with lots of water and essential fatty acids from seeds and their oils.

Supplements   Vitamin A, all antioxidants (vitamins A, C and E, zinc and selenium), gamma-linolenic acid (GLA) from borage or evening primrose oil.

Skin treatments   Use a cream containing significant amounts of vitamins A, C and E in forms that can penetrate the epidermis (such as retinyl palmitate, ascorbyl palmitate and vitamin E acetate – see Resources, page 526).

The way to perfect skin

Many common nutritional factors are involved in a wide variety of skin problems. To prevent these problems and keep your skin healthy here are some key diet and supplement guidelines:

Diet

- Limit alcohol, caffeine, chemical additives, salt, saturated fat, sugar and smoking.

- Eat plenty of fresh fruit and vegetables, preferably organic.

- Eat some seeds, nuts or their cold-pressed oil every day. Take either a heaped tablespoon of ground seeds, or a tablespoon of a blended seed oil containing cold-pressed flax, pumpkin, sesame and sunflower oil.

- Drink at least a litre of water a day, either neat or in herb teas or added to juice.

Disorder	Factors to consider	Possible solution	Diet recommendations	Supplements
Acne	Poor digestion, constipation, dairy sensitivity, hormone imbalance, stress	Gut cleanse, balance hormones, balance blood sugar levels	2 litres water daily, increase fibre, avoid sugar, limit animal fats	Vitamin A, zinc, chromium
Cellulite	Sluggish detoxification, constipation, lack of exercise	Gut and liver cleanse, exercise, lymphatic drainage massage, skin-brushing	Avoid all chemicals and processed foods, limit alcohol and sugar	Gotu kola
Cold sores	Viral infection, lowered immunity	Support immunity	Avoid foods high in arginine e.g. nuts, chocolate, soya	L-lysine, vitamin C, garlic
Eczema	Food allergies, leaky gut, essential-fat deficiency, contact sensitivity	Identify allergens, support digestion and heal gut	Experiment with eliminating foods (under guidance from nutritionist), e.g. milk, eggs, nuts; increase oily fish, nuts (if not allergic) and seeds	Fish or evening primrose oil, flavonoids, e.g. quercetin

Supplements

- Take a good, all-round vitamin and mineral supplement plus extra antioxidant nutrients – vitamins A, C and E. An ideal daily intake is 2,250mcg of vitamin A, 2,000mg of vitamin C and 400mg of vitamin E.

- If you are prone to dry skin or skin inflammation, supplement borage oil or evening primrose oil to give the equivalent of 200mg of gamma-linolenic acid (GLA).

Skin creams

- Use a cream containing significant amounts of vitamins A, C and E in forms that can penetrate the epidermis (such as ascorbyl palmitate, retinyl palmitate and vitamin E acetate – see Resources, page 526).

Other recommendations

- Limit your exposure to strong sunlight and use a sunblock.

- Wash your skin with a gentle, oil-based cleanser, not soap.

> **Dig deeper** by reading my book *Solving Your Skin Problems* co-authored with Natalie Savona.

Part 4

The Benefits of Optimum Nutrition

chapter 28.

Improving Intelligence, Memory and Mood

Most people believe that intelligence is something you are born with and there is nothing you can do to change it. While there is clearly an inherent component to intelligence, psychologists tell us that we use less than 1 per cent of our intellectual capacity and that every day we think thousands of thoughts, the vast majority of which are repeats! Imagine what would happen if we could focus all our mental energy on the task at hand and tap into our full potential.

The brain and nervous system, our mental 'hardware', consist of a network of neurons, special cells that are each capable of forming tens of thousands of connections with others. Thinking and feeling represent a pattern of activity across this network. The activity, or signals, involve neurotransmitters, chemical messengers in the brain. When we learn we actually change the wiring of the brain. When we think or experience emotions we change the activity of neurotransmitters. Both brain and neurotransmitters are derived from nutrients and are therefore affected by what you eat and drink.

Neurotransmitters such as serotonin, which is involved in mood, or adrenalin which gives you motivation, or acetylcholine which is vital for good memory, are made from the amino acids in the protein you eat. However, their production in the brain depends on vitamins and minerals. These micronutrients help turn glucose into energy, amino acids into neurotransmitters, simple essential fats into more complex fats like GLA or DHA and prostaglandins, and choline and serine into phospholipids.

They help build and rebuild the brain and nervous system and keep everything running smoothly. They are your brain's best friends.

Knowing this, we decided to test what would happen to the intelligence of schoolchildren if given an optimal intake of vitamins and minerals. Gwillym Roberts, a schoolteacher and nutritionist from the Institute for Optimum Nutrition, and Professor David Benton, a psychologist from Swansea University, put sixty schoolchildren on a special multivitamin and mineral supplement designed to ensure an optimal intake of key nutrients.[1] Without their knowledge, half these children were placed on a placebo.

After eight months on the supplements, the non-verbal IQs in those taking the supplements had risen by over 10 points! No changes were seen in those on the placebos. This study, published in the *Lancet* in 1988, has since been proven many times in other studies. Most have used RDA levels of nutrients, much lower than those in our original study, but they still show increases in IQ averaging 4.5 points. In other words, optimum nutrition levels of vitamins and minerals work twice as well as RDA levels. Don't think it's just kids who get smarter with optimum nutrition. It works for adults and old people too.

Dr Chandra from the Memorial University of Newfoundland in Canada decided to test whether supplementation with vitamins and trace elements in modest amounts could improve memory and mental performance in healthy, elderly subjects. He gave ninety-six such men and women, all over the age of sixty-five, either a daily supplement of trace elements and vitamins or a placebo for twelve months. The participants' blood nutrient levels were measured at the beginning and at the end of the study, as was their immediate and long-term memory, abstract thinking, problem-solving ability and attention. Of the eighty-six people who completed the year, those taking supplements showed a highly significant improvement in all cognitive tests except long-term memory recall. He also found that the lower the blood nutrient levels, the worse the mental performance.[2]

But why do vitamins and minerals raise IQ? The answer is that you can think faster and can concentrate for longer with an optimal intake of vitamins and minerals.

The ultimate head start

The sooner you start optimally nourishing your brain, the better. Of course, that puts the responsibility on mothers while pregnant and breastfeeding. A sixteen-year study by the Medical Research Council shows just how critical optimum nutrition is in the early years. They fed 424 premature babies either a standard or an enriched milk formula containing extra protein, vitamins and minerals. At eighteen months, those fed standard milk 'were doing significantly less well' than the others, and at eight years they had IQs up to 14 points lower![3]

Improving learning difficulties

Even more convincing are the results of optimum nutrition strategies on children with learning difficulties (currently about one in every ten children) including children with Down's syndrome, the result of a genetic defect. When researcher Dr Ruth Harrell heard of a case in which the IQ of a Down's syndrome child rose from 20 to 90 points after nutritional intervention, she decided to explore the idea that many mentally retarded children might have been born with increased needs for certain vitamins and minerals.[4]

In her first study Dr Harrell took twenty-two mentally retarded children and divided them into two groups. One group received vitamin and mineral supplements, the other placebos. After four months, the IQ in the group taking the supplements had increased by between 5 and 9.6 points; those on placebos showed no change. For the next four months, both groups of children were given the supplements and the average improvement rose to 10.2 points. Six of the children showed improvements of between 10 and 25 IQ points. While not all researchers have been able to replicate these results, there have now been a substantial number of well-documented cases of Down's syndrome children having IQ shifts of 10 to 40 points.

Autistic children and those with learning difficulties have also shown great improvements in intelligence. In a study by Dr Colgan on sixteen children with learning and behavioural difficulties, each child had his or her individual nutrient needs determined. Half the children were then given supplements. Each child attended a remedial reading course designed to improve his or her reading age by one year. Over the next twenty-two weeks teachers carefully monitored the reading age, IQ and behaviour of the children. Those not taking supplements showed an average increase in IQ of 8.4 points and in reading age of 1.1 years. However, the group on supplements had an improvement in IQ of 17.9 points and their reading age went up by 1.8 years.

A 5 per cent shift in IQ score would get a substantial number of children currently classified as educationally subnormal back into regular school, saving millions of pounds spent on special education. Isn't it time schoolchildren were given free vitamins at a fraction of this cost? This might also reduce aggressive behaviour and crime.

Curbing aggressive tendencies

Bernard Gesch, a social worker who became convinced of the link between diet, crime and delinquency, ran a double-blind trial on young offenders in

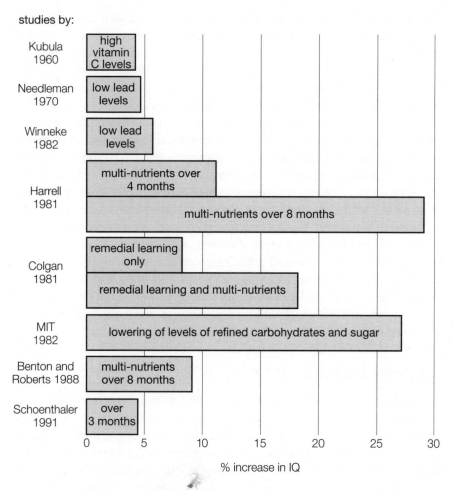

studies by:

Effects of optimum nutrition on intelligence

a maximum-security prison in Aylesbury, giving them either a multi-nutrient containing vitamins, minerals and essential fatty acids, or a placebo. The results, published in the *British Journal of Psychiatry*, showed a staggering 35 per cent decrease in acts of aggression after only two weeks.[5] Since prison diets are, if anything, better than those most young offenders eat, this shows just how important optimum nutrition is for reducing violent and deviant behaviour. When the trial was over and the supplements were stopped, there was a 40 per cent increase in offences in the prison.

Brain fats

Particularly important for brain development are the essential fatty acids and phospholipids that form part of the structure of brain cell membranes.

Low levels of essential fatty acids are also associated with lower levels of intelligence. This is thought to be the reason why, by the age of seven, children who were breast-fed as babies have been shown to have higher IQs. Breast milk contains DHA, an essential Omega 3 fatty acid crucial for brain development. EPA, the other important Omega 3 fatty acid, has also been shown to be highly effective in children with dyslexia.

Many studies have shown that an optimal intake of essential fats, especially Omega 3 fats, improves intelligence, reduces aggression and enhances mood. One study in America gave severely depressed patients, who were already on anti-depressants, a concentrated supplement of EPA. By the third week, the depressed patients were showing major improvement in their mood, while those on placebo were not.[6] Similar results are now being reported in Britain. Dr Basant Puri from London's Hammersmith Hospital decided to try EPA on one of his patients, a twenty-one-year-old student who had been on a variety of anti-depressants, to no avail. He had a very low sense of self-esteem, sleeping problems and little appetite, found it hard to socialise and often thought of killing himself. After one month of supplementing the Omega 3 fats he was no longer having suicidal thoughts and after nine months he no longer had any depression.[7]

Mummy I shrank your brain

The richest dietary source of EPA and DHA is fish, which is also full of another important family of brain nutrients – phospholipids. The brain and nervous system of a foetus use up more than half the available nutrients supplied during development in the womb and around a quarter this during adult life. The brain is very dependent on glucose, with almost half of all the available glucose powering it, and on essential fats and phospholipids. Research at the Royal Postgraduate Medical School in London shows that women's brains shrink during pregnancy. It seems to be the size of the cells, not the number, that changes, and one possible explanation is that the foetus takes supplies of essential fats and phospholipids from the mother if there are not enough to go around. If this proves to be so, it highlights the importance of getting a sufficient quantity of these essential brain nutrients.

Acetylcholine – the memory molecule

Probably the most important phospholipid is phosphatidyl choline, which also supplies the brain nutrient choline; the latter is needed to make acetylcholine, a vital neurotransmitter for memory, control of sensory input signals and muscular control. Acetylcholine deficiency results in poor memory, lethargy, decreased dreaming and a dry mouth. This is thought to be one of the major causes of senile dementia, which affects one in every seven people over the age of seventy-five. Research on rats at Duke University Medical Center in the US demonstrated that giving choline during pregnancy creates the equivalent of superbrains in the offspring.

The researchers fed pregnant rats choline halfway through their pregnancy. The infant rats whose mothers were given choline had vastly superior brains with more neuronal connections and, consequently, improved learning ability and better memory recall, all of which persisted into old age. This research showed that giving choline helps restructure the brain for improved performance.[8]

Acetylcholine is made by the action of an enzyme dependent on vitamin B5 called choline. The combination of B5 and choline has proved effective in enhancing memory and mental performance. The best supplemental source of choline is lecithin, which also supplies phospholipids. Lecithin is an emulsifier which is also used in some foods. All health food stores stock it, either as capsules or as granules that can easily be sprinkled on food. However, not all lecithin is the same. Look at the label before you buy, and make sure the product contains more than 30 per cent phosphatidyl choline.

One problem with supplementing any form of choline is that it does not readily enter brain cells. This is why large quantities – around a tablespoon of lecithin granules a day – are needed to have an effect.

Another nutrient found in fish, particularly in anchovies and sardines, is DMAE (dimethylaminoethanol), which does pass easily into the brain and can be converted into choline to make acetylcholine. DMAE has been shown to elevate mood, improve memory, increase intelligence and physical energy, and extend the life of laboratory animals. One of the pioneers of DMAE therapy, Dr Carl Pfeiffer, found it to be an excellent slow-acting stimulant and an alternative to anti-depressants. It is now prescribed in the US (although not in the UK), often under the name Deaner or Deanol, for learning problems, hyperactivity, reading and speech difficulties, and behavioural problems in children, and it is currently being researched for its effects on extending lifespan. As one person on DMAE said, 'I am more awake when I'm awake, and more sound asleep when I'm asleep. Not only does my memory improve, but I have an easier time daydreaming when I want to, and concentrating on real-world tasks when I want to.'

The positive effects of supplementing another important phospholipid, phosphatidyl serine (PS), are equally amazing. In one study, supplementing PS improved the subjects' memories to the level of people twelve years younger. Dr Thomas Crook from the Memory Assessment Clinic in Bethesda, Maryland, gave 149 people with age-associated memory impairment a daily dose of 300mg of PS or a placebo. When tested after twelve weeks, the ability of those taking PS to match names to faces (a recognised measure of memory and mental function) had vastly improved.[9]

Smart nutrients

The buzzword in brain enhancement is 'nootropics' – substances derived from an amino acid called pyroglutamate which is found in fruit and vegetables. The discovery that the brain and cerebro-spinal fluid contain large amounts of pyroglutamate led to its investigation as an essential brain nutrient. Doctors prescribe nootropic drugs, which are chemical variations of pyroglutamate, to millions of people every year for memory-deficit problems. Their basic effect is to improve learning, memory consolidation and memory retrieval, all without toxicity or side effects.

One extraordinary finding was that nootropics promote the flow of information between the right and left hemispheres of the brain. The left brain is associated with analytical, logical thinking and the right brain with creative, relational thinking. This is thought to be a possible reason why nootropics have proved helpful in the treatment of dyslexia. A study published in 1988 by Dr Pilch and colleagues suggests that nootropics may increase the number of acetylcholine receptors in the brain, thereby improving the brain's efficiency.[10] Older mice were given piracetam, a pyroglutamate derivative, for two weeks. The researchers found that these mice subsequently had a 30–40 per cent higher density of receptors. This suggests that pyroglutamate-like molecules not only maximise mental performance but also may have a regenerative effect on the nervous system.

The synergy factor

The effects of enhancing mental performance through supplementation of 'smart nutrients' such as Omega 3 fats, phosphatidyl choline, PS, pantothenic acid, DMAE and pyroglutamate are likely to be far greater when these substances are taken in combination than when they are taken individually. In one study in 1981, a team of researchers led by Raymond Barrus gave choline and piracetam to elderly laboratory rats, which are noted for age-related memory decline.[11] They found that 'rats given the piracetam/choline combination exhibited [memory] retention scores several times better than those with piracetam alone'. Only half the dose was needed when piracetam and choline were combined.

I supplement a brain-food formula every day that gives me all of these – phosphatidyl choline, PS, DMAE, pyroglutamate and pantohenic acid, as well as Omega 3 fats. I also eat fish and organic or free-range eggs from chickens fed Omega-3-rich feed. You can find these Omega-3-rich eggs in most supermarkets.

The brain drain

While 'good' chemicals and nutrients can improve mental function, 'bad' chemicals can and do reduce your intelligence. Alcohol is a prime example. Coffee, while commonly thought to improve concentration, actually diminishes it. A number of studies have shown that the ability to remember lists of words is made worse by caffeine. According to one researcher, Dr Erikson, 'Caffeine may have a deleterious effect on the rapid processing of ambiguous or confusing stimuli', which sounds like a description of modern living! The combination of caffeine and alcohol slows reaction time and, in one study, made subjects more drunk than alcohol alone. Caffeine is present in coffee, tea, chocolate, Lucozade, cola drinks and the herb guarana.

A diet high in sugar and refined carbohydrates, as discussed earlier, is another factor that reduces intelligence. Researchers at the Massachusetts Institute of Technology found that the higher the intake of refined carbohydrates, the lower the IQ. In fact, the difference between the high-sugar consumers and the low-sugar consumers was a staggering 25 points![12] Sugar has been implicated in aggressive behaviour,[13] anxiety,[14] hyperactivity and attention deficit,[15] depression,[16] eating disorders,[17] fatigue,[18] learning difficulties[19] and PMS ratings.

Heavy metals such as lead, cadmium and aluminium accumulate in the brain and have been clearly demonstrated to reduce intelligence, concentration, memory and impulse control. Therefore keeping pollution to a minimum, which includes not smoking, is another prerequisite to boosting your brainpower.

Here are some simple guidelines for improving your memory and mental performance:

- Reduce your intake of stimulants such as coffee, tea, chocolate and cola, and of sugar and refined foods.

- Minimise your exposure to pollution and cigarettes.

- Make sure you are 'well oiled' with regular fish, seeds, their oils or essential-fat supplements.

- Eat Omega 3-rich eggs – at least four a week.

- Ensure that you achieve optimum nutrition through your diet and by taking a high-dose multivitamin and mineral supplement.

● Take daily supplements of smart nutrients: pantothenic acid 100-500mg; choline 500-1,000mg (or as one heaped teaspoon of high-phosphatidyl-choline lecithin granules); phosphatidyl serine (PS) 30-100mg; DMAE 100-500mg; pyroglutamate 250-750mg.

Dig deeper by reading my book *Optimum Nutrition for the Mind*.

chapter 29

Increasing Your Energy and Resistance to Stress

A s a nutritionist the two most common complaints I hear from my clients are that they lack energy and are under too much stress. The net result is tiredness, exhaustion, lethargy, apathy, poor concentration, lack of motivation – whatever expression you use, the feeling is the same. Many people turn to sugary food, coffee or cigarettes, or become 'adrenalin junkies' with high-powered jobs or exhilarating pastimes, to regain this feeling of energy. Yet often these attempted solutions only generate more stress, and soon they feel out of control and stressed out on the roller-coaster of life. Stress is one of the most common health problems, associated with a wide variety of illnesses and accounting for the loss of forty million working days a year in the UK. But what has it got to do with nutrition?

One surprising result which emerged from a survey of patients seen at the ION clinic was that, before consulting a nutritionist, 54 per cent of them scored high on a questionnaire concerning their ability to cope with stress, yet within six months of starting their optimum nutrition regimes only 28 per cent still had a high stress rating. For the rest, whatever happened during those six months improved their ability to cope.

The chemistry of stress

Your body chemistry changes fundamentally every time you react stressfully. Stress starts in the mind. We perceive a situation as requiring our immediate attention – a young child stepping into the road, a car driving too close to us, a hostile reaction from a colleague, a financial crisis, an impossible deadline. Rapid signals stimulate the adrenal glands to produce adrenalin. Within seconds your heart is pounding, your breathing changes, stores of glucose are released into the blood, the muscles tense, the eyes dilate, even the blood thickens. You are ready for fight or flight – the average adrenalin rush of a commuter stuck in a traffic jam is enough to keep him or her running for a mile. That represents how much glucose is released, mainly by breaking down glycogen held in muscles and the liver.

To get the fuel into the body, the pancreas releases two hormones, insulin and glucagon. Insulin, aided by a substance released from the liver, glucose-tolerance factor, helps to carry the fuel out of the blood; glucagon tops up the blood sugar if its levels get too low. All this happens as a result of a stressful thought. Where, you might wonder, does all this extra energy and increased alertness come from? The answer is from a diversion of energy from the body's normal repair and maintenance jobs such as digesting, cleansing and rejuvenating. So every moment you spend in a state of stress speeds up the ageing process in your body. It is stressful just thinking about it!

The effects of prolonged stress are even more insidious than that. Imagine your pituitary, adrenals, pancreas and liver perpetually pumping out hormones to control blood sugar that you do not even need. Like a car driven too fast, the body goes out of balance and parts start to wear out. Levels of the anti-ageing adrenal hormone start to fall, as do those of cortisol, and before long your body simply cannot respond to stress as it used to.

The blood sugar blues

As a consequence your energy level drops, you lose concentration, get confused, suffer from bouts of 'brain fag', fall asleep after meals, get irritable, freak out, cannot sleep, cannot wake up, sweat too much, get headaches ... sounds familiar? In an attempt to regain control, most people turn to stimulants. Legal stimulants include coffee (containing theobromine, theophylline and caffeine), tea (containing caffeine), cola drinks (containing caffeine), chocolate (containing caffeine and theobromine), cigarettes (containing nicotine) and psychological stimulants such as horror films or bungee jumping – something to put you on the edge. Illegal stimulants include amphetamines and other 'uppers', cocaine, crack and crime. Naturally it becomes increasingly difficult to relax while living on stimulants, so most people learn to use relaxants such as alcohol, sleeping pills, tranquillisers, cannabis and so on.

Addicted to stress

Of course, you cannot live like this for ever, so most people burn out and have to head for the beach to recover. Yet as they wait in the airport, what better way to relax than by reading a paperback thriller? The cover promises 'murder, mystery, greed, lust, gripping suspense'. Sounds good. Backed up by a cup of coffee, a glass of wine and a stressful journey, they arrive ready for the beach. Then, after two blissful hours engrossed in raunchy pulp fiction on the beach, it is time for some excitement – windsurfing, water-skiing, something exhilarating. The point is that most people become addicted to stress, because without it they come crashing down, revealing their true state of adrenal exhaustion. This is why people feel exhausted or get ill when they take time off.

■ Test your stress – symptoms linked with adrenal imbalance

- **Hard to get up in the morning**
- **Tired all the time**
- **Craving certain foods**
- **Anger, irritability, aggressiveness**
- **Mood swings**
- **Restlessness**
- Poor concentration
- Poor sleep patterns
- Rapid or pounding heartbeat
- Prone to catching flu or colds
- Muscle and joint aches
- Spotty skin
- Allergies
- Hair loss
- Yeast overgrowth
- Hard-to-shift fat around waist
- Hungry all the time
- Difficulty in making decisions
- Poor memory
- **Energy slump during the day**
- **Regular feelings of weakness**
- **Apathy**
- **Depression**
- **Feeling cold all the time**
- Headaches
- Hyperactivity
- Frequent sore throats
- Poor wound-healing
- Water retention
- PMT
- Watery or itchy eyes
- Excessive sweating
- Bloated feeling
- Faintness

If you have three or more of the symptoms printed in **bold** type you may have an adrenal hormonal imbalance. If you also have five or more of the other symptoms, this warrants investigation by a nutritionist.

Energy-consumers

Yet in a very real sense all stressors and stimulants consume our energy. The 'high' is literally energy leaving the system, like a wave that breaks and seems for a few seconds to be full of energy. Yet a few seconds later there is no wave at all – likewise the energy is gone.

In an article on drug abuse, psychologist and philosopher Oscar Ichazo says, 'Drugs (all of them) can be characterised as "energy consumers", consuming energy at a rate much greater than our natural ability to replace it. As drugs burn all our accumulated vitality in short periods of time, the brief exaltation is inevitably followed by depletion of vital energy, felt as the "down", the depressant effect of drugs. Nothing can replace a natural, clean body capable of producing natural and clean vital energy.' He rates the drugs most damaging to our vital energy, in descending order of harmfulness, as alcohol, heroin and opiates, tobacco, cocaine, barbiturates, anti-depressants, amphetamines, marijuana and caffeine.[20]

But what does it mean to 'consume energy'? It means that body cells are starved of fuel nutrients like glucose, and catalyst nutrients like B vitamins, which drive the enzyme systems necessary to release energy from fuel nutrients. The nutrients necessary to make messenger molecules like neurotransmitters, or carrier molecules like insulin, are also depleted. So every moment you spend in a stressful state you are using up valuable nutrients. Consider this. Have you ever had a massage, after which you felt as if a whole load of muscular tension had gone? Every single muscle cell that you hold in tension, often for decades, even when you are asleep, is consuming energy, B vitamins, vitamin C, calcium and magnesium – to name but a few – just to stay in that state of tension. If you could relax all the muscles in your body, think how much you would save in nutritional supplements! Conservative estimates suggest that you double your need for vitamins when you are in a stressed state.

The energy equation

If you want to maximise your available energy for life, and to retain that energy rather than burning out, the nutritional message is simple:

- Eat slow-releasing carbohydrates – ones that release their 'fuel' slowly.

- Ensure you have optimal intakes of all essential nutrients – vitamins, minerals and others.

- Avoid stimulants and depressants.

The resultant increase in energy will help you to cope with the stresses and strains of life. The optimum nutrition approach is both a way of breaking energy-consuming patterns that keep depleting us, and a method of regenerating energy for breaking the mental habits that initiate a stress response in the first place. So let's examine what stress-busting optimum nutrition actually means.

The anti-stress diet

Fast-releasing sugars create a state of stress in the body, stimulating the release of cortisol. So avoid eating white bread, sweets, and breakfast cereals or other foods with added sugar. Slow-releasing carbohydrates, on the other hand, provide an 'even keel' of consistent energy. Scientists have investigated exactly what effect different sources of carbohydrates have on blood sugar, energy and mood. In general these are fruit, whole grains, beans, lentils, nuts and seeds; a complete list of these foods is given in Chapter 10. Contrary to the rules of classic food combining (see page 168), recent research has found that eating some protein with carbohydrate provides additional adrenal support by reducing the stimulation of cortisol. So if you are stressed out, eat your fruit with some nuts, or brown rice with fish. Nuts, seeds, beans and lentils already contain both protein and carbohydrate and are therefore good anti-stress foods.

The energy nutrients

Energy nutrients include vitamin B6 and zinc, which help insulin to work; vitamin B3 and chromium, which are part of the glucose-tolerance factor and now available as a complex called chromium polynicotinate; and a whole host of nutrients required to turn glucose within cells into energy. These include vitamins B1, B2, B3 and B5, co-enzyme Q10, vitamin C, iron, copper and magnesium. Vitamin B12 is required to make adrenalin, while B5 (pantothenic acid) is required to make another class of adrenal hormones called glucocorticoids. Muscle and nerve transmission, the end result of turning fuel into energy, requires yet more B5 and large amounts of the semi-essential nutrient choline, plus the minerals calcium and magnesium. Choline is also needed to produce stress hormones. Amino acids, the building blocks of protein, are also the building blocks of stress hormones and neurotransmitters. Methionine, an amino acid that is commonly deficient, is required to make adrenal hormones. Insulin is a complex of fifty-one amino acids and zinc. Adrenalin is synthesised from the amino acids phenylalanine or tyrosine.

The ideal quantity to take in supplement form to provide top-level support for stressed people, and to maximise energy, depends very much on individual circumstances. Optimal daily requirements, however, are likely to be in the ranges shown in the following table.

■ Daily supplement to deal with stress

B1 (thiamine)	25–100mg
B2 (riboflavin)	25–100mg
B3 (niacin)	50–150mg
B5 (pantothenic acid)	50–300mg
B6 (pyridoxine)	50–150mg
B12 (cyanocobalamin)	5–100mcg
Folic acid	50–400mcg
Choline	100–500mg
Co-enzyme Q10	10–50mg
Vitamin C	1,000–5,000mg
Calcium	150–600mg
Magnesium	250–450mg
Iron	10–20mg
Zinc	10–25mg
Chromium	50–200mcg

Stimulants and their alternatives

Consumption of coffee, tea, sugar or chocolate is associated with an increased risk of diabetes. In the short term it may give a boost, but in the long term high stimulant consumption can kill you prematurely. Try this simple experiment. Give up all these stimulants for one month, and notice what happens. The more damage the stimulants are doing to you, the greater the withdrawal effect such as headaches, lack of concentration, fatigue and nausea.

(Fortunately, by eating slow-releasing carbohydrates and taking energy nutrients as supplements you can minimise the withdrawal symptoms, which usually last no more than four days.) Then start again and notice what happens with your first cup of tea or coffee, your first spoonful of sugar or bite of chocolate. You will experience what stress expert Dr Hans Selye called the 'initial response' – in other words a true response to these powerful chemicals (a pounding head, hyperactive mind, fast heartbeat, and insomnia, followed by extreme drowsiness). Keep on the stimulants and you will adapt (phase 2). Keep doing this long enough and eventually you hit exhaustion (phase 3). This happens to everybody. The only variation is how long it will take you to get to the exhaustion phase.

Recovery is not only possible, it is usually rapid. Most people experience substantially more energy and ability to cope with stress within thirty days of cutting out stimulants and simultaneously taking nutritional support. Coffee, tea and chocolate are best omitted from your diet altogether, since even decaffeinated coffee and tea still contain stimulants. Nowadays there are plenty of coffee alternatives and herb and fruit teas. Health food stores also have sugar-free 'sweets' and bars. Check the label for hidden sugar.

It is best to reduce the sugar content of your diet slowly. Gradually get used to less sweetness. For example, sweeten breakfast cereal with fruit. Dilute fruit juices 50:50 with water. Avoid foods with added sugar. Limit your intake of dried fruit. Eat fruits like bananas that contain fast-releasing sugars with slow-releasing carbohydrates such as oats.

Natural stimulants

If you still need a boost, especially during the first week off caffeine, you can do it the natural way. The body makes adrenalin, and its cousins the 'feel-good' neurotransmitters dopamine and noradrenalin, directly from an amino acid called tyrosine. Supplementing 1,000mg of tyrosine on an empty stomach or with some carbohydrate, such as a piece of fruit, gives a positive lift. This is well worth it in the week you're quitting caffeine.

In addition to tyrosine there are a number of 'adaptogenic' herbs. These include Asian ginseng, Siberian ginseng, reishi mushrooms and rhodiola. While rhodiola was a favourite in Siberia, Reishi mushroom is one of the most respected tonics in Chinese medicine. In Asia it has been revered for as long as 5,000 years. These herbs are called adaptogens because they help to even out and maintain normal levels of another energy-giving adrenal hormone called cortisol. These are all available as herbal supplements, and you can also find them combined with tyrosine (see Resources, page 528).

The exercise factor

Exercise plays an essential role in both energy and stress resistance, but it has to be the right kind. Becoming muscle-bound doesn't necessarily enable vital energy to flow easily in the body; nor does an unfit body, or a body full of tension. This tension literally eats up our energy – it takes a lot of energy to keep muscle cells in tension. Conversely, being unfit and overweight places a strain on the body, again depleting vital energy.

Strength, suppleness and stamina

Somewhere in the middle there is an optimal balance where the body is relaxed but strong, supple, with good posture, and sufficiently fit to have the stamina necessary for physical tasks. Remember the three Ss – strength, suppleness and stamina. The body produces energy when carbohydrate foods react with oxygen from the air we breathe. Oxygen is the most vital nutrient of all, yet most of us breathe shallowly and use only a third of our lung capacity. Deeper breathing not only energises the body; it also clears the mind. Mastering the right way to breathe is the first step in most forms of meditation, yoga and t'ai chi. Most types of exercise ignore this, so you get out of breath. The resultant oxygen deficiency allows toxic substances to build up, generating tension in the body. If you feel exhausted or stiff after exercising, something is unbalanced in your exercise programme.

If you could develop stamina, suppleness, strength and a beautiful body by spending fifteen minutes a day on an exercise system that anyone can do anywhere, that leaves you feeling physically energised, emotionally balanced and mentally clear, would you do it? Such an exercise system exists. It is called Psychocalisthenics®, and was developed by Oscar Ichazo, founder of the Arica Institute, a School of Knowledge.* The word means strength (*sthenos*) and beauty (*kallos*) through the breath (*psyche*), and involves a unique series of twenty-two exercises that develop the three Ss and oxygenate the whole body. Psychocalisthenics is suitable for anyone, young or old, and takes only a day to learn. Classes take place all over the UK and US (for details see Resources, page 526), or you can do it by yourself accompanied by a CD or DVD.

Too much exercise can elevate levels of the stress hormone cortisol and is not recommended if you are stressed out. On the other hand, Psychocalisthenics, yoga, t'ai chi, walking for half an hour or meditation can help to rebalance stress hormones.

Meditation is as important to the mind as food is to the body. While food makes the body, thoughts make the mind. For maximum energy, eat pure food and have pure thoughts. Meditation is a time you set aside to sit in silence, focusing on something simple (the breath, a mantra, a prayer), letting go of your endless stream of thoughts and tapping into the source of energy within every human being, from which come creativity, joy, natural humour and lightness.

I like to start each day with fifteen minutes of meditation, followed by fifteen minutes of Psychocalisthenics, followed by Get Up and Go, my special breakfast made from high-energy whole foods plus energy nutrients. (Get

---

*Psychocalisthenics is a registered trademark of Oscar Ichazo. Used by permission.

Up and Go is available from health food stores, or by mail order, see Resources, page 531.) The result is a consistent level of energy and resistance to stress.

Action plan for high-energy living

Before breakfast

- Meditation (fifteen minutes), then Psychocalisthenics, yoga, t'ai chi (fifteen minutes).

Breakfast (never miss it)

- Get Up and Go drink, mixed with berries and soya milk, or oat flakes with fruit and ground seeds.
- One high-strength multivitamin and mineral, one essential Omega 3 plus Omega 6 supplement, 1,000mg vitamin C.

Mid-morning snack

- Fresh organic fruit plus some almonds or seeds.

Lunch

- Lots of raw or lightly cooked vegetables with rice, beans, lentils, quinoa, tofu, buckwheat noodles or fish.
- One high-strength multivitamin and mineral, one essential Omega 3 plus Omega 6 supplement, 1,000mg vitamin C.

Afternoon snack

- Fresh organic fruit plus some almonds or seeds.

After work, every other day

- Thirty minutes' exercise (walking, jogging, swimming, cycling, aerobics).

Dinner (eat early, at least two hours before bedtime)

- Vegetable steam-fry: select from carrots, broccoli, cauliflower, mangetout, broad beans, water chestnuts, soaked almonds, organic or shiitake mushrooms, bamboo shoots, green peppers, courgettes, tofu and braised tofu. Cut into pieces, wash, put in a pan, cover with a tight lid and steam for five minutes maximum. Add one of the following four sauces. Chinese: soy sauce, water, lemon juice, ginger, fresh coriander and garlic. Thai: coconut milk and Thai spices. Mexican: watered down Mexican spice sauce (versions are available in supermarkets, but check chemical additives). Mediterranean: tomato sauce with peppers, mushrooms and herbs. Serve with brown rice, quinoa or buckwheat noodles. Alternatively, use other combinations of raw or lightly cooked vegetables with rice, beans, lentils, quinoa, tofu, buckwheat noodles or fish.

Dig deeper by reading my book *Beat Stress and Fatigue*.

chapter 30

Achieving Peak Physical Performance

No top-class athlete can afford to ignore optimum nutrition. Capable of increasing speed, endurance and strength, the right diet and supplements can mean the difference between winning and losing.

My first experience of the power of optimum nutrition in the context of sport was with Mick Ballard, a veteran cyclist who, after changing his diet and starting to take supplements, broke the record for the ten-mile time trial by an astonishing thirty-seven seconds. 'I'm convinced that my tremendous improvement in times and recovery is due to my special vitamin programme,' said Ballard. Then, at the insistence of her coach, I advised Susan Devoy, rated amongst the top ten women squash players of her day. She did not think it would make any difference. It did. She became the UK and world number 1 for much of the next ten years. Athletes on optimum nutrition programmes consistently report increased endurance and more rapid recovery.

These findings confirm those of Dr Michael Colgan, who advises many US Olympic athletes including US mile record-holder Steve Scott, twice world triathlon champion Julie Moss and Howard Doerffling of the US cycle team. Colgan also found substantial time improvements in controlled trials on long-distance runners.

Muscle power

Optimum nutrition has been shown to increase not only endurance, but also sheer muscle power, as Hollywood actor Sylvester Stallone will testify.

An ardent follower of optimum nutrition, he takes handfuls of supplements every day and watches his diet carefully.

The ability to increase strength is best illustrated in a study by Dr Colgan in which two experienced weightlifters were given a special supplement programme, and another two were given placebos.[21] After three months, those on supplements had increased the maximum weight they could lift by about 50 per cent. The others, on dummy tablets, had only a 10–20 per cent increase. During the following three months the supplements and the placebos were swapped around. Those previously on placebos caught up with the other weightlifters.

The right fuel

Maximising physical performance depends on giving the body the right fuel. During sustained, less strenuous 'aerobic' exercise (jogging, tennis, swimming, walking, for example) carbohydrates yield twice as much energy as fat. During short bursts of strenuous or 'anaerobic' exercise (sprinting, for example) the body can really use only carbohydrate, making carbohydrate yield five times more energy than fat. Carbohydrates, not fat, are the premier fuel for performance. Also, carbohydrates can be stored as glycogen, while fat cannot. Glycogen is a short-term store of energy, held in muscles and the liver, which can be called on during extended physical performance. That is why endurance athletes eat rice or pasta or other complex carbohydrates some hours before an event to increase their glycogen stores.

Contrary to popular opinion, increasing protein intake does not improve athletic performance. Even body-builders who are going for maximum muscle gain need little more than the recommended 15 per cent of total intake of calories in the form of protein. Consider this equation: to gain 9lb (4kg) of muscle in a year requires less than 2lb (less than 1kg) of protein, since muscle is 22 per cent protein. Divide that by 365 days and all you need is ½oz (2.4 g) of protein a day. That is less than a teaspoonful, or the amount provided by a few almonds or a teaspoon of tuna. Difficulty in building muscle is rarely due to a lack of protein and often the result of not taking in enough muscle-building vitamins and minerals such as zinc and vitamin B6, which help to digest and use dietary protein.

While fat is not the best fuel for the body, sources of essential fats have many important benefits for athletes. They help transport oxygen and keep red blood cells, the oxygen-carriers, healthy. They are vital for the immune system, which is often taxed in people who take a great deal of exercise. They are a back-up source of energy and, according to Dr Udo Erasmus, an expert on fat, actually increase metabolic rate. So nuts, seeds and their oils form an important part of a high-performance diet.

Water – the forgotten nutrient

Probably the most important item in the diet of sportsmen and -women is water. Muscles are 75 per cent water. A loss of only 3 per cent of this water causes a 10 per cent drop in strength and an 8 per cent loss of speed. During athletic performance thirst sensors are inhibited, so it is easy for athletes to become dehydrated. This leads to an increase in body temperature, and energy is diverted away from muscles to cool the body down. During endurance sports it is best to drink water to allow the body to sweat and cool down this way. However, it is even more important to hydrate the body in advance by drinking a glass of water every fifteen minutes for one to four hours before the event, depending on its length. Eating plenty of carbohydrate also helps to store water because each unit of carbohydrate, stored as glycogen, is bound with nine units of water. As the glycogen is liberated to provide energy for muscles, so too is the water.

Supplementary benefit

A considerable body of research has produced results that support the benefits of nutrient supplementation in sport. While studies testing single nutrients have often shown little or no effect, multi-nutrient studies using optimal, rather than RDA, levels of nutrients consistently show improvement in athletic performance. As well as vitamins and minerals, semi-essential nutrients such as co-enzyme Q10 are an important part of a winning formula; ideal levels are 60–100mg a day. The ideal amount of each nutrient to take varies from person to person and is likely to be in the same range as those given for maximising energy and reducing stress (see page 260).

However, if you do regular endurance exercise such as running or cycling it is important to increase your intake of antioxidant nutrients such as vitamins A, C and E. These help the body to use oxygen and detoxify the by-products of making energy, which reduces the stress of endurance sports.

Many competitive sports people supplement creatine. Creatine is a substance in the body made of three amino acids – arginine, methionine and glycine. Not surprisingly, meat is naturally rich in it. Creatine is also sold as a supplement, and it's a top seller among sports people because it promotes muscle regeneration and recovery after exercise, as well as improving energy during intensive exercise.

Normally muscle cells derive energy by breaking down ATP (adenosine triphosphate) to ADP. When supplies of ATP are exhausted, for example in a sprint, creatine can quickly replace the phosphate needed to 'reload' the cell. Because muscles can work harder with extra creatine, the extra activity also results in more muscle growth as well as increased muscle size as creatine increases water concentration in muscles. And here's a caution. If you take creatine, it is essential to drink plenty of water, as some people experience high blood pressure if they don't. Others also get diarrhoea. While there is good evidence supporting the fact that creatine can give you the edge, it is ideally suited for athletes participating in sports in which every second counts. To this end you need 2 to 5g a day, although some nutritionists recommend 'loading up' for five days before an event with 20g.

General dietary guidelines for a sportsman or -woman are:

- Eat plenty of complex carbohydrates such as whole grains, fruit, vegetables, beans and lentils, and 'load up' before a long event.

- Have some protein with your carbohydrate foods, e.g. nuts with fruit, fish with rice.

- Avoid eating too much protein, but do make sure you get enough.

- Drink plenty of water before and, where possible, during events.

- Take a personalised supplement programme on an ongoing basis, perhaps with extra co-enzyme Q10.

- Consider creatine if you are competing.

chapter 31.

Turning Back the Clock

The quest for immortality, or at least extended lifespan, is nothing new. Since the beginning of history, myths and legends about magic potions and immensely long-lived people have abounded. Now, however, many scientists and gerontologists (gerontology is the study of ageing) are predicting that a lifespan of 110 years will soon be commonplace.

To date, the oldest person ever recorded is Madame Jeanne Calmant from Arles in France who died in 1997 at the age of 122, thus breaking the record of a Japanese fisherman named Izumi, who died at the age of 120 having been essentially healthy and active until he was 113. A bit of a rogue as far as healthy living is concerned, Madame Calmant was not a health fanatic, gave up smoking at the age of 117 and drank two glasses of port every day until her last decade. With most of her relatives and family living to ripe old ages, scientists think she was genetically strong and maintained a good mental attitude, resisting stress and depression. However, the most significant factor in increasing your chances for a long and healthy life is what you eat – or do not eat.

Preventing premature death

The vast majority of people die from preventable diseases. The US Surgeon General states that 'of the 2.2 million Americans who die each year 1.8 [million] die from diet-related diseases'. Three-quarters of all deaths are caused by cancer, heart disease, bronchial infections, Alzheimer's or accidents. Eradicate these and you instantly extend your probable healthy lifespan by ten to twenty-five years, the key words being 'healthy lifespan'. By preventing these diseases, and all the degenerative changes that lead up to them, through optimum nutrition, you effectively turn back the clock and slow down the ageing process.

However, the challenge that has occupied gerontologists is not how to prevent the diseases responsible for premature ageing and death, but to discover what determines the maximum possible lifespan. Why, for example, can an elephant live a hundred years or more, while insects have a lifespan of days? The big question, of course, is how we can extend the maximum possible lifespan.

Extending your maximum lifespan

While the likely maximum lifespan of a human being is in the region of 110 to 120 years or more, you may be surprised to know that a proven method already exists for extending this length of time. It is, at least, proven in all animal species so far tested, and it is achieved by restricting calorie intake while providing optimum nutrition.

Pioneered by Dr Roy Walford, calorie restriction has been shown to promote health, reduce disease and extend lifespan by 10 to 300 per cent. Studies with fish have achieved a remarkable 300 per cent extension, while with rats the maximum increase has been 60 per cent.[22] Although this effect has been proved in many species by US government-backed research groups it is too soon to complete human trials, but there is little doubt that the same approach will produce results. The unknown factor is: how much calorie restriction, and at what level, is required to produce a result? Even a 10 per cent extension means increasing maximum lifespan to over 130 years – a concept now accepted by many gerontologists, although considered fantasy twenty years ago.

Ongoing research is aimed at discovering why optimum nutrition with calorie restriction is so effective, and the answer to this question, once found, will probably shed light on the process of ageing. Current theories focus on the energy factories within cells, called mitochondria. The mitochondria are responsible for the rate of metabolism or energy production. The harder they work, the more oxidising free radicals are produced (see Chapter 00), which in turn age the mitochondria and have the potential to damage the cell's DNA, the blueprint for new cells.

Ron Hart from the National Institute of Health has demonstrated that the ageing of species is also linked to the ability to repair DNA. According to Professor Denham Harman, from the University of Nebraska Medical School, the 'chances are 99 per cent that free radicals are the basis for ageing'. There is growing consensus that the process of ageing hinges on declining ability to repair the damage caused by free radicals.

This also means that the key to longevity lies in reducing our exposure to free radicals and increasing the body's protection against them by increasing our intake of antioxidants. When animals are given very high-quality, low-calorie diets this is exactly what is achieved. They receive exactly what they need in the way of fuel, so there is no wasted 'burning' by the body – this process is the major generator of free radicals, the toxic by-product of energy metabolism. By being provided with optimum nutrition, especially a high intake of antioxidant nutrients, the animals have both maximum protection from free radicals and all the co-factor nutrients necessary to make sure that energy metabolism takes place as efficiently as possible.

While the roles of antioxidant vitamins A, C and E are well known, there are other important antioxidant nutrients. Two of these are lipoic acid and carnitine. Studies involving the feeding of these to old rats have shown amazing reversals of ageing.[23] Professor Bruce Ames, a molecular biologist at the University of California, who led this research, said of the animals who had been on supplements of lipoic acid plus acetyl-l-carnitine, 'The brain looks better, they are full of energy – everything we looked at looks like a younger animal. It's the equivalent of making a seventy-five- to eighty-year-old person act middle-aged.'

But can we apply all this to humans? To date, the circumstantial evidence is remarkably consistent across a wide variety of species and there is no reason to believe that humanity will be any different. Longevity, or the risk of mortality, correlates very well with blood levels, or dietary intakes of vitamin C, vitamin E, vitamin A and betacarotene.

For example, in a study published in the *American Journal of Clinical Nutrition*, which followed 11,178 people between the ages of 67 and 105 over ten years, the overall risk of death was reduced by 42 per cent for those who took supplements of both vitamin C and vitamin E.[24] This is a remarkable finding that confirms earlier studies. What is not known, however, is how much of the reduction is due to the prevention of premature death from disease and how much to the extension of the maximum lifespan.

In practical terms there is only one way to maximise your lifespan, having reduced the risk of dying prematurely from disease. Restrict calories and nourish yourself optimally, especially where antioxidants are concerned.

Eat less, live longer

It is more than likely that the leaner you are the longer you will live. Calorie restriction, however, is not the same as malnutrition. It is about giving the body exactly what it needs and no more. Many foods in today's diet provide 'empty' calories – sugar or saturated fat, but none of the micronutrients needed to process them. These foods are out if you want to extend your lifespan. Nutrient-dense foods such as organic carrots, apples, nuts and seeds provide as many nutrients as calories plus, in the case of fresh fruit and vegetables, plenty of essential and calorie-free water.

One way to restrict calories is simply to eat less. Another is to fast or have a modified fast one day a week. This may mean, for example, just eating fruit. I keep my overall calorie intake low by eating a substantial breakfast and dinner but a small lunch (sometimes no lunch at all) and snacking on fruit throughout the day. Life insurance companies are well aware of the correlation between weight and longevity. Weight charts give an ideal weight range for your height; generally, the ideal weight for increased life expectancy is at the low end of this range. What really counts is keeping down the percentage of your body weight that consists of fat.

Lower your homocysteine

Ageing isn't determined just by oxidation, which damages cells. It's also determined by methylation. This fundamental process, explained in Chapter 16, is vital for repairing DNA in your cells and picking up the right information in the first place. How good you are at methylation, which is best reflected by measuring your homocysteine level, determines how long you'll live.

In Chapter 16 I told you about the extraordinary findings of a comprehensive research study at the University of Bergen in Norway, published in 2001.[25] The researchers measured the homocysteine levels of 4,766 men and women, aged 65 to 67 in 1992, and then recorded any deaths over the next five years, during which 162 men and 97 women died. They then looked at the risk of death in relation to their homocysteine levels. They discovered that 'a strong relation was found between homocysteine and *all* causes of mortality'. In other words, homocysteine is an accurate predictor of death, whatever the cause.

What they found was that the chances of a person of 65 to 67 years dying from any cause increased by almost 50 per cent for every 5-unit increase in homocysteine! This strongly reflects how central homocysteine and methylation are to the underlying causes of the common diseases that kill most of us prematurely in the twenty-first century. Turn this equation around and what it suggests is that if, for example, your H score was 15, and you drop it to 6 units or less and maintain it there, you can probably add around ten years to your life! And it will be a lively decade because, as you will see, if you lower your homocysteine level below 6 units with the proper balance of diet and supplementation, and alleviate your methylation problems, your cells will age more slowly, you'll have increased vitality and you'll feel younger than your years. In practical terms this means eating more greens and beans and supplementing B vitamins. See Chapter 16 for the full strategy for keeping your hymocysteine score low.

Exercise keeps you young

Regular exercise can add seven years to your lifespan, conclude Dr Rose and Dr Cohen of the Veterans' Administration Hospital in Boston. But the exercise must be continued late into life and must be aerobic – that is, your heart rate must reach 80 per cent of its maximum for at least twenty minutes. Cycling, swimming and running are good; weightlifting and strengthening exercises, on the other hand, do little to extend your life. Aerobic exercise reduces blood cholesterol levels, pulse rate and blood pressure, promoting better cardiovascular health as well as increasing mental function. It also helps you to maintain proper blood sugar control and is therefore especially helpful for diabetics.

Keeping cool

One method of extending lifespan in animals has yet to prove practical or popular: it involves lowering the body temperature. Certain drugs have the ability to do this, but have undesirable side effects.

Keeping cool in terms of avoiding stress, however, may prove to be an important life-extension factor. Prolonged stress causes depletion of the adrenal hormone DHEA. Low DHEA levels are associated with an increased risk of many killers, including Alzheimer's, cancer and heart disease, and of ageing in general. DHEA also helps the body to burn fat and stay lean. DHEA levels, if low, can be restored by supplementation. Nutrition consultants can determine your DHEA status through analysis of saliva samples. Although freely available in the US, DHEA is not available over the counter in the UK, where it is classified as a medicine.

In summary, if you want to maximise your healthy lifespan:

● Follow all the advice in this book for preventing killer diseases.

● Ensure optimum nutrition through diet plus supplements.

● Stay away from avoidable sources of free radicals – fried or browned food, exhaust fumes, smoke, strong sunlight and so on.

- Eat plenty of antioxidant-rich fruit and vegetables.

- Take extra antioxidant nutrients – including vitamins A, C and E, selenium and zinc, plus lipoic acid and acetyl-l-carnitine.

- Eat plenty of greens and beans.

- Supplement B vitamins.

- Reduce your calorie intake to exactly what you need to stay fit and healthy.

- Keep fit with a moderate (not excessive) amount of aerobic exercise.

- Avoid stress.

- Have your DHEA levels checked if you are over 50.

chapter 32

Conquering Cancer

C ancer is the second greatest cause of death in the Western world. In the UK one in three people is diagnosed with cancer during their life and one in four currently dies from it. Cancer occurs when cells start to behave differently, growing, multiplying and spreading. It is like a revolution in the body, where a group of cells stop working for the good of the whole and run riot. The odd revolutionary cell is a common occurrence and the body's immune system isolates and destroys such offenders. However, in cancer, the immune system is overcome and the damage spreads.

Yet it may surprise you to know that cancer is, for the large part, a twentieth-century invention. The top five cancers – lung, breast, stomach, colorectal and prostate – were basically unheard of before the beginning of the twentieth century. The growth in the incidence of cancer parallels the industrialisation and chemicalisation of our world. The more developed a country, the more prevalent is cancer. The higher the income per capita, the higher the incidence of cancer.[26]

Conventional treatments see cancer very much as the enemy and cut it out, burn it out through radiation or drug it out with chemotherapy. All these treatments weaken the body. Advances in them only concern less damaging ways of applying them and cannot be considered breakthroughs. Although 'five-year survival rates' have slightly improved, this is more due to more advanced methods of detection rather than to successful treatment.

What causes cancer?

Most cancers are primarily the result of changes that humans have made to the total chemical environment – what we eat, drink and breathe. According to one of Britain's top medical scientists, Sir Richard Doll, 90 per cent of all cancers are caused by such environmental factors. At least 75 per cent of cancers are associated with environmental and lifestyle factors, say even the most conservative cancer experts.

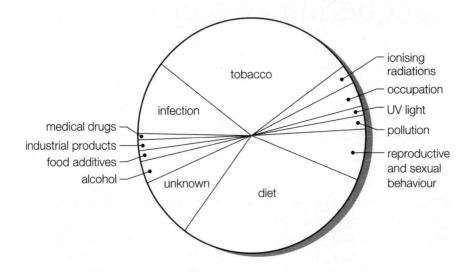

What causes cancer?

In the space of two generations, we have invented ten million new chemicals and unwittingly released thousands of them into the environment. What's more, our diet and lifestyle have exposed us to many more, from oxidants in cigarettes to the tumour-promoter 'IGF1', in cow's milk. Many are known as carcinogens, that is they are capable of causing cancer; others are cancer-promoters, that is they may not cause cancer but they accelerate its growth. We take in these substances in our food, air and water. Many are easily avoidable – but some are not.

We have, it seems, been unwittingly digging our own graves with a knife and fork. Today's diet, laced with chemicals and devoid of nutrients as a result of food-refining, is now thought to be the greatest single contributor to cancer risk. Conversely, by eating the right diet you can cut your risk of cancer by up to 40 per cent, says the World Cancer Research Fund, having reviewed some 5,000 studies linking diet and cancer.[27] The European Commission has estimated that a quarter of a million lives could be saved each year across the original twelve member states through dietary changes alone. According to the Cancer Research Campaign, 'At least three out of four of all cancers are potentially preventable, but will only be avoided if the messages get through at a young age.' Meanwhile, in the US, according to a statement issued by sixty-nine highly respected and prominent medical and scientific experts, 'Over the last decade some five million Americans died of cancer and there is growing evidence that a substantial proportion of these deaths were avoidable.'[28]

An area where considerable advances have been made, however, is in understanding the underlying causes and risks for many types of cancer. At least 85 per cent of cancers are associated with lifestyle factors including diet, smoking and drinking alcohol. This figure has been arrived at from both ends, so to speak – firstly by looking at the link between cancer and causative agents, and secondly by looking at identical twins to see whether they get the same cancers. The twin research has shown clearly that no more than 15 per cent of cancers are considered to be inherited, some part of which is our genetic inheritance. This is not to say, however, that 15 per cent of cancer cases are genetic. Even people with 'cancer genes', such as the BCRA1 gene for breast cancer, won't develop cancer without the environmental insults that tip the scales from healthy into abnormal cell growth. Other risk factors include hormonal imbalance, often induced by exposure to hormone-disrupting chemicals such as HRT, exposure to radiation or ultraviolet light, pollution, food additives, drugs and infections.

However, of all risk factors diet is the greatest, a fact that is backed up by the great progress being made in both the treatment and the prevention of cancer with nutritional therapy. This is because an underlying cause in many types of cancer seems to be one of three things:

- Free-radical damage to the DNA of cells, triggering their altered behaviour, or exposure to hormone-disrupting chemicals. Risk factors such as smoking and radiation encourage free-radical activity, while a good intake of antioxidant nutrients from fruit, vegetables and also antioxidant supplements provides a measure of protection.

- Over-exposure to hormone-disrupting chemicals in food and water. Eating a diet low in hormone-disrupting chemicals and high in phytoestrogens is another important protection factor, especially for hormonal cancers such as breast and prostate.

- Poor methylation, resulting in high homocysteine and increased damage to DNA. The solution to this is more B vitamins.

Let's explore these three underlying causes.

Antioxidant protection

While there was already substantial evidence a decade ago of the protective effect of antioxidant nutrients vitamin A, betacarotene, C and E vitamins and selenium against certain types of cancer in animals, as every year unfolds we are seeing data from long-term human trials that support the role of nutritional therapy. We have also learnt how nutrients work in synergy to disarm oxidants against cancer (see Chapter 15) and hence protect against cancer.

High levels of vitamin A (retinol) in the blood have long been associated with reduced risk. Recent research has shown that two metabolites of retinol, 13-cis-retinoic acid and trans-retinoic acid, are powerful anti-cancer agents. A study by Dr Huang found that trans-retinoic acid puts acute myeloid leukaemia into complete remission.[29] Another study, by Dr Wann Ki Hong and Dr Scott M. Lippman, found that 13-cis-retinoic acid suppressed carcinomas of the neck and head.[30] They gave forty-nine patients 13-cis-retinoic acid, and after a year only 4 per cent had developed another tumour, compared with 24 per cent of fifty-one patients on a placebo.

Betacarotene, which can be converted into vitamin A, is also anti-cancer. A Japanese study involving 265,000 people found a significant correlation between low betacarotene intake and the incidence of lung cancer.[31] In fact, the risk of lung cancer was the same for those who smoked and has good antioxidant levels as it was for non-smokers with low antioxidant levels.

Betacarotene – does it prevent or promote cancer?

While almost all studies involving dietary betacarotene and cancer have proven its protective effect, and while the vast majority of studies involving using betacarotene supplements have either proven it to be positive or ineffective, but not harmful, three studies *have* found an increased risk of cancer with betacarotene. One study by the National Cancer Institute gave smokers betacarotene and reported a 28 per cent increase in the incidence of lung cancer.[32] Confusing, isn't it? A closer look at the figures shows that this 'trend', which sounded dramatic, represented the difference between five cases of cancer in a thousand people and six in a thousand people – people who had smoked for years and probably had undetected cancer before starting the trial. Hidden in the figures was an unreported finding. Among those who gave up smoking during the trial and took betacarotene there were 20 per cent fewer cases of lung cancer. Does this mean that betacarotene has moral powers and gives smokers cancer but protects those who give up? In truth, what it shows is that giving one antioxidant on its own to smokers, ignoring the principle of synergy, could make matters slightly worse, not better.

The other study that found a trend towards increased risk gave male smokers vitamin E, vitamin E and betacarotene, or betacarotene on its own. The first two groups showed no significant change, but the betacarotene-only group showed an increased risk.[33] Why? A recent trial, published by the National Cancer Institute, may shed some light on this.

In this trial people with a history of colorectal adenomas were given 25mg of betacarotene and/or both 100mg of vitamin C and 400mg of vitamin E, versus placebo. While there was less recurrence of colorectal adenomas in those who took either the betacarotene or vitamins C and E or both, there was a modest increase in cancer recurrence among those who took only betacarotene supplements and both smoked and drank alcohol every day.[34]

My instinct tells me that what these studies are showing is that the oxidants in cigarettes are oxidising betacarotene and, in the absence of other synergistic vitamins such as vitamins C and E, this does more harm than good. My advice is not to take betacarotene on its own if you are a heavy smoker or drinker – and to stop smoking and drinking! Many other studies that have either given betacarotene supplements with other antioxidants, or provided it through betacarotene-rich food, which naturally contains other antioxidants, show clear reduction of cancer risk. Even among smokers a high dietary intake of betacarotene is not associated with increased risk.[35] So, keep eating the carrots!

Cancer patients live four times longer on vitamin C

Nobel laureate Dr Linus Pauling and cancer expert Dr Ewan Cameron first demonstrated vitamin C's amazing anti-cancer properties in the 1960s. They gave terminally-ill cancer patients 10 grams a day and showed that they lived four times longer than patients not on vitamin C.[36] Many studies have since been performed.

A review of vitamin C research concluded that 'evidence of a protective effect of vitamin C for non-hormone cancers is very strong. Of the forty-six studies in which a dietary vitamin C index was calculated, thirty-three found statistically significant protection.' These kinds of strong associations are being confirmed the world over. When Dr Gladys Block, from the University of California, looked at a grand total of ninety studies, she came to the conclusion that the evidence was strong for a protective effect against cancers of the mouth, oesophagus, stomach and pancreas, and substantial for colorectal, breast and lung cancers.[37] The evidence for a protective effect against prostate cancer, however, is not strong.

As well as being an antioxidant and able to disarm free radicals, vitamin C can disarm a number of other carcinogens (cancer-causing agents), such as nitrosamines. These can occur when chemicals called nitrates combine with amines. Nitrate levels are high in vegetables grown with nitrate-based fertilisers, as well as in water, owing to soil residues leaching into water sources. Nitrates are also added to some cured meats such as ham, sausages, bacon and pies. Seventy per cent of our intake comes from vegetables grown with artificial fertilisers, 21 per cent from water and 6 per cent from meat. Vitamin C may be especially effective against cancers of the digestive tract because of its ability to disarm these carcinogens, as well as its proven immune-boosting properties.

The synergy of vitamins C and E and selenium

A ten-year study on over 11,000 people, completed in 1996, found that those who supplemented both the antioxidants vitamin C and vitamin E halved their overall risk of death from all cancers and heart disease.[38] Vitamin C is water-soluble, while vitamin E is fat-soluble. Together they can protect the tissues and fluids in the body. What is more, when vitamin C has disarmed a carcinogen it can be reloaded by vitamin E, and vice versa, so their combined presence in diet and in the body has a synergistic effect. Vitamin E is a powerful anti-cancer agent, especially in combination with selenium. While high blood levels of vitamin E alone are associated with a significant reduction in cancer risk, studies in Finland by Dr Jukka Salonen found that combined low levels of vitamin E and selenium increase cancer risk more than ten times.[39]

The mineral selenium has long been known to protect against cancer. Studies in the region of Quidong in China, where liver cancer rates are among the highest in the world, have found a strong correlation between low selenium intake and cancer risk, with other risk factors being hepatitis B infection, exposure to the dietary carcinogen aflatoxin and a genetic predisposition.[40] The researchers then began a large-scale selenium study in which an entire village of 20,000 people took a selenium supplement, which was added to their salt. In the following years there was a significant drop in the incidence of both hepatitis B and liver cancer. Professor Gerhard Schrauzer, an expert on selenium and cancer, recommends a supplement of 200–300mcg of selenium for those who want optimal protection.

■ Which nutrient for which type of cancer?

The following antioxidant vitamins and minerals have so far been proved effective in medical research against the types of cancer indicated.

Type	Vitamin A	Betacarotene	Vitamin C	Vitamin E	Selenium
Bladder		*			*
Breast		*	*	*	*
Cervix	*		*	*	*
Colon	*	*	*		*
Head and neck	*	*			
HIV-related			*		
Kidney			*		
Leukaemia			*		*
Liver					*
Lung	*	*	*	*	
Lymphoma	*				
Oesophagus			*		*
Oral	*	*	*		*
Pancreas			*		
Prostate	*				*
Skin	*		*		*
Stomach	*		*	*	*

As you might expect, supplementing all these cancer-protective nutrients reduces risk. French researchers at the Scientific and Technical Institute for Nutrition and Diet in Paris carried out a large study involving 13,000 men and women between the ages of thirty-five and sixty to investigate the effects of a pill containing a number of antioxidant vitamins and minerals.

Half the study volunteers were given a placebo pill and the other half were give a supplement pill containing small amounts of betacarotene (6mg), vitamin C (120mg), vitamin E (30mg), selenium (100mcg) and zinc (20mg). The participants were followed up over a seven-and-a-half-year period. Over the course of the follow-up, 103 men and 71 women died. Cancer affected 562 people and was the major cause of death. There was a highly significant 31 per cent reduction in the risk of all cancers in men, plus the overall death rate in men was 37 per cent lower in those taking the supplement. Surprisingly the results weren't statistically significant for women. It isn't clear exactly why only men seemed to benefit from the supplements, although it's suggested that perhaps they had a poorer diet to start with. Another explanation is that cancer in women (they were affected primarily by breast cancer) may not be so responsive to antioxidant intake.[41]

Hormone-related cancers

While antioxidant nutrients have a protective effect in many cancers, free-radical damage is unlikely to be the major cause in all of them. Evidence is accumulating that the high incidence of cancer of the breast and ovaries in women, and of the prostate and testes in men, may be related to disturbed hormone signals in the body. All of these body tissues are sensitive to hormones and hormone-disrupting chemicals, and excess oestrogen, a hormone that stimulates cell growth, may play a key role in these cancers.

Research shows that if oestrogen levels are increased, the proliferation rate of breast cells increases by over 200 per cent, more than twice the normal rate. On the other hand, if progesterone is given and the level in breast tissue is raised to normal levels, the rate of cell multiplication falls to 15 per cent of that in untreated women.[42]

This study, undertaken on healthy, pre-menopausal women, shows that oestrogen will promote the proliferation of breast cancers, while progesterone is protective. This may explain why the risk of breast cancer doubles for women who take oestrogen HRT for five or more years and why the risk of ovarian cancer is 72 per cent higher in women given oestrogen HRT, according to a 1995 study by the Emery University School of Public Health, which followed 240,000 women over eight years.[43]

On the basis of this and many other studies, I've been advising women for the past decade not to have HRT. However, it wasn't until the 'million women study', published in the British Medical Journal in 2002, confirmed a doubling of breast-cancer risk that HRT was effectively banned for the treatment of osteoporosis. This study, involving 1,084,110 women in Britain, confirmed that the risk of invasive breast cancer among HRT users goes up by 66 per cent and that the risk of death goes up by 22 per cent. The biggest risk by far was seen in women on combined oestrogen/progestin HRT preparations. In these women the incidence of breast cancer doubled, compared with a 30 per cent increase among those on oestrogen-only HRT, which is generally given only to women who have had a hysterectomy since oestrogen given on its own increases the risk of womb cancer. The researchers estimate that in Britain alone, the use of HRT by women aged fifty to sixty-four has resulted in an estimated 20,000 extra cases of breast cancer in the last decade alone![44]

The increased incidence of hormone-related cancers cannot, however, be attributed solely to oestrogen dominance due to HRT, especially in men, for whom prostate cancer is the fifth-largest cause of death, affecting one in ten men. Hormone expert Dr John Lee believes that many factors are contributing to oestrogen dominance and progesterone deficiency, which in his opinion is the major cause of these cancers. 'Stress, for example, raises cortisol which competes with progesterone. Xenoestrogens from the environment have the ability to damage tissue and this leads to increased cancer in later life. There are also nutritional and genetic factors to consider.' He recommends a plant-based diet, excluding sources of oestrogen such as meat and milk, high consumption of which is strongly associated with increased cancer incidence, particularly of the colon, breast and prostate.

Countries that have low or no consumption of dairy produce and the meat of dairy animals have remarkably low incidences of both breast and prostate cancer, as well as other hormone-related cancers. The fact that the incidence of breast cancer in China is 1 in 100,000 women, compared with our incidence of 1 in 10 women, and that prostate cancer, which affects 1 in 7 men in Britain, is virtually unheard of in China, points a strong finger at diet. The major difference between diets in Western countries and China is that the Chinese do not consume dairy produce or meat from dairy animals, and eat more fruit and vegetables and more beans, especially soya.

In case you are wondering whether there's something inherently different in Asian people, their risk goes up when they immigrate to the US or the UK. Within three generations their risk, and presumably their diet, becomes just as bad.

The other possible causes of cancer are hormone-disrupting chemicals. We've invented some 100,000 of them, 30,000 of which are in use in foods, food packaging, household products, toiletries and industry. Some of these damage DNA, some disrupt hormone signals and some mimic oestrogen. These xenoestrogens from the environment come from pesticide residues, industrial residues and plastics, which contaminate water and get into the food chain. Even cosmetics, skin products and your sofa may be a problem! A recent study found parabens, used in underarm deodorants, present in breast tumours and there is now clear evidence that widely used flame-retardants, called PBDEs (polybrominated di-ephenyl ethers), required on many fabric-covered furnitures, are carcinogenic. Research has shown that the combination of tiny amounts of these hormone-disrupting chemicals, equivalent to the levels found in human blood, are carcinogenic and trigger breast cells to proliferate.

The first step is to avoid sources of hormone-disrupting chemicals as much as possible. This means eating organic and drinking pure water (mineral water, filtered water or distilled water). As far as diet is concerned, my advice is to also to avoid fried, browned and burnt foods, which are sources of free radicals; to cut out or cut down on meat, especially beef, and milk, which are sources of natural oestrogen and IGF1, a hormone-disruptor that is becoming strongly linked to both breast and prostate cancer.

Other possible steps are to avoid HRT containing either oestrogens or synthetic progestins. Natural progesterone, however, helps to counter the potentially damaging effects of oestrogen. Under medical guidance, progesterone, which is given as a transdermal skin cream, can both help to balance hormones and reverse cancer risk.[45]

Homocysteine and cancer

If oxidation is one of the principal ways in which DNA becomes damaged, high homocysteine and associated abnormal methylation is another (see Chapter 16). DNA is always being damaged, often by oxidants, and therefore needs to be constantly repaired. It also needs to be copied, encoding new cells that we make at an extraordinary rate of tens of millions per minute. Methylation controls both the synthesis and the repair of DNA, putting homocysteine, and the key homocysteine-lowering nutrients such as B12, folate, vitamin B6, B2 and TMG smack in the middle of the whole cancer process. Any lack of these B vitamins is already well established to increase the risk of certain cancers.

Does a high hymocysteine score increase your risk for cancer? This is a key question and one that is only starting to be explored. As in the case of heart disease, having accurate markers for cancer helps in its diagnosis, prevention and treatment. Such markers can not only identify someone at risk, but also encourage immediate preventive steps and even measure the success of a cancer treatment.

Dr Lily L. Wu and colleagues at the University of Utah's Health Science Center wondered whether homocysteine might act as a tumour marker, so they decided to measure homocysteine along with other known tumour markers in cancer patients undergoing treatment.[46]

They found that when the other tumour markers went up, the homocysteine went up, and when the tumour markers went down, the homocysteine went down. They also observed that homocysteine proved to be a better marker than the other more conventional indicators. Remarkably, homocysteine levels also reflected much more accurately whether cancer therapy was going successfully or not. If the cancer was growing larger and therefore not responding to therapy, homocysteine increased at the same time; if the cancer was becoming smaller with therapy, homocysteine levels also decreased. Among the tumour markers, only homocysteine revealed the success of cancer therapy in this way. Although it's in the early days of research, this study certainly indicates that homocysteine levels may prove to be a very useful indicator of the existence of cancer as well as of the success or failure of cancer therapies.

To date, the cancers most associated with high homocysteine are skin cancer, leukaemia, dysplasia, colon cancer and, to a lesser extent, breast cancer. It is well known that colon-cancer risk is strongly linked to a poor diet – diets high in cooked, especially burnt, meat and low in fibre, fruit and vegetables – but that taking in large amounts of folate, a key nutrient in vegetables, is highly protective.[47] It is highly likely that, as the spotlight focuses in on homocysteine as the marker for methylation problems, and with methylation problems being seen as part of the root cause of many cancers, we will start to see an association between homocysteine and many different types of cancer.

For now, we can only say that there is reasonable evidence that having a high homocysteine level increases cancer risk, especially of colon cancer, skin cancer, leukaemia and the dysplasias, including cervical dysplasia. For these cancers, and probably others, an optimal diet plus supplements may reduce risk.

Cancer-fighting foods

Eating certain kinds of foods is associated with a decreased risk of cancer. While the evidence accumulates, adding the following foods to your diet cannot hurt, and is likely to help.

- Fruit and vegetables are top of the anti-cancer foods. These are good sources of vitamins A and C. A study in Japan on 265,000 people found that those with a low intake of betacarotene, which is found in fruit and vegetables, had a high risk of lung cancer.[48] Other studies have produced the same result for colon, stomach, prostate and cervical cancers. Betacarotene is found in particularly large amounts in carrots, broccoli, sweet potatoes, cantaloupe melons and apricots. There is lots of vitamin C in fresh vegetables and fruit.

- Garlic, used liberally, may keep cancer away. A National Cancer Institute study carried out in China in 1989 discovered that provinces where garlic was used liberally in their cooking had the lowest rate of stomach cancer.[49] Garlic contains sulphur compounds that help deal with toxins and free radicals.

- Soya beans have been associated with a lower risk of breast cancer. In Japan and China, women who get most of their protein from soya bean foods – tofu, soya beans themselves and soya milk – have lower rates of breast cancer. These results have been confirmed in animal studies. A list of phytoestrogen-rich foods is given in Part 9.

- Yoghurt may protect against colon cancer. The bacterium *Lactobacillus acidophilus*, found in many live yoghurts, slows down the development of colon tumours, and yoghurt-eaters have a lower incidence of colon cancer than those who do not eat yoghurt, as do those whose calcium intake is high.[50] Abnormal cell divisions in the colon have also been shown to slow right down when calcium intake is increased to 2,000mg a day. Of course, non-dairy yoghurt would be best.

- Sesame and sunflower seeds are rich in selenium, vitamin E, calcium and zinc. Eat a spoonful every day to keep your antioxidant army in top condition.

Dig deeper by reading my book *Say No to Cancer*.

chapter) **33.**

Fighting Infections Naturally

Prevention is better than cure and, as Louis Pasteur said on his deathbed, the host is more important than the invader. Medical scientists are increasingly finding that we succumb to bugs only when we are run down, so your best line of defence is to keep your immune system strong so that it is ready to attack when an invader comes along (read Chapter 24 on boosting the immune system). Invaders come in many shapes and sizes: there are bacteria, viruses and fungi, as well as parasites. It is important to know which you are dealing with, as each requires slightly different treatment. A cold, flu, herpes and measles are all viruses. Most ear infections, stomach aches and chest and sinus infections (usually a follow-on to a cold) are bacterial. Thrush and athlete's foot are fungal infections.

Immune-boosting nutrients are good all year round, especially if you are run down or exposed to people with infections. During an infection both the invader and our own immune army produce free radicals to destroy each other. We can mine-sweep these dangerous chemicals with antioxidant nutrients, which are good for everybody at any time. Anti-viral, anti-bacterial and anti-fungal agents are best increased when dealing with a specific invader. Judging by the results of research on vitamin C, it would be wrong to believe that immune-healthy people get no infections. They just have 'pre-colds' that are all over in twenty-four hours, where less healthy people end up horizontal for a week. So the aim is to boost your immune system by giving it the right food and the right environment, so that it can adapt quickly to attempted invasions.

While vitamin C's main strength is against viruses, grapefruit seed extract, for example, is anti-bacterial or 'antibiotic'. The table below shows which natural remedies work best against different kinds of invaders (see also the A to Z of natural infection-fighters on page 291).

■ **Which invaders, which natural remedy?**

Nutrients	Antioxidants	Immune boosters	Anti-viral	Anti-bacterial
Vitamin A	✳	✳	✳	
Betacarotene	✳	✳	✳	
Vitamin C	✳	✳	✳	✳
Vitamin E	✳	✳		
Selenium	✳	✳		
Zinc	✳	✳	✳	
Iron	✳	✳		
Manganese	✳			
Copper	✳			
B vitamins	✳	✳		
L cysteine	✳			
N-a-cysteine	✳			
Glutathione	✳			
Lysine			✳	
Aloe vera		✳	✳	✳
Astragalus	✳	✳		
'Power' mushrooms		✳	✳	
Echinacea		✳	✳	
St John's wort		✳		✳
Garlic	✳	✳	✳	✳
Grapefruit seed			✳	✳
Silver			✳	✳
Tea tree				✳
Artemisia				✳
Bee pollen				✳
Cat's claw	✳	✳	✳	
Goldenseal				✳

Get in fast

The best form of defence is attack, and the quicker you get in there the more chance you have of restoring your health before an infection sets in. All invaders produce toxins as part of their weapons of war. If you wake up feeling more tired than usual, perhaps with bloodshot eyes, a slight headache, itchy throat, slightly blocked nose or foggy brain – and you haven't been drinking the night before – you are probably under attack! Just as when you have consumed alcohol, these are signs that your body is trying to eliminate an undesirable agent. If the war is raging, turn up the heat.

The immune system works best in a warm environment, which is why the body creates a fever to turn up the temperature. So keep yourself warm and get plenty of rest. One day taking it easy can make all the difference, especially if you boost your immune army with natural remedies. Lack of sleep depletes your energy reserves. Also avoid all the other ways in which we habitually dissipate energy: alcohol consumption, exposure to smoky atmospheres, strong sunlight and stress, overeating, engaging in arguments, over-exertion, having sex and taking antibiotics. You can tilt the balance in your favour by reducing these energy-robbers.

There is some truth in the old wives' saying 'Starve a fever, feed a cold'. During an infection listen to your body. It is fine not to eat for a day, but if an infection goes on for a long time your immune system does need a number of nutrients, plus protein, to replenish the troops. It is best to eat lightly – small meals made from high-energy natural foods, raw or lightly cooked. During an infection the body fights hard to eliminate the waste products of war, so drink plenty of water or herb tea to help your body detoxify and reduce mucus. Avoid salt and mucus-forming and fatty foods, such as meat, eggs and dairy produce.

How to kill a cold

There is some dispute among nutritionists about the effect of vitamin C on the common cold. At an amount below 1 gram of vitamin C a day there is little evidence of substantial reduction in colds. At 1 gram a day some studies show fewer colds, and most studies show shorter or less severe colds.[51] I estimate that the optimal daily intake of vitamin C for cold prevention, especially if you are over forty, have a stressful lifestyle, live in a city and meet lots of people, is 2 grams a day.

While 1 or 2 grams of vitamin C a day helps to reduce the severity and incidence of colds, achieving 'tissue saturation' during a cold has even greater results. In order to take hold, a cold virus must get inside cells and reprogramme them to make more cold viruses, which then infect other cells. However, if the body's tissues are high in vitamin C the virus cannot survive. Tissue saturation is more likely to be achieved by taking in around 10–15 grams a day, or 2 grams every four hours, which is 250 times the RDA! Fortunately, vitamin C is one of the least toxic substances known to man. A daily intake of 2–3 grams, spread out through the day, may be sufficient to maintain a high level of immune protection.

Viruses get into body cells by puncturing their walls with tiny spikes made of a substance called hemagglutinin. According to research by virologist Madeleine Mumcuoglu, working with Dr Jean Linderman, who discovered interferon, an extract of elderberry disarms these spikes by binding to them and preventing them from penetrating the cell membrane.[52] 'This was the first discovery,' says Mumcuoglu. 'Later I found evidence that elderberry also fights flu virus in other ways. Viral spikes are covered with an enzyme called neuraminidase, which helps break down the cell wall. The elderberry inhibits the action of that enzyme. My guess is that we'll find elderberry acts against viruses in other ways as well.'

In a double-blind controlled trial she tested the effects of the elderberry extract on people diagnosed with any one of a number of strains of flu virus. The results, published in 1995, showed a significant improvement in symptoms – fever, cough, muscle pain – in 20 per cent of patients within twenty-four hours, and in a further 73 per cent of patients within forty-eight hours. After three days 90 per cent had complete relief from their symptoms compared with another group on a placebo, who look at least six days to recover. While this is the first published trial of elderberry extract, I have heard many success stories from my clients who have successfully speeded up recovery from colds and flu by taking elderberry extract.

Immune-boosting herbs

More and more immune-boosting herbs are being discovered to help fight infections. Four excellent ones, covered in greater detail in the list below, are cat's claw, echinacea, garlic and grapefruit seed extract. Cat's-claw tea tastes good with added blackcurrant and apple concentrate, and one cup a day helps maintain immune power. If you have a sore throat or stomach upset, add four slices of root ginger. Echinacea is the original Native American snakeroot, which later became known as snake oil. The great advantage of grapefruit seed extract is that it has a similar effect to antibiotics but without damaging beneficial gut bacteria as conventional antibiotics do. Even if you are taking probiotics like acidophilus it is best to take them separately from grapefruit seed extract.

In summary, the following steps will help you to fight an infection (for more specific information on dosages see the list further below):

● Eat lightly, making sure you get enough protein, which is needed to build immune cells, and keep warm. If you have a mucus-related infection, avoid dairy products.

- Increase your intake of vitamin C to 3 grams every four hours.

- Drink cat's-claw tea and consider adding ginger and echinacea drops and taking garlic capsules or cloves.

- If you have a cold, take one dessertspoon of Sambucol four times a day.

- If you have a bacterial, fungal or parasitical infection take ten drops of grapefruit seed extract (citricidal) two or three times a day.

- Find out what your infection is and, if necessary see your doctor, especially if you are not better within five days.

- Consider other remedies in the A to Z of natural infection fighters below.

A to Z of natural infection-fighters

Two doses are given below: the first for pulling out the plug when under attack, the second for general maintenance. Once an invasion is over, wait forty-eight hours before going on to the maintenance dose. Some natural remedies have no maintenance dose and are recommended only to fight an infection.

Vitamin A

Vitamin A is one of the key immune-boosting nutrients. It helps to strengthen the skin, inside and out, and therefore acts as a first line of defence, keeping the lungs, digestive tract and skin intact. By strengthening cell walls it keep viruses out. Vitamin A can be toxic in large doses, so levels above 3,000mcg are recommended only on a short-term basis.

Fighting infections 3,000 to 7,500mcg (one week only) a day.
   Maintenance 2,250mcg a day.

Aloe vera

Has immune-boosting, anti-viral and antiseptic properties. It is a good all-round tonic, as well as a booster during any infection. Daily dose as instructed on the bottle.

Antioxidants

Substances that detoxify free radicals. These include vitamins A, C, E and betacarotene, zinc, selenium and many other non-essential substances, including silymarin (milk thistle), pycnogenol, lipoic acid, bioflavonoids and bilberry extract. It is best to take an all-round antioxidant supplement during any infection.

Artemisia

A natural anti-fungal, anti-parasitical and anti-bacterial agent, often used alongside caprylic acid for the treatment of candidiasis or thrush.

Fighting infections **100 to 1,000mg a day.**

Astragalus

A Chinese herb renowned for all-round immunity boosting. It is high in beneficial mucopolysaccharides.

Fighting infections **1 to 3 grams a day.**
    Maintenance 200mg a day.

Betacarotene

The vegetable source of vitamin A and an antioxidant in its own right. Red, orange and yellow foods and fresh vegetables are the best sources. Drinking carrot or watermelon juice is a great way to boost your levels of this all-round infection-fighter.

Fighting infections **3,000 to 7,500mcgREs a day.**
    Maintenance 2,500mcgREs a day.

Vitamin C

Vitamin C is an incredible anti-viral agent. Viruses cannot survive in a vitamin C-rich environment. To achieve this you need to take 3 grams of vitamin C immediately and then 2 grams every four hours. Alternatively, mix 6 to 10 grams of vitamin C powder in fruit juice diluted with water and drink throughout the day. Vitamin C is non-toxic but too much can cause loose bowels. Decrease the dose if this becomes unacceptable.

Fighting infections **6 to 10 grams a day.**
    Maintenance 1 (1,000mg)–3 grams a day.

Bee pollen

A natural antibiotic. It is probably better as a general tonic than as a specific treatment. Be careful if you are pollen-sensitive.

Fighting infections **1 to 2 dessertspoons a day.**
 Maintenance 1 teaspoon a day.

Caprylic acid

An anti-fungal agent derived from coconuts, primarily used for eliminating the *Candida albicans* organism responsible for thrush. Anti-candida programmes are best carried out under the supervision of a qualified nutrition consultant.

Fighting infections **1 to 3 grams a day.**

Cat's claw

A powerful anti-viral, antioxidant and immune-boosting agent from the Peruvian rainforest plant *Uncaria tomentosa*. It contains chemicals called alkaloids, one of which is isopteridin, which has been proved to boost immune function. It is available as a tea or in supplements.

Fighting infections **2 to 6 grams a day.**
 Maintenance 2 grams a day.

Cysteine

See Glutathione and cysteine.

Vitamin E

Vitamin E is the most important fat-soluble antioxidant. You will find it in nuts, seeds, wheat germ and their cold-pressed oils, but make sure they are fresh. Vitamin E is best supplemented every day during an infection.

Fighting infections **300 to 600mg a day.**

Echinacea

A great all-rounder with anti-viral and anti-bacterial properties. The active ingredients are thought to be specific mucopolysaccharides. It comes in capsules and in extracts, taken as drops.

Fighting infections **2 to 3 grams a day (or 15 drops of concentrated extract three times a day).**
 Maintenance 1 gram a day.

Elderberry extract (also called Sambucol)

Reduces the duration of colds and flu by preventing the virus from taking hold.

Fighting infections **1 dessertspoon three times a day.**

Garlic

Contains allicin, a substance that is anti-viral, anti-fungal and anti-bacterial. It also acts as an antioxidant, being rich in sulphur-containing amino acids. There is no doubt that it is an important ally in fighting infections, and a wise inclusion in your diet as garlic-eaters have the lowest incidence of cancer. Consider a clove or capsule equivalent for an easy guide to your daily dose.

Fighting infections **2 to 6 cloves a day.**
   Maintenance 1 clove a day.

Ginger

Particularly good for sore throats and stomach upsets. Put six slices of fresh root ginger in a thermos with a stick of cinnamon and fill up with boiling water. Five minutes later you have a delicious, throat-soothing ginger and cinnamon tea. You can add a little lemon and honey for taste.

Glutathione and cysteine

These are both powerful antioxidant amino acids. You will find them in many all-round antioxidant supplements. During a prolonged viral infection they get depleted and it may be worth taking a supplement. The most usable forms are reduced glutathione or N-acetyl-cysteine.

Fighting infections **2 to 3 grams a day.**
   Maintenance 1 gram a day.

Goldenseal

A natural anti-bacterial agent containing specific alkaloids that are particularly helpful for mucus-membrane problems. Can be used in douches or in gargles as an antiseptic and be taken internally for a healthy digestive system.

Fighting infections **200 to 500mg a day.**

Grapefruit seed extract (also called citricidal)

A powerful natural antibiotic, anti-fungal and anti-viral agent. It comes in drops and can be swallowed, gargled with or used as nose drops or eardrops, depending on the site of infection.

Fighting infections **20 to 30 drops a day.**
   Maintenance 5 drops a day.

Lysine

An amino acid that helps get rid of the herpes virus. (During an infection it is best to limit arginine-rich foods such as beans, lentils, nuts and chocolate.)

Fighting infections **1 to 3 grams a day.**
  Maintenance 1 gram a day.

Mushrooms

Shiitake, maiitake, reishi, ganoderma and other mushrooms were traditionally believed by Chinese Taoists to confer immortality. All have been shown to contain immune-boosting polysaccharides. You will find them added to some immune-boosting supplements and tonics, or you can buy shiitake fresh in the supermarket or dried in health food stores.

Probiotics

Unlike antibiotics, these are beneficial bacteria that promote health. It is best to supplement them during a bacterial infection and after a course of antibiotics. The two most important types are *Lactobacillus acidophilus* and *Bifidobacteria*. These have been shown to halve the recovery time from a bout of diarrheoa.

Dosage Follow instructions on the supplement you choose.

St John's wort (hypericum)

Particularly good for anything that penetrates the skin, such as a wound or skin infection. It is a good general tonic for the immune system.

Fighting infections **50 to 500mg a day.**

Selenium

An immune-enhancing mineral that also acts as an antioxidant. It is abundant in seafood and seeds, especially sesame, and is included in most antioxidant supplements.

Fighting infections **200 to 300mcg a day.**
  Maintenance 100mcg a day.

Tea tree oil

An Australian remedy with antiseptic properties. Great for rubbing on the chest or using in the bath, steam inhaling, or to help keep mosquitoes away. Take as instructed on the bottle. Lozenges are also available.

Zinc

The most important immune-boosting mineral. There is no doubt that it helps fight infections. Zinc lozenges are available for sore throats. You will also find it included in most antioxidant supplements.

Fighting infections **25 to 50mg a day.**

   Maintenance 15mg a day.

Dig deeper by reading my book *Boost your Immune System* co-authored with Jennifer Meek.

chapter 34

Unravelling Allergies

An estimated one in three people has an allergy.[53] Some of these are to airborne substances such as pollen (hay fever), house-dust mite or cat's fur, others to chemicals in food, household products or the environment. But the most common category of allergy-provoking substances is the food you eat. In a survey of 3,300 adults 43 per cent said that they experienced adverse reactions to food. [54]

If you get three or more of the symptoms shown below, you probably have an allergy and most likely to something you are eating. The most common allergy-provoking foods are:

Cow's milk	Gluten grains – wheat, rye, barley, oats
Yeast	Nuts
Eggs	Beans
Wheat	White fish
Gliadin grains – wheat, rye, barley	Shellfish

If you eat any one of these foods two or three times a day and would find them difficult to give up, it may be worth testing to see if you're allergic to them.

What is an allergy?

The classic definition of an allergy is 'any idiosyncratic reaction where the immune system is clearly involved'. The immune system, which is the body's defence system, has the ability to produce 'markers' for substances it doesn't like. The classic markers are antibodies called IgE (immunoglobulin type E). These attach themselves to 'mast cells' in the body. When the

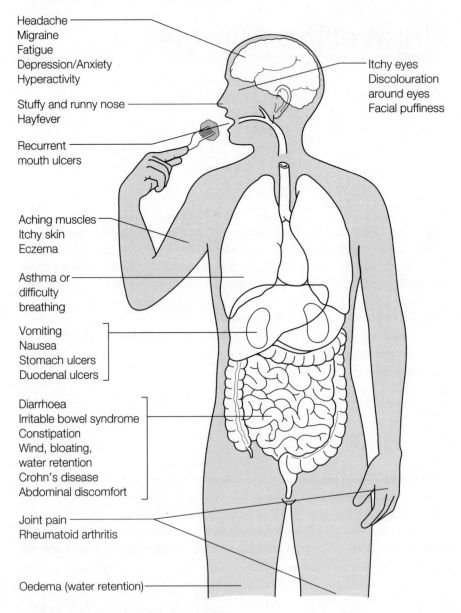

Headache
Migraine
Fatigue
Depression/Anxiety
Hyperactivity

Stuffy and runny nose
Hayfever

Recurrent
mouth ulcers

Itchy eyes
Discolouration
around eyes
Facial puffiness

Aching muscles
Itchy skin
Eczema

Asthma or
difficulty
breathing

Vomiting
Nausea
Stomach ulcers
Duodenal ulcers

Diarrhoea
Irritable bowel syndrome
Constipation
Wind, bloating,
water retention
Crohn's disease
Abdominal discomfort

Joint pain
Rheumatoid arthritis

Oedema (water retention)

Symptoms associated with food allergy

offending food, called an allergen, complexes (combines) with its specific IgE antibody, the IgE molecule triggers the mast cell to release granules containing histamine and other chemicals that cause the symptoms of classic allergy – skin rashes, hay fever, rhinitis, sinusitis, asthma and eczema. Severe food allergies to shellfish or peanuts, for example, can cause immediate gastrointestinal upsets or swelling in the face or throat. All these reactions are immediate, severe, inflammatory reactions, and are known as Type 1 allergic reactions.

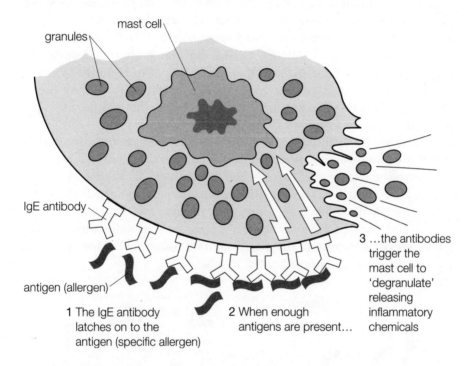

granules

mast cell

IgE antibody

antigen (allergen)

1 The IgE antibody latches on to the antigen (specific allergen)

2 When enough antigens are present…

3 …the antibodies trigger the mast cell to 'degranulate' releasing inflammatory chemicals

How IgE-based allergic reactions happen

Hidden allergies

However, most allergies are not IgE-based. There is a new school of thought and a new generation of allergy tests designed to detect allergies not based on IgE antibody reactions, but probably involving another marker, known as IgG. Allergy expert Dr James Braly, who pioneered the current state-of-the-art test, the IgG ELISA test, for allergies says, 'Food allergy is not rare, nor are the effects limited to the air passages, the skin and digestive tract. Most food allergies are delayed reactions, taking any-where from an hour to three days to show themselves, and are therefore much harder to detect. Delayed food allergy appears to be simply the inability of your digestive tract to prevent large quantities of partially digested and undigested food from entering the bloodstream, to which the body reacts.'

IgG antibodies were first discovered in the 1960s. The IgG antibodies may serve as 'tags' but don't initiate such a severe, immediate reaction. However, a large build-up of IgG antibodies to a particular food indicates a chronic, long-term sensitivity, or food intolerance. It is now well established that many if not the majority of food intolerances do not produce immediate symptoms, but have a delayed, cumulative effect. This, of course, makes them hard to detect by observation. Dr David Hill, Director of the Department of Allergy at the Royal Children's Hospital in Melbourne, researching in Australia, found that the majority of food-sensitive children reacted to foods two or more hours after eating them. In contrast, IgE reactions are immediate, suggesting that a build up of IgG antibodies may be a primary factor in food sensitivity.

According to Dr Jonathan Brostoff, consultant in medical immunology at the Middlesex Hospital Medical School, certain ingested substances can cause the release of histamine and invoke a classic allergic symptom without involving IgE. These include lectins (in peanuts), shellfish, tomatoes, pork, alcohol, chocolate, pineapple, papaya, buckwheat, sunflower, mango and mustard. He also thinks it is possible that undigested proteins could directly affect mast cells (which contain histamine) in the gut, causing the classic symptoms of allergy.

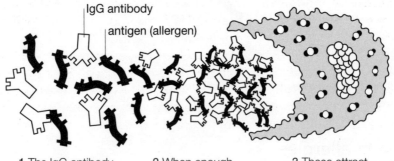

IgG antibody

antigen (allergen)

1 The IgG antibody latches on to the allergen

2 When enough antigens are present, immune complexes are formed

3 These attract phago-cytic cells like neutrophils which eat them up, enlarging and sometimes bursting

How IgG allergic reactions happen

One common cause of allergic reactions is a substantial production of antibodies (mainly IgG) in response to an allergen in the blood. This results in large immune complexes. 'It is the sheer weight of numbers that causes a problem,' says Brostoff. 'These immune complexes are like litter going round in the bloodstream.' The litter is cleaned up by cells, principally neutrophils, which act like vacuum cleaners.

Why food allergy?

Have you ever wondered whether the food you eat actually wants to be eaten? In most cases it appears that it does not. Most foods try their best to protect themselves from predators – with spikes, thorns and chemical toxins. The idea that food is 'good' is far from the truth. Most foods contain numerous toxins, as well as beneficial nutrients. Omnivores like us have a risk-high return strategy as far as food is concerned. We try different foods and if we don't get sick then it's OK. But this shortsighted test has failed in many instances. Indeed, even today, the average diet kills most people in the long run.

Some foods are designed to be eaten. For example, many fruit rely on animals' eating them to spread the growth of their species. The idea is that the animals, such as us human beings, eat the fruit and deposit the seed some distance from the original tree with a rich manure starter kit. However, the fruit has to protect itself from unwanted scavengers such as bacteria or fungi that simply rot the seed. Seeds are often hard to crack and toxic, such as apricot kernels which contain cyanide compounds. For protective reasons, wild food contains a massive and often selective chemical arsenal to ward off specific foes. Food and humans have been fighting for survival since the beginning of time.

So why do food intolerances occur? Are they simply a reaction to less desirable toxins in food? It is unlikely to be that simple. After all, we too have evolved over millions of years to protect ourselves from chemical poisons by developing complex detoxification processes which occur mainly in the liver. A number of theories exist, some of which have good supporting evidence.

Leaky gut syndrome?

The best place to start in unravelling the true cause of allergies is the digestive tract. The textbooks tell us that large food molecules get broken down into simple amino acids, fatty acids and simple sugars. Only these get into the body. Anything larger is considered a foe. Could it be that undigested food, or leaky gut walls, could expose the immune system to food particles that trigger a reaction? This might explain why frequently-eaten foods are more likely to cause a reaction. Indeed, recent research shows that people with food allergies do tend to have leaky gut walls.

Consumption of alcohol, frequent use of aspirin, deficiency in essential fatty acids or a gastrointestinal infection or infestation (such as candidiasis) are all possible contributors to leaky gut syndrome that need to be corrected in order to reduce a person's sensitivity to foods. A lack of key nutrients such as zinc can also prevent proper integrity of the gut wall.

Digestive enzymes

These problems may be particularly severe in people who don't produce enough of the right digestive enzymes, which results in large amounts of big, undigested food molecules reaching the gut wall. One research study of people with a sensitivity to man-made chemicals showed that 90 per cent of them produced inadequate amounts of one digestive enzyme, compared with 20 per cent of healthy control subjects. Undigested food may increase the chances of a localised reaction, increase the amount of large molecules entering the blood, or simply provide food for undesirable bacteria in the gut, which then multiply prolifically. Often, supplementation with digestive enzymes reduces symptoms associated with food allergy and intolerance. Zinc supplementation can also be helpful as deficiency is extremely common among allergy sufferers. Zinc is not only needed for protein digestion, but also essential for the production of hydrochloric acid in the stomach.

Cross-reactions

Another contributor to food sensitivity is exposure to inhalants that provoke a reaction. For example, it is well known that, when the pollen count is high, more people suffer from hay fever in polluted areas than in rural areas, despite lower pollen counts in cities. It is thought that exposure to exhaust fumes makes a pollen-allergic person more sensitive. Whether this is simply because their immune system is weakened from dealing with the pollution, and therefore less able to cope with the additional pollen insult, or due to some kind of 'cross-reaction' is not known. In the US, where ragweed sensitivity is common, a cross-reaction with bananas has been reported. In other words, one sensitivity sensitises you to another. A similar cross-reaction may occur with pollen, wheat and milk for hay-fever sufferers.

The emerging view, shared by an increasing number of allergy specialists, is that food sensitivity is a multi-factorial phenomenon possibly involving poor nutrition, pollution, digestive problems and over-exposure to certain foods. Removing the foods may help the immune system to recover, but other factors need to be dealt with in order to have a major impact on long-term food intolerance.

Food addiction or allergy?

One interesting finding among people with food allergies is that they often become hooked on the very food that causes a reaction, which can lead to bingeing on the foods that harm them most. Many people describe the foods as leaving them feeling drugged or dopey. In some cases the foods induce a state of mild euphoria. In this way, the food can act as a psychological escape mechanism from uncomfortable situations. But why do some foods cause drug-like reactions? When pain no longer serves a purpose as part of a survival mechanism, chemicals called endorphins are released. These are the body's natural painkillers; they make you feel good. The way they do this is by binding to sites that turn off pain and turn on pleasant sensations. Opiates such as morphine are similar in chemical structure and bind to the same sites, which is why they suppress pain.

These endorphins, whether made by the body or taken as a drug, are peptides. Peptides are small groups of amino acids bound together – smaller than a protein and larger than an amino acid. When the protein that you eat is digested, it first becomes peptides and then, if the digestion works well, single amino acids. In the laboratory, endorphin-like peptides have been made from wheat, milk, barley and corn using human digestive enzymes. These peptides have been shown to bind to endorphin receptor sites. Preliminary research does seem to show that certain foods, most commonly wheat and milk, may induce a short-term positive feeling, even if, in the long-term, they are causing health problems.

Too often, the foods that don't suit you are the foods you 'couldn't live without'. This is exactly what happens in the case of many food allergies. If you stop eating the suspect food you may get worse for a few days before you get better. Some things are addictive in their own right such as sugar, alcohol, coffee, chocolate and tea (especially Earl Grey, which contains bergamot). You can react to these foods without being allergic. Wheat and milk could be added to this list on the basis of their endorphin-like effects.

Reducing your allergic potential

There are several possible reasons why a person becomes food-allergic. Among these are lack of digestive enzymes, leaky gut, frequent exposure to foods containing irritant chemicals, immune deficiency leading to hypersensitivity of the immune system, micro-organism imbalance in the gut leading to leaky gut syndrome, and no doubt many more. Fortunately, tests exist to identify deficiencies in digestive enzymes, leaky gut syndrome, and the balance of bacteria and yeast in the gut. These tests can be done at home,

As well as identifying and avoiding foods that cause a reaction, in order to allow the gut and immune system to calm down, there is a lot you can do to reduce your allergic potential.

- Digestive enzyme complexes that help digest fat, protein and carbohydrate (lipase, amylase and protease) are well worth trying. Since stomach acid and protein-digesting enzymes rely on zinc and vitamin B6, it may help to take 15mg of zinc and 50mg of B6 twice a day, as well as a digestive enzyme with each meal.

- Leaky guts can heal. Cell membranes are made out of fat-like compounds. One fatty acid – butyric acid – helps to heal the gut wall. The ideal daily dose is 1,200mg. Vitamin A is also crucial for the health of any mucous membrane including the gut wall. Having 5 grams of glutamine powder in water before bed also helps heal the gut.

- Beneficial bacteria such as *Lactobacillus acidophilus* or *Bifidobacteria* can also help to calm down a reactive digestive tract if the reaction and reduce allergic potential.

- Boosting your immune system (see Chapter 24) also helps to reduce any hypersensitivity it may have.

How to test for allergies and intolerances

There are two ways to find out what you are allergic to. The first we could call 'educated trial and error'. It involves avoiding suspect foods for fourteen days and noting what happens. How to do this is explained below.

The pulse test

Most people are free of symptoms within fourteen days of avoiding an allergy-provoking food. Most react on reintroducing such a food within forty-eight hours, although some may have a delayed reaction of up to ten days. Delayed reactions are much harder to test. For some, symptoms improve considerably when they leave out offending foods, while for others, noticeable changes are slight.

One simple method of identifying possible suspects is the pulse test. This requires avoiding all suspect foods for fourteen days, then reintroducing them, one by one, with a forty-eight-hour gap in between each item to be tested. Take your resting pulse sitting down, before you eat the food, then after ten minutes, thirty minutes and sixty minutes. If you have either a marked increase in pulse rate of more than 10 points, or any symptoms of ill health, including weight gain, avoid the food and wait twenty-four hours before testing the next food.

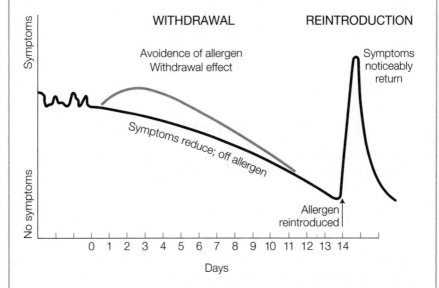

The avoidance/reintroduction test for allergies. If you avoid a food you are allergic to, you may notice an improvement in how you feel within fourteen days. If you then reintroduce the food you may notice a return of symptoms.

While day-to-day changes in symptoms are hard to pin down to specific causes, avoidance of suspect foods for fourteen days often lessens symptoms, which then increase significantly on reintroduction. This way it is possible to notice which foods or drinks make you worse. It is very important to observe symptoms accurately because you may have preconceived ideas about what you do or don't react to, perhaps because of what somebody told you, including me, or because you dread being allergic to certain foods that you're addicted to.

(If you have ever had a severe or life-threatening allergic reaction I recommend you to do this avoidance/reintroduction test only under the supervision of a suitably qualified practitioner.)

Suspect food	Pulse				Symptoms
	Before	10 mins	30 mins	60 mins	
E.g.					
Wheat					
Milk					
Yeast					

IgG allergy testing – the gold standard

Quite apart from the fact that many food reactions are delayed in avoidance/reintroduction tests, they may not always be picked up for two reasons:

- You do not suspect the food and do not avoid it.

- You suspect one food you might be allergic to, but not another, so you continue to have a background of allergic reactions and cannot notice the difference when you take only one allergen out of your diet.

The best test for detecting which foods you are sensitive to is what is called a quantitative IgG ELISA test. 'Quantitative' means that the test shows not only if you are allergic, but also how strong your allergic reaction is. Many of us live quite healthily with minor allergies. But stronger allergies can create all sorts of problems, including weight gain. 'ELISA' is the technology used. You don't need to know the details but trust me, it is the most accurate system used by almost all the best allergy laboratories in the world. To explain how the test works, and why it is so good, I need to explain a bit about your immune system.

Your immune system can produce tailor-made weapons that latch on to specific substances to help escort them out of your body. They are like bouncers on the lookout for, say, wheat, if you are allergic to it. The bouncers are called immunoglobulins, or Ig for short. There are different types. The real heavies are called IgE, although most allergies involve IgG reactions. IgE reactions tend to more immediate and severe. However, most 'hidden' allergies that may be insidiously causing you to gain weight are IgG-based. In an ideal world you test both; however, I normally start by testing a person for IgG sensitivity to food.

The good news is that you can now do this using a home test kit. This involves a clever device that painlessly pricks your finger; the blood is absorbed into a tiny tube and then sent to the laboratory. You then get an accurate reading of exactly what you are allergic to. Your body doesn't lie. Either you have IgG bouncers tagged for wheat or you don't. Your diluted blood is introduced to a panel of liquid food 'testers', and if you've got IgG for that food, a reaction takes place. (See Resources, page 527, for further details.)

Main allergy-inducing foods

These are the most common foods people react to:

Cow's milk   An allergy to cow's milk is the most common food allergy of all. Cow's milk is in most cheeses, cream, yoghurt and butter, and is hidden in all sorts of food, sometimes called 'casein' which is milk protein. Logically, this should not be surprising since cow's milk is a highly specific food, containing all sorts of hormones designed for the first few months of a calf's life. However, it's not the lactose, the sugar in milk, that causes the allergic reaction. It's the protein. If you react to cow's milk it doesn't necessarily mean you react to goat's milk or sheep's milk. However, many people do. It's often best to eliminate all dairy food for the first three months, and then try goat's milk or cheese or yoghurt.

Yeast   This substance is included not only in bread as baker's yeast, but also in beer and, to a lesser extent, wine. Beer and lager are fermented with brewer's yeast. If you've noticed that you feel worse after beer or wine than after spirits, the cleanest being vodka, then you may be yeast-sensitive. Does this mean you can't drink? Not at all. Just stick to spirits and champagne! Champagne is made by a double-fermentation process, which means that it includes much less in the way of yeast. Some people think they are allergic to wheat because they feel worse after eating bread. If you've noticed this – perhaps you feel sluggish, tired or blocked up after eating bread – but feel fine after eating pasta, you may not be allergic to wheat but be reacting to the yeast in the bread.

Wheat More people react to this grain than to any other. It contains gluten, a sticky protein also found in rye, barley and oats. Gluten sensitivity occurs in about one in 100 people according to research by the University of Maryland in the US,[55] but is medically diagnosed in fewer than one in 1,000 people. So, there's a 90 per cent chance that your doctor won't pick this up. However, there's something in gluten, called gliadin, which some so-called gluten-sensitive people react to. There's no gliadin in oats, so some people feel fine when eating oats, but not when they are eating wheat, rye and barley. Rice, buckwheat, millet and corn are all gluten-free, although some people react to corn. The only way to know for sure is to have a food-intolerance test.

Alcohol As well as causing allergies in some people, alcohol irritates the digestive tract in everyone, making it more permeable to undigested food proteins, increasing the chances of an allergic reaction to anything. This is why some people feel worst when they both eat foods they are allergic to and drink alcohol. For example, you might be only mildly allergic to wheat and milk and feel fine after either. But when you have both, plus alcohol, you don't feel great.

The good news about IgG-based allergies is that if you avoid the offending food strictly for three to six months you will no longer be allergic to it. This is because there will no longer be any IgG antibodies to that food in your system and the body will have forgotten that it was allergic to it. This isn't the case with IgE-based reactions. The body, it seems, never forgets these.

In summary, if you suspect you have allergies:

- Avoid suspect foods for fourteen days and reintroduce them one by one, noting your symptoms, or have an allergy test.

- Avoid foods you test allergic to for three months while improving your diet to allow your digestive system to heal and desensitise.

- Even if you don't have a dairy allergy, reduce the amount of cow's milk produce you eat, substituting goat cheeses and soya produce and just drinking less milk.

- Even if you don't react to gluten, reduce the amount of wheat you eat, substituting other grains like oats, rye and rice.

- Reintroduce allergy-provoking foods one by one after three months, eating them infrequently, ideally no more than every four days, to minimise the chance of becoming allergic to the food once more.

chapter 35

Detoxing Your Body

Throughout the centuries, health experts have extolled the value of spring-cleaning the body. In much the same way as you need a holiday, a break from your work, your body, too, needs a break from its work. One of the traditional methods of purifying the body is fasting. The fact that many people report feeling so much more vital after fasting is a testimony to the fact that making energy is as much a result of improving the body's ability to detoxify as it is about eating the right foods.

However, not everyone feels better as a result of fasting and not always right away. Once the body starts to liberate and eliminate toxic material, if the liver isn't up to the job, symptoms of intoxication can result. So modern-day detox regimes tend to use modified fasts in which the person is given a low-toxin diet, plus plenty of the key nutrients needed to speed up the body's ability to detoxify. Doing this once a year, for a week, can make a major difference to your energy levels.

Prevention, however, is better than cure, so if you are basically healthy and want to promote and maintain optimal liver function, the best advice is to cut down on your intake of toxic substances, eat an optimal diet and take a balanced nutrition supplement programme.

■ Check your detox potential

Complete this questionnaire to discover whether you need to improve your detoxification potential:

☐ Do you often suffer from headaches or migraine?

☐ Do you sometimes have watery or itchy eyes or swollen, red or sticky eyelids?

☐ Do you have dark circles under your eyes?

☐ Do you sometimes have itchy ears, earache, ear infections, drainage from the ears or ringing in the ears?

☐ Do you often suffer from excessive mucus, a stuffy nose or sinus problems?

☐ Do you suffer from acne or skin rashes or hives?

☐ Do you sweat a lot and have a strong body odour?

☐ Do you sometimes have joint or muscle aches or pains?

☐ Do you have a sluggish metabolism and find it hard to lose weight, or are you underweight and find it hard to gain weight?

☐ Do you often suffer from frequent or urgent urination?

☐ Do you suffer from nausea or vomiting?

☐ Do you often have a bitter taste in your mouth or a furry tongue?

☐ Do you have a strong reaction to alcohol?

☐ Do you suffer from bloating?

☐ Does coffee stay in your system for a long time?

If you answer 'yes' to seven or more questions you need to improve your detox potential.

If you answer 'yes' to between four and seven questions you are beginning to show signs of poor detoxification and need to improve your detox potential.

If you answer 'yes' to fewer than four questions, you are unlikely to have a problem with detoxification.

How the body detoxifies

If eating the right food is one side of the coin, detoxification is the other. From a chemical perspective, much of what goes on in the body involves substances being broken down, built up and turned from one thing into another. A good 80 per cent of this involves detoxifying potentially

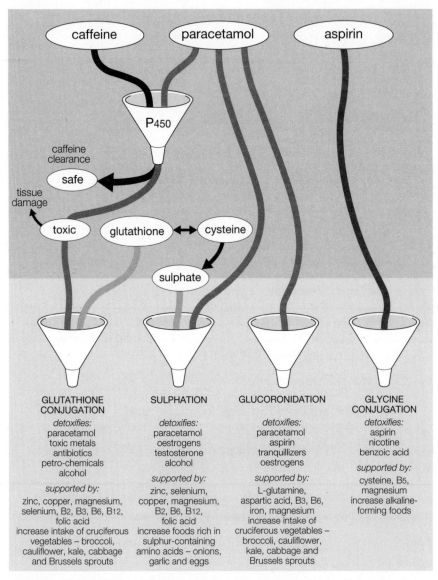

How the body detoxifies. The body processes toxins in the liver using different chemical pathways. Shown here are examples of what the liver does with caffeine, paracetamol (acetaminophen) or aspirin. These different pathways, such as glutathione conjugation or sulphation, need different nutrients to work properly.

harmful substances. Much of this is done by the liver, which represents a clearing house able to recognise millions of potentially harmful chemicals and transform them into something harmless or prepare them for elimination. It is the chemical brain of the body – recycling, regenerating and detoxifying in order to maintain your health.

External toxins, or exo-toxins, that are taken in from the environment represent just a small part of what the liver has to deal with; many toxins are made within the body from otherwise harmless molecules. Every breath and every action can generate toxins. These internally created toxins, or endo-toxins, have to be disarmed in just the same way as exo-toxins do. Whether a substance is bad for you depends as much on your ability to detoxify it as on its inherent toxic properties.

Disarming the toxins

The liver detoxifies substances by sticking things on to them so that they are ready to be eliminated from the body in a process called conjugation. The four main types of conjugation are: glutathione conjugation, sulphation, glucoronidation and glycine conjugation. To optimise each of these particular processes, it is essential to have an adequate supply of the nutrients fundamental for them to work, plus an ensured intake of all vitamins and minerals (from a multi-supplement), a range of which is needed enhance the four processes.

The keys to enhancing these are taking glutathione and sulphur supplements. In addition, eat plenty of cruciferous vegetables, such as broccoli, cauliflower, kale, cabbage and Brussels sprouts. These vegetables are rich in a family of nutrients called glucosinolates, which are particularly supportive of glutathione conjugation and glucoronidation. The final key factor in supporting the detoxification pathways is maintaining the right acid–alkaline balance in the body – that is, it should not be too acid. In order to ensure that you are doing this, take a formula that contains alkalising minerals such as potassium bicarbonate, in addition to including plenty of fresh fruit and vegetables in your diet.

Liver problems or health problems?

Having a liver's-eye view on disease processes often sheds new light on the health problems and solutions of the early twenty-first century. Just about any allergic, inflammatory or metabolic disorder may involve or create sub-optimum liver function, including eczema, asthma, chronic fatigue, chronic infections, inflammatory bowel disorders, multiple sclerosis, rheumatoid arthritis and hormone imbalances.

Substances that interfere with proper liver function include caffeine, alcohol, recreational and medicinal drugs, the Pill and HRT, dioxins, cigarette smoke, exhaust fumes, high-protein diets, organophosphate fertilisers, paint fumes, saturated fat, steroid hormones and charcoal-barbecued meat. Needless to say, you should try to avoid any of these you can and minimise your exposure to the rest.

The good news is that, with a good diet, lifestyle, regular detoxification and the right supplements you can restore and maintain optimal liver function.

Protect yourself with antioxidants

We are threatened by internal toxins as well as external ones. For example oxygen, the basis of all plant and animal life, is our most important nutrient, needed by every cell every second of every day. It is also chemically reactive and highly dangerous. In normal biochemical reactions oxygen can become unstable and capable of 'oxidising' neighbouring molecules. This can lead to cellular damage that triggers cancer, inflammation, arterial damage and ageing. Known as 'oxidants', this equivalent of 'nuclear waste' must be disarmed to remove the danger. Oxidants are made in all combustion processes including smoking, exhaust-fume emissions, radiation, frying or barbecuing food and normal body processes. Antioxidants disarm these harmful oxidants (see Chapter 15).

The balance between your intake of antioxidants and exposure to oxidants may literally be the difference between life and death. You can tip the scales in your favour by making simple changes to your diet and taking antioxidant supplements. The key fact to remember, though, is that none of these nutrients works in isolation in the body. Vitamin C, which is water-soluble, and vitamin E, which is fat-soluble, are synergistic: together they can protect the tissues and fluids in the body. What's more, when vitamin E has 'disarmed' an oxidant, the vitamin E can be 'reloaded' by vitamin C, which is then recycled by glutathione, which itself is recycled by anthocyanidins, so their combined presence has a synergistic effect.

Detox supplements

It is wise to make sure that your daily supplement programme contains significant quantities of antioxidants, especially if you are older, live in a polluted city or have any other unavoidable exposure to oxidants.

The easiest way to do this is by taking a comprehensive antioxidant supplement, in addition to a good multivitamin and mineral. Most reputable supplement companies produce formulas containing a combination of the following nutrients. The kind of total supplementary intake (which may come in part from a multivitamin and extra vitamin C) to aim for is:

Vitamin A (retinol/betacarotene)	2,500mcgRE (7,500iu)	to	6,600mcgRE (20,000iu)
Glutathione (reduced)	25mg	to	75mg
Vitamin E	66mg (100iu)	to	330mg (500iu)
Vitamin C	1,000mg	to	3,000mg
CoQ10	10mg	to	50mg
Lipoic acid	10mg	to	50mg
Anthocyanidin source	50mg	to	250mg
Selenium	30mcg	to	100mcg
Zinc	10mg	to	20mg

There are several other supplements that really help boost your detoxification. An increasingly popular one is MSM (methyl sulphonyl methane) – a form of sulphur – which is particularly helpful in supporting the sulphation process in the liver. Aloe vera juice is also a great all-round tonic for boosting the cleansing processes in the digestive tract. Blended with a range of herbs, aloe vera juice is a great basis for any cleansing programme (see Supplement resources, page 528).

My seven-day detox

- **Begin your detox at the weekend** or during a time when you don't have too much going on.

- **Walk for at least fifteen minutes every day.**

- **Drink at least 2 litres of water a day** – purified, distilled, filtered or bottled. You can also drink dandelion coffee or herb teas.

- **Have half a pint of fruit or vegetable juice a day** – either carrot and apple juice (you can buy these two separately and combine them with one-third water) with grated ginger, or fresh watermelon juice. The flesh of the watermelon is high in betacarotene and vitamin C. The seeds are high in vitamin E and antioxidant minerals zinc and selenium. You can make a great antioxidant cocktail by blending flesh and seeds in a blender.

- **Eat in abundance:**
  Fruit – the most beneficial fruits with the highest detox potential include fresh apricots, all types of berry, cantaloupe, citrus fruits, kiwi, papaya, peaches, mango, melons and red grapes.

Vegetables – especially good for detoxification are artichokes, peppers, beetroot, Brussels sprouts, broccoli, red cabbage, carrots, cauliflower, cucumber, kale, pumpkin, spinach, sweet potato, tomato, watercress and bean and seed sprouts.

- **Eat in moderation:**
  Grains – brown rice, corn, millet, quinoa: not more than twice a day.
  Fish – salmon, mackerel, sardines, tuna: not more than once a day.
  Oils – use extra-virgin olive oil for cooking and in place of butter, and cold-pressed seed oils for dressing.
  Nuts and seeds – one handful a day of raw, unsalted nuts and seeds should be included. Choose from almonds, Brazil nuts, hazelnuts, pecan nuts, pumpkin seeds, sunflower seeds, sesame seeds and flax seeds.

- **Supplement** two multivitamins/minerals, 2 grams of vitamin C, two antioxidant complexes and 2 grams of MSM every day. Also have a shot of aloe vera juice.

- **Avoid** all wheat products, all meat and dairy produce – milk and all dairy products, eggs and meat, salt – and any foods containing them, hydrogenated fats, artificial sweeteners, food additives and preservatives, fried foods, spices, dried fruit.

- **Limit** potatoes to one portion every other day and bananas to one every other day.

Don't be surprised if you feel worse for a couple of days before you feel better. This is especially likely if you are eliminating foods to which you are allergic or upon which you are dependent.

chapter 36

Breaking the Fat Barrier

Every day in Britain 1,000 people become obese, joining the 20 per cent of the currently obese population. More than one in two people are overweight. Once a person is obese their risk for diabetes goes up seventy-seven times, and once diabetic their risk for heart disease goes up eight times. Obesity is a serious health issue that is costing the National Health Service close to £1 billion and accounting for more than 30,000 premature deaths and 20 million lost working days a year. Yet the startling fact is that it is relatively easily solved by tackling the true underlying cause – by restoring blood sugar control.

Most people believe that eating too many calories causes weight gain. Yet the average calorie intake in Britain has consistently dropped over the last fifteen years, while the incidence of obesity has increased. On top of this, people in countries where obesity is extremely rare, like China, eat substantially more calories (2,630kcals a day) than the obesity capital of the world, America (2,360kcals). In Britain we average around 2,000kcals. Different levels of activity can explain part of this, but this isn't the whole story. The big difference is the quality of what we eat. Contrary to popular opinion, it isn't fat that's the main culprit. Like our calorie intake, our dietary percentage of fat has steadily declined. We eat too much sugar and refined carbohydrates.

Your weight is a burning issue

The missing link in the calorie equation is metabolism – how the body turns food into fat. And the key is to maintain an even blood sugar level.

According to Professor Gerald Reaven of Stanford University in California, one in four people in the Western world now has 'insulin resistance', which means an inability to keep their blood sugar level even. Among obese people this figure rises to nine in ten. Put simply, if you can't keep your blood sugar level even, it goes up and down like a yo-yo. When it's too high, you turn the excess sugar into fat, and when it's too low you feel lethargic. The end result of insulin resistance is diabetes.

Whenever your blood sugar level rises, your body produces the hormone insulin, which helps to transport the sugar out of your blood into your cells, converting any excess sugar into fat. The more often your blood sugar rises, the more insulin you produce. And as more insulin is produced, more sugar is turned into fat. Over time, your body's cells become less responsive (or resistant) to insulin, causing even more insulin to be produced. Eventually cells become so non-responsive that diabetes results. For these people, even the slightest indulgence means extra weight gain.

This, by the way, is why high-protein diets like the Atkins diet work for some people. Dr Atkins proposed that turning fat and protein into energy was so difficult that you used up calories doing it, and hence lost weight. This has been proven to be untrue. He also proposed that the by-products of running on fat and protein, ketones, would be another route to losing calories, since these ketones, which have a calorific value, are excreted in the urine. Again, this is untrue. No appreciable amount of calorie loss occurs via ketone excretion. However, what is true is that by eating a high-protein, low-carbohydrate diet your appetite decreases. The reason for this is simple. By having more protein in a meal and less carbohydrate, your blood sugar level doesn't go shooting up, so your body doesn't have to make more insulin to carry the excess sugar out of the bloodstream, which would then get dumped as fat. Blood sugar is the key to appetite and to weight control. There are, however, easier, less restrictive and healthier ways to reduce insulin secretion and control blood sugar.

Eat low-GL foods

Low-carbohydrate diets limit the *quantity* of carbohydrate you eat. This tells you little to nothing about what the carbohydrate is doing to your blood sugar. Instead of avoiding carbohydrates I recommend that you eat what are called low-GL (glycemic load) carbohydrates.

As explained in Chapter 10, the glycemic load of a food is derived from knowing both the *quantity* of the food that is carbohydrate and the *quality* of the carbohydrate – fast or slow releasing (which is determined by the 'glycemic index' of the food). If you want to lose weight and feel great, eat no more than 40 GL units of carbohydrate a day, preferably with protein. This means roughly 10 points for breakfast, 10 for lunch, 10 for dinner and 5 in each of two snacks, mid-morning and mid-afternoon. If you choose the good, low-GL foods you'll be able to eat more food. If you choose the bad, high-GL foods you'll be able to eat much less. The chart on pages 501–13 shows you which foods are the best.

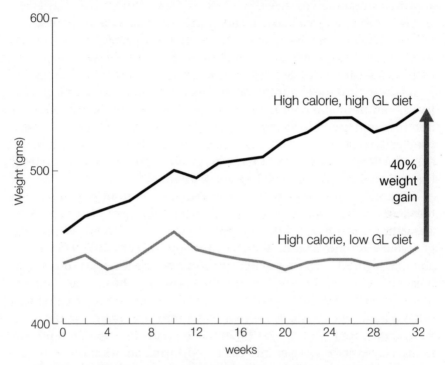

What diet works best? This chart shows weight change on high-GL and low-GL diets of equal calories and fat/protein/carbohydrate percentage.

To understand how powerful controlling the GL of your diet is, consider this animal experiment. Two groups of rats were given the identical amount of calories, with the identical balance of protein, fat and carbo-hydrate. The only difference was in the type of carbohydrate. One group ate high-GL carbs, the other low-GL carbs. The high-GL carb group gained weight, while the low-GL group lost weight on the same calories.[56] Similar results have been shown in human studies.[57] One of the reasons why diets with balanced carbohydrates work better than very low-carbohydrate diets is that they promote serotonin.

Serotonin controls your appetite

In Chapter 28 I extolled the virtues of a particular amino acid, 5-hydroxytryptophan (5-HTP). It's the daughter of tryptophan and the mother of serotonin, the brain's 'happy' neurotransmitter. Many people have low levels of this essential brain chemical and feel depressed as a result. This is especially true of people on weight-loss diets, which are notoriously low in tryptophan. But that isn't all. Serotonin controls appetite. The more you have, the less you eat. Anyone who has taken Ecstasy, which causes a massive and dangerous release of serotonin, will tell you they have no desire to eat. Similarly, most people eat more when they are depressed (and low in serotonin). This may be why people eat more in the winter. The less light you get, the less serotonin you make.

If you are low in serotonin one of the quickest ways to restore normal levels, and normal mood, is to supplement 5-HTP. Two studies, one on non-insulin-dependent diabetics, and the other on non-diabetic obese people, have clearly shown that supplementing 5-HTP causes an immediate reduction in appetite, and less craving for sugar and carbohydrates.[58] (Animal studies have proven the same thing.)

Why the reduced carving for carbohydrates? In front of you are two breakfast choices. One is an Atkins-style bacon and eggs, high in protein. The other is cornflakes with chopped banana and a muffin. Which will give your serotonin a boost, thereby satisfying you the most? If you think about it logically, you'd say the protein-rich, hence tryptophan-rich, breakfast. But you'd be wrong. It's the cornflakes, banana and muffin breakfast. Why? Even though the bacon and eggs do contain tryptophan, it has a hard time getting from your blood into your brain – it just doesn't compete well with all the other amino acids in these high-protein foods. However, it does get into the bloodstream. So, what drives it into your brain? The answer is insulin. It is released by a high-carbohydrate breakfast, carries tryptophan into the brain and gives you a mood boost. What this means is that when you are feeling tired, hungry and a little blue, you crave something sweet, not a sausage. Sounds familiar?

One great big secret of successful weight loss is to a) ensure you that have enough serotonin, so you have less desire to eat in excess, and b) keep your blood sugar level and insulin release even so you don't have increased appetite due to blood sugar dips. Remember, too much insulin drives blood sugar into body fat, but too little results in you not making serotonin, which controls your appetite.

The modern approach to fat-burning

The trick to losing weight is to eat a diet that keeps your blood sugar level even, not to overeat and to exercise more. While this all sounds very familiar, there have been some important scientific developments that, in combination, provide a much more effective way to lose weight and regain weight control. In practical terms, this boils down to five key steps:

1. **Eat the right kind of carbohydrates to achieve a better blood sugar balance.** This means selecting foods that have little effect on raising blood sugar levels, such as fresh vegetables, beans, lentils, whole grains and fish. You should also avoid refined foods, fruit juices and other sugary, sweet foods. The best single measure of a food's effect on your blood sugar and hence weight is the GL of a food (see the chart, pages 501–13). My book *The Holford Diet* limits your carbohydrate intake to no more than 40 GL points.

2. **Eat only low-GL carbohydrates and eat them only *with* protein-rich foods.** This reduces hunger as well as your tendency to store fat. This means eating fish with rice, tofu with vegetables or beans with pasta.

3. **Increase the amount of essential fats you eat, but keep down your saturated-fat intake.** Yes, the right fats actually help you burn fat. One of the greatest myths in conventional weight control is that 'a calorie is a calorie'. This is untrue. A calorie of saturated fat has a very different outcome from a calorie of an essential fat that is used by the brain, immune system, skin, hormone system and cardiovascular system. Moreover, Omega 3 essential fats, principally from fish and flax seeds, actually counteract some of the negative effects of insulin resistance. Therefore dieting strategies that incorporate significant amounts of Omega 3 fats help to promote weight loss. In practical terms, this means eating a 4oz serving of fish three times a week and a tablespoonful of flax seed a day, or supplementing Omega 3 fats every day. You should also reduce your intake of cream, high-fat cheese and red meat.

4. **Cut down on stimulants such as tea, coffee, chocolate, cigarettes and alcohol.** Sugar and refined carbohydrates aren't the only substances that disturb blood sugar control. So do stimulants that affect both energy and weight control. This means minimising alcohol and caffeine intake.

5. **Eat three meals a day, especially breakfast – and snack on fruit.** Snacks are a big no-no on many diets that try to curb people's eating patterns by focusing on consuming fewer calories. Yet one of the most effective ways to stabilise blood sugar and control weight and appetite is to eat the right kind of foods little and often. The easiest way keep your blood sugar level even is to have three meals a day, never miss breakfast and have a mid-morning and mid-afternoon fruit snack with some almonds. It shouldn't be just any fruit. Apples, pears and berries have a much lower glycemic index than other fruit, and if you eat them with twelve almonds your blood sugar level won't peak.

    If you don't need a snack don't have one – but don't fool yourself. If you are hungry it's better to have some fruit (but not bananas, grapes, raisins or dates) than pig out because your blood sugar has dipped so low that your cravings become stronger than your common sense.

How to do all this exactly is explained in my book *The Holford Diet*, which suggests simple breakfasts, lunches and dinners to help you lose weight without getting hungry. I lost a stone in weight in less than two months when I did this. I haven't gained (or lost) more than 3lb in twenty years since. When you find your perfect fat-burning diet you can eat plenty, feel satisfied, lose weight when you need to and keep your weight stable if you don't.

Fat-burning vitamins and minerals

The ability to turn food efficiently into energy instead of fat depends upon hundreds of enzymes which, in turn, depend upon vitamins and minerals. To tune up your metabolism for fat-burning, it is essential to consume optimal amounts of these nutrients. For example, your body needs zinc and vitamin B6 to make insulin, while insulin's ability to control blood sugar levels is helped by chromium, an essential mineral that in helping to stabilise blood sugar levels helps control weight. Finally, to turn glucose into energy rather than fat, you need the B vitamins, vitamin C and magnesium.

Unfortunately, most people don't get enough of these fat-burning nutrients from their diet. In addition to supplementing with these specific nutrients, you should strive to increase your intake of foods rich in them. For example, most seeds contain high amounts of zinc and magnesium, and almost all fruit and vegetables are rich sources of B vitamins and vitamin C. Chromium is found in whole wheat flour, bread or pasta, as well as in asparagus, mushrooms, beans, nuts and seeds.

Hydroxycitric acid

Although it isn't a vitamin, hydroxycitric acid (HCA) could help you lose weight. Originally developed by the pharmaceutical giant Hoffmann-LaRoche, HCA has proven to slow down the production of fat and reduce appetite. HCA has no apparent toxicity or safety concerns. It is extracted from the dried rind of the tamarind (*Garcinia cambogia*) fruit, which has been used as a spice and preservative in the East for hundreds of years and is thought to be the richest source of HCA. HCA works by inhibiting the enzyme ATP citrate lyase which converts sugar into fat.

In one study, half the participants were given 750mg of HCA, while the others received a placebo. Those on the HCA reported an average weight loss of more than 11lb per person, compared with just over 4lb per person in the placebo group.[59] HCA is likely to prove a useful addition to reduced-calorie diets rich in slow-releasing carbohydrates and low in saturated fat. It is widely available as a supplement, often found in combination with chromium. If you are interested in using HCA – it's available in any health food store – I recommend taking 750mg a day.

Fat-burning exercises

The good news about exercise is that you really do not have to be fanatically fit to lose weight. The reason why, once again, is not calories but metabolism. According to calorie theory, exercise does little to promote weight loss. After all, running a mile burns up only 300 calories – equivalent to two slices of toast or a piece of apple pie. But this argument misses a number of key points.

The first is that the effects of exercise are cumulative. Running a mile may burn up only 300 calories, but if you do that three days a week for a year, that makes 22,000 calories, equivalent to a weight loss of 11lb! Also, the amount of calories you burn up depends on how fat or fit you are to start with. The more fat and unfit you are, the more benefit you will derive from small amounts of exercise.

Contrary to popular belief, moderate exercise also decreases your appetite. It appears that a degree of physical activity is necessary for appetite mechanisms to work properly. People who take no exercise have exaggerated appetites, so the pounds pile on.

The most important reason why exercise is a key to weight loss is its effect on your metabolic rate. According to Professor William D. McArdle, exercise physiologist at City University, New York, 'Most people can generate metabolic rates that are eight to ten times above their resting value during sustained cycling, running or swimming. Complementing this increased metabolic rate is the observation that vigorous exercise will raise metabolic rate for up to fifteen hours after exercise.' Surveys do show that leaner people tend to exercise more.

Benefits of my Fatburner Diet compared with high-protein diets

As opposed to conventional low-fat diets – which emphasise low calorie intake and as little fat as possible – the Fatburner Diet emphasises a radical move away from fast-releasing carbohydrates such as sugar and white bread, towards slow-releasing carbohydrates such as oats and whole rye bread, and less saturated fat, but more essential fats from seeds and fish.

Thanks to recent trials published in top medical journals we can make a comparison. To compare like with like, the studies featured here all involved people who, given the diets to follow, said they followed them 'as best they can'.

Let's first look at high-protein diets versus conventional low-calorie, low-fat diets. Two trials carried out at the University of Pennsylvania Medical Center showed that after six months, those on the high-protein diets had lost between 10lb and 12.7lb, versus 4lb to 4.5lb on a conventional low-fat diet. However, after twelve months there was no significant difference in weight loss in either diet in either study.[60]

Why do Atkins-type diets lead to short-term weight loss? A review of all studies to date on low-carbohydrate diets concludes that 'weight loss was principally associated with decreased calorie intake'.[61] So although the research in these studies implies that high-protein diets work, it finds the results aren't that spectacular and are probably due simply to eating less.

A study in Ireland compared my Fatburner Diet with a conventional low-calorie, low-fat diet with support group meetings. The average weight loss after three months was 13.7lb on the Fatburner Diet, versus 2lb on the conventional low-calorie diet, despite the extra support.[62]

Not only do Fatburner dieters appear to lose *more* weight in half the time of the average high-protein dieters, but also they feel better and have none of the risks of bone[63] or kidney problems[64] or cancer associated with high-protein diets, or the risks of dry skin and essential-fat deficiency associated with low-fat diets.

This, in brief, is how to slim without suffering:

● Follow a low- to medium-calorie diet (1,000–1,500 calories), high in fibre, low in fat and balanced for fat, protein and carbohydrate.

● Eat no more than 40 GLs of carbohydrates a day, preferably with protein.

● Avoid sugar, sweetened foods, coffee, tea, cigarettes and alcohol, or at least reduce your intake of them as much as possible.

● Take aerobic exercise at least twice a week – running, swimming, brisk walking, low-impact aerobics, dance classes and so on.

● Supplement your diet with vitamins and minerals. Most important are the B vitamins, vitamin C and the minerals zinc and chromium. Also consider taking a daily 750mg of HCA, often found in supplements together with chromium, and/or 100mg of 5-HTP if you crave sweet foods.

Dig deeper by reading my book *The Holford Diet*.

chapter 37

Solving the Riddle of Eating Disorders

Eating disorders are complex mental health conditions characterised by a 'definite disturbance of eating habits or weight-control behaviour'.[65] Figures from the Eating Disorders Association estimate that eating disorders may affect as many as 1.15 million people in the UK. Eating disorders rank fifteenth among the top twenty causes of disability in women.[66] The *average* length of time for recovery is five to six years.

Anorexia nervosa and bulimia nervosa are probably the best known of the conditions. Whilst both involve restricted food intake, anorexia is characterised by extreme weight loss, whilst bulimia is characterised by episodes of binge eating and purging to control weight. There is also a further category, 'eating disorder not otherwise specified' (EDNOS). This is something of a catch-all term for situations where someone has many of the features of an eating disorder, but either not severely enough, or not for long enough, to justify a diagnosis of anorexia or bulimia. Many people with eating problems probably fall into this category

Eating disorders often feature prominently in the media and are surrounded by many myths, having been described as slimming diseases, developmental teenage fads, attempts to avoid growing up, obsessions with food and weight and so on. Anorexia nervosa was first described as a separate disorder by Dr William Gull in 1874. It has the highest mortality rate for any psychiatric condition, from the effects of starvation or from suicide. Bulimia nervosa was first categorised as a distinct condition by Dr

Gerald Russell in 1979. It is perhaps the most common of the disorders, although it is also the easiest to hide.

Isn't anorexia just about zinc deficiency?

In the 1970s, a number of researchers noticed that the symptoms of anorexia were similar in some respects to those of zinc deficiency, giving rise to a hypothesis that zinc supplementation might be useful for treating anorexia and possibly also bulimia. During the 1980s and 1990s a number of small trials were carried out to supplement zinc for patients with anorexia as they started to eat and gain weight. There were some positive results, with improvements in weight gain, mood, emotional state and menstrual function. The researchers concluded that individuals with anorexia and bulimia may have zinc deficiency. However, the complexity of treating eating disorders clearly indicates that while zinc deficiency may be a contributing factor in the conditions, it is neither the whole story nor the root cause. [67]

Biochemical and physiological imbalances

People with eating disorders often eat nutrient-poor food, skip meals or eat very erratically. This may result in a number of underlying biochemical and physiological imbalances that can contribute to many of the associated symptoms. The following are important areas to consider:

- **Blood sugar imbalance and insulin resistance**   Dieting, skipping meals and bingeing on foods high in sugar and refined carbohydrates disrupt blood sugar leading to low blood sugar levels, cravings and desensitisation of cells to insulin.[68] Chromium, an important mineral for blood sugar control, is also excreted when the diet is high in sugars. Reliance on caffeine to boost energy blocks the production of both serotonin and melatonin and can result in tiredness, irritability and feelings of anxiety and depression. The solution is to follow the kind of diet recommended in this book.

- **Neurotransmitter imbalance**   When neurotransmitters are present in sufficient amounts, mood and emotions are stable. When they are depleted, or 'out of balance', individuals may overeat (particularly sweet and starchy foods) or starve simply to try and manage mood.[69]

    In eating disorders there may be a particular link to disturbed serotonin metabolism. Serotonin is a neurotransmitter that plays a role in controlling carbohydrate intake, promoting sleep and managing impulsive and obsessional behaviours. Serotonin is made from tryptophan, an amino acid found in foods such as milk, cottage cheese, poultry, turkey and chicken, eggs, red meats, soya beans, tofu and almonds. Vitamin B6, zinc and insulin are also needed for serotonin production. Chapter 28 explains how to promote serotonin through nutrition and lifestyle changes.

Dieting has been shown to deplete levels of tryptophan very quickly, particularly in women.[70] In one study, when bulimics were deprived of tryptophan, their serotonin levels dropped and they binged on an average of 900 additional calories each day.[71] This led to a large increase in serotonin production and release within the brain, temporarily reducing stress and depression. However, the serotonin 'fix' was followed by overwhelming feelings of guilt and low self-esteem, triggering the powerful need to purge. Vomiting also depresses serotonin levels as the body loses the essential nutrients needed to make serotonin.

Low serotonin may also give rise to some of the personality traits commonly seen with bulimia – depression, impulsiveness, irritability and mood swings. One further study showed that even years into recovery, bulimics can have a return of their cravings and mood problems after only a few hours of tryptophan depletion.[72]

- **Hormone imbalances**   The sex hormones oestrogen, progesterone and testosterone interact with neurotransmitters to stimulate many of the brain's mood sites. Low oestrogen has been linked to low serotonin and an increase in cravings. Low progesterone can lead to infertility, anxiety and PMS, while too much can lead to lethargy, increased appetite, weight gain and depression – common symptoms in people with eating problems.

  An eating disorder places considerable stress on the body and on the adrenal glands which are responsible for producing most of the stress hormones. Adrenal stress can easily disrupt other hormones, particularly in the thyroid and the ovaries. Where the diet is low in good-quality protein, for instance in some vegetarian and vegan diets, the risk of adrenal exhaustion may be even greater owing to a lack of amino acids for hormone production. Vegetarianism is much more common in those with eating disorders (particularly anorexia nervosa) than in the general population.

- **Food allergies and intolerances**   Certain foods may have a mood-altering effect in some people; for instance, refined carbohydrates and sugar impact serotonin and endorphin production, increase blood sugar and stress the adrenal glands. Wheat (plus rye, oats and barley) contains gluten which can interfere with the absorption of nutrients and affect neurotransmitter production and thyroid function. People with gluten intolerance may also be low in serotonin and this may give rise to depression. Casein, a milk protein found in dairy products, and lactose, a milk sugar, may also result in similar problems. Soya can depress thyroid function because its phytate content blocks the uptake of iodine and the absorption of thyroid hormones. Low thyroid function in people who binge eat may contribute to weight gain or obesity.

- **Deficiency of essential fatty acids (EFAs)** People with eating disorders are often 'fat-phobic'. Low-fat diets have been associated with depression and irritability partly because essential fats are crucial for brain function and for the production of sex and stress hormones. Blood sugar levels can also drop very rapidly in the absence of fat.

- **Gastrointestinal disturbance** A diet high in sugars and refined carbohydrates may result in yeast overgrowth in the gut. This can contribute to constipation, bloating, slow gastric emptying and malabsorption, as well as to mental and emotional symptoms. The mechanisms and hormones that control hunger and fullness can also be disrupted.

Optimum nutrition for eating disorders

There have always been differing views as to whether nutritional approaches or psychological treatments hold the key to successful recovery from an eating disorder. Although more research is needed into the efficacy of nutritional approaches, there appears to be growing recognition that the disorders do have nutrition-related aspects and that approaches combining both nutritional and psychological treatment may offer the best possibility for recovery.[73]

It must, however, be remembered that eating disorders are complex mental health conditions with potentially serious consequences. Care must include psychological treatments, regular medical monitoring, and possibly medication. Nutritional counselling should not be offered as a sole treatment, but it may form part of a multi-disciplinary approach. Hospitalisation should be considered where people do not respond to outpatient treatment, if weight is very unstable or extremely low, if there are serious physical complications or if there is risk of suicide.

Dig deeper by reading my book *Optimum Nutrition for the Mind.*

chapter 38.

Mental Health – the Nutrition Connection

L ife in the twenty-first century is stressful. Some of us are rising to the challenge, but most of us are struggling to keep up and are living with tiredness, anxiety, stress, depression and sleeping problems as a result. Some people tip over the edge into mental health problems – from attention deficit disorder to Alzheimer's disease and schizophrenia. In fact, the world over, there's been a massive increase in the incidence of mental health problems, especially among young people. The incidences of autism, sui-cide, violence and depression are on the increase, according to the World Health Organization. Mental health problems, they say, are fast becoming the number-one health issue, with one in ten people suffering at any point in time, and one in four people suffering at some point in their lives.[74]

If you've got a strange set of physical symptoms, your doctor is proba-bly going to run a basic biochemical screening blood test to see if anything abnormal shows up. The same is rarely done for those with mental health problems, as the belief is that biochemical imbalances don't manifest as psychological symptoms. Of course, the reverse is true. The brain is far more sensitive to biochemical imbalances and nutritional deficiencies than any other organ of the body.

The very fact that most treatment of mental illness involves chemical drugs is an indication of the direct link between a person's biochemical state and their psychological state. We also know that deficiencies in nutrients, and excesses in 'anti-nutrients' such as lead or chemical addi-tives, can cause mental health symptoms.

There's more to it than that, however. Having worked with thousands of people with mental health problems I'm convinced that most have one, or more, of a combination of thirteen common biochemical imbalances that if left untreated can lead to mental illness.

So, if you do have mental health problems, it is well worth checking out these imbalances, each of which has a clear set of symptoms. If you have some or all of the symptoms, then an objective biochemical test can be run to confirm whether or not this imbalance is present. Then, a nutritional strategy can be implemented to help solve the problem.

A new diagnosis of mental health problems

The diagnosis of mental health problems should be based on the observation of symptoms, objectively measured in questionnaire tests, and on physical and biochemical tests that help determine if any of the many kinds of biochemical imbalances are causing, or contributing to, a person's problems. Here are some of the more common biochemical imbalances that can result in symptoms of mental illness.

1. Blood sugar imbalance

The most common underlying imbalance in many types of mental health problem is fluctuating blood sugar levels, called disglycemia. If you've got this, the chances are you crave sweet foods or stimulants such as tea, coffee and cigarettes, all of which affect your blood sugar level. Here are the most common symptoms:

- Difficulty concentrating
- Heart palpitations
- Fainting, dizziness or trembling
- Excessive sweating or night sweats
- Excessive thirst
- Chronic fatigue
- Frequent mood swings
- Forgetfulness or confusion
- Tendency to depression
- Anxiety and irritability
- Feeling weak
- Aggressive outbursts or crying spells

- Cravings for sweets or stimulants

- Drowsiness after meals

If you've got five or more of these symptoms, you are likely to have disglycemia. The best way to confirm this is by a blood test that measures 'glycosylated haemoglobin'. As more and more people are becoming disglycemic, the incidence of related conditions such as obesity, age-related memory loss, Alzheimer's disease, heart disease and diabetes is also on the increase.

Here are a few simple steps you can take to help balance your blood sugar:

- Avoid sugar and foods containing sugar.

- Break your addiction to caffeine by avoiding coffee, tea and other caffeinated drinks for a month, while improving your diet. Once you are no longer craving caffeine, the occasional cup of weak tea and very occasional coffee is not a big deal.

- Break an addiction to chocolate, if you have one.

- Always have something substantial for breakfast, such as an unrefined oat-based cereal; unsweetened live yoghurt with banana, ground sesame seeds and wheat germ; or an egg.

- Eat a high-fibre diet rich in fresh vegetables and fruit. Fibre helps keeps your blood sugar level even.

- Certain vitamins and minerals can help regulate your blood sugar level and minimise the withdrawal effects of stimulants. These include vitamin C, vitamin B complex, especially vitamin B6, and the minerals magnesium and chromium.

2. Stimulant and drug dependence

Although many people know that drinking and eating stimulants is not good for their health, it is not assumed that it can make them crazy. This is far from the truth. Excessive intake of stimulants (tea, coffee, alcohol, sugar, cola, caffeine pills, cigarettes) can bring on symptoms of mental illness. The symptoms are very similar to those for dysglycemia, coupled with cravings for any of these substances. In addition, you can experience extreme anxiety, paranoia and depression through the excessive use of some of these substances. Complete the stimulant inventory in Chapter 11 and take the necessary steps to reduce your stimulant load.

3. Food and chemical allergies and intolerances

If you suffer from daily mood swings, or are fine at some times and not at others, for no apparent reason, one possibility is that you are reacting to something you're eating. The most common single food that's been linked to mental health problems is wheat, which is a rich source of gluten. Other foods that can cause allergic reactions include milk products, oranges, eggs, grains other than wheat, foods with yeast, shellfish, nuts, beef, pork and onions. Food colourings such as tartrazine and other chemical additives can also cause problems. Some people develop intolerances to tea and coffee, while alcohol, which irritates the gut wall and makes it more leaky, often increases allergic sensitivity to anything eaten. Check yourself out on the symptoms below:

- Childhood history of colic, eczema, asthma, rashes or ear infections
- Daily mood swings
- Deep depressions for no particular reason
- Frequent, rapid colds or blocked nose
- Difficulty sleeping
- Facial puffiness, circles or discoloration around the eyes
- Hyperactivity
- Dyslexia or learning difficulties
- Aggressive outbursts or crying spells

If you score five or more, or know you feel better when you avoid certain foods, then food or chemical allergies/intolerances may be contributing to your problem. The best advice is to see a nutritional therapist, who can show you how to do a two-week 'avoidance' and 'challenge' test with your suspect foods. Alternatively, have a quantitative IgG ELISA allergy test using a simple home test kit (see Resources, page 527). This involves a pinprick of blood from which you can be tested for allergy to over a hundred different foods and chemicals.

4. Underactive or overactive thyroid

If your mind and body feel sluggish most of the time, you may have an underactive thyroid, referred to as hypothyroidism. If your thyroid is clinically underactive your doctor may prescribe thyroid hormones. However, blood tests are often unable to detect sub-clinical hypothyroidism, so it may be better to go by the symptoms. You can test your thyroid function your-self with the Broda Barnes Temperature Test. If your temperature before you rise in the morning is consistently below 36.5°C, this suggests your thyroid may be underactive. Below are the typical symptoms of hypothyroidism:

- Physical or mental fatigue or lethargy

- Depression or irritability

- Dry skin and/or hair

- Intolerance to cold or cold hands and feet

- Constipation, gas, bloating or indigestion

- Weight gain

- Painful periods

- Muscle pain

- Poor memory

- Sore throat or nasal congestion

If you score five or more, an underactive thyroid may be contributing to your problem. Get it tested by your doctor and also see a nutritional ther-apist, who can show you which foods to eat and which foods to avoid to support your thyroid. Chronic stress can deplete thyroid function, as the stress hormone, cortisol, inhibits it. Thyroid health is also dependent on specific nutrients in the diet, most importantly iodine – which is abun-dant in seafood and seaweed – zinc, selenium and tyrosine, an amino acid found in all protein-rich foods.

Having an overactive thyroid can lead to mania, overactivity and a fast metabolism, so it is not common for people with this condition to be overweight. If these symptoms are present ask your doctor to check your thyroid function.

5. Niacin (B3), pyridoxine (B6), folic acid or B12 deficiency

These four B vitamins are your brain's best friends. They 'oil the wheels' of the brain's neurotransmitters, especially dopamine, adrenalin, nora-drenalin and serotonin. These neurotransmitters are the brain's chemicals of communication, sending messages from one brain cell to another. Without enough of these essential B vitamins the brain can produce chemicals that make you feel crazy. This is because they help to control methylation, a chemical process that goes on throughout the brain and body, helping to turn one neurotransmitter into another. Some people need a lot more B vitamins than others, so it's best to be guided by symptoms, rather than by blood tests. Here are the more common symptoms of a deficiency in these vitamins:

- Feeling 'unreal'
- Hearing your own thoughts
- Anxiety and inner tension
- Inability to think straight
- Suspicion of people
- Good pain tolerance
- Seeing or hearing things abnormally
- Having delusions or illusions
- Loose bowels or skin problems at onset of mental health problems
- Difficult sexual orgasm
- Tendency to gain weight
- Frequent mood swings

If you have five or more of these symptoms, it may be worth your while increasing your intake of these nutrients for two months. As a recommendation try 100mg of B3, 100mg of B6, 1,000mcg of folic acid and 100mcg of B12.

6. Essential fatty acids – deficiencies and imbalances

Your brain is 60 per cent fat, if you take out all the water. This fatty tissue needs replenishing, but it's crucial to know which fats will feed your brain the best. Essential fatty acids known as Omega 3 and Omega 6 are intimately involved in brain function, and deficiencies or imbalances in brain fats are now known to be associated with everything from dyslexia, hyperactivity and depression to schizophrenia and manic depression.

Most authorities agree that of our total fat intake, no more than one-third should be saturated (hard) fat, and at least one-third should be polyunsaturated oils providing the two essential fats Omega 3 and Omega 6. These two essential fats also need to be roughly in balance – in other words 1:1, which is the ratio our pre-Industrial Revolution ancestors achieved. Nowadays, an average balance is more like 1:20 in favour of Omega 6. It may not be just gross deficiency in these fats, but also the gross imbalance between the two types, that is contributing to the mental and other health problems we see today.

Why is the modern diet likely to be more deficient in Omega 3 fats than in Omega 6? It's all because the grandmother of the Omega 3 family, alpha linolenic acid, and her metabolically active grandchildren EPA (eicosapentaenoic acid) and DHA (docasahexaenoic acid), are more unsaturated and so more prone to damage by cooking, heating and food processing. In fact, the average person today eats a mere one-sixth of the Omega 3 fats found in the diets of people living in 1850. This decline is partly due to food choices, but mainly to food processing.

In short, it is important to assess your need for essential fats if you have a mental health problem. Common symptoms of deficiency or imbalance include:

- Excessive thirst

- Chronic fatigue

- Dry or rough skin

- Dry hair, loss of hair or dandruff

- Pre-menstrual syndrome (PMS) or breast pain

- Eczema, asthma or joint aches

- Dyslexia or learning difficulties

- Hyperactivity

- Depression or manic depression

- Schizophrenia

If you have five or more of these symptoms and you have a mental health problem, it might be a good idea to have a blood test to determine your essential-fat status. The best foods for brain fats are:

Omega 3: flax seeds (linseeds), hemp seeds, pumpkin seeds, walnuts, salmon, mackerel, herring, sardines, anchovies, tuna and eggs.

Omega 6: sunflower seeds, sesame seeds, pumpkin seeds, maize, soya beans and wheat germ.

As far as supplements are concerned, for Omega 3 take fish oils (at least 200mg of EPA and 200mg of DHA), or one to two tablespoons of flax seed oil. For Omega 6 take starflower oil, 500 to 1,000 mg a day, or evening primrose oil, 1,000mg a day.

7. Heavy-metal toxicity

Heavy metals are so commonplace in our modern environment that the average person has body levels 700 times higher than those of our ancestors. Although high levels of lead are less common since the advent of lead-free petrol, some people have very high copper levels, mainly from copper plumbing in soft-water areas. Copper, although an essential mineral, can also be a toxic one when levels are elevated. High levels of cadmium are often found in smokers, as tobacco is relatively rich in it. Mercury from dental fillings can result in memory loss, and aluminium from cookware and foil is associated with senility. Check yourself out on the symptoms below:

- Anxiety, extreme fears or paranoia
- Phobias
- Poor concentration or confusion
- Poor memory
- Angry or aggressive feelings
- Hyperactivity
- Emotional instability
- Headaches or migraines
- Joint pain
- Nervousness

If you have five or more of these symptoms, a hair-mineral analysis is suggested, to test whether you've got an excess of toxic minerals. This inexpensive, non-invasive test can also highlight deficiencies in important minerals such as zinc, magnesium and manganese. A nutritional therapist can arrange this test for you.

8. Pyroluria and porphyria

Some people produce more of the protein-like chemicals kryptopyrroles and porphyrins than is healthy. An excess is linked to mental illness. The madness of King George III, for example, was almost certainly caused by porphyria. This, and probably pyroluria, are genetically inherited tendencies which increase a person's need for zinc. Stress also depletes zinc. So, if your mental health problems are strongly stress-related and the symptoms below apply to you, you may be pyroluric, or even porphyric, although the latter is much less common.

- Nausea or constipation

- White spots on fingernails

- Pale skin that burns easily

- Frequent colds and infections

- Stretch marks

- Irregular menstruation

- Impotency

- Crowded upper front teeth

- Poor tolerance of alcohol or drugs

- Poor dream recall

If you score five or more you may be pyroluric. You can test this by having a urine test for kryptopyrroles. If your level is high, you need more zinc and vitamin B6. Try 25mg of zinc and 100mg of B6 a day.

9. Histamine imbalance

Histamine is an often-overlooked neurotransmitter. Some people are genetically pre-programmed to produce too much histamine, a condition known as histadelia, and this can make a person excessively compulsive and obsessive. High-histamine types have a faster metabolism and therefore use up nutrients at a fast rate. Without good nutrition, they can easily become deficient, which can precipitate patches of deep depression. These are some of the symptoms associated with excess histamine:

- Headaches or migraines

- Sneezing in sunlight

- Crying, salivating or feeling nauseated easily

- Easy sexual orgasm

- Abnormal fears, compulsions, rituals

- Light sleep

- Fast metabolism

- Depression or suicidal thoughts

- Producing a lot of body heat

- Little body hair and lean build
- Large ears or long fingers and toes
- Good tolerance of alcohol
- Inner tension or 'driven' feeling
- Shyness or over-sensitivity as a child
- Seasonal allergies (e.g. hay fever)
- Obsessive or compulsive tendencies

If you have five or more of these symptoms you may be a high-histamine type. You can confirm this by having a blood test for histamine. If your blood levels are high you will benefit from supplementing vitamin C. Since histamine is detoxified by methylation, check your homocysteine level (see page 136).

Low levels of histamine are associated with the same kind of symptoms as B3, B12 and folic acid deficiency (see point 5, page 333), and respond well to supplementing of these nutrients. Histamine levels can also be determined as part of an overall neurotransmitter screening test.

10. Serotonin imbalance

A deficiency of the neurotransmitter serotonin is one of the most common findings in people with mental health problems. It is associated with sleeping problems, mood disturbance and aggressive and compulsive behaviour. Check yourself out on the symptoms below:

- Depression, especially post-menopausal
- Anxiety
- Aggressive or suicidal thoughts
- Violent or impulsive behaviour
- Mood swings, including PMS
- Obsessive or compulsive tendencies
- Alcohol or drug abuse
- Sensitivity to pain (low pain threshold)
- Craving for sweet foods
- Sleeping problems

If you have scored five or more you may be low in serotonin. A neuro-transmitter screening test can help confirm this.

Anti-depressant drugs like Prozac work by stopping the body from breaking down serotonin, thereby keeping more circulating in the brain. The trouble is that these kinds of drugs can induce unpleasant side effects. If you're low in serotonin, the natural alternative to take is 5-hydroxytryptophan (5-HTP). This is a precursor to serotonin and can help restore normal levels.

11. Adrenal imbalance

The adrenal glands and the brain produce three motivating neurotrans-mitters called dopamine, adrenalin and noradrenalin. The adrenal glands also produce cortisol. An excess of adrenalin can result in a state of high stress and anxiety, while a deficiency can result in the opposite – low energy, no motivation and poor concentration. There is evidence that some people may abnormally turn excessive amounts into toxins that induce disperceptions and even hallucinations. Check yourself out on the symptoms below:

- Irritability

- Nervousness or anxiety

- Extreme fears

- Raised blood pressure

- Rapid or irregular heartbeat

- Insomnia

- Cold hands and feet

- Excessive sweating

- Teeth-grinding

- Headaches or migraine

- Muscle tension

- Restlessness

- Seeing or hearing things

If you can relate to five or more of the symptoms you may have excessive levels of adrenalin or cortisol. If, on the other hand, the symptoms below sound like you, you may have adrenal insufficiency:

- Depression

- Difficulty concentrating

- Short attention span

- Lack of drive or motivation

- Difficulty in initiating or completing tasks

- Frequent tiredness

- Inability to deal with stress

- Social withdrawal

Both excess and deficiency can be tested either with an adrenal stress index, using saliva samples, or as part of a neurotransmitter screening test. For high adrenalin levels, cut back on stimulants and sugar and up your intake of vitamins B and C. If you have low adrenalin levels, you may benefit from supplementing the amino acid tyrosine. 'Adaptogenic' herbs such as Asian or Siberian ginseng or rhodiola can also help.

12. Acetylcholine imbalance

Acetylcholine is the brain's learning neurotransmitter. Low levels are associated with memory loss and even Alzheimer's disease. Levels tend to decline with age, but they don't have to if you are optimally nourished. Check yourself out on the symptoms below:

- Poor dream recall

- Infrequent dreaming

- Difficulty visualising

- Dry mouth

- Poor memory or forgetfulness

- Mental exhaustion

- Poor concentration

- Difficulty learning new things

If you score five or more on the symptom list, the chances are that you might be low in acetylcholine. A neurotransmitter screening test can help confirm this. Alternatively, you can simply supplement brain-friendly nutrients, such as a combination of phosphatidyl choline, serine, DMAE (dimethylaminoethanol), pyroglutamate and pantothenic acid (vitamin B5).

13. High homocysteine

A high level of homocysteine is very strongly linked with depression, schizophrenia, memory decline and Alzheimer's disease. For example, having a high homocysteine level doubles a person's risk for developing Alzheimer's disease, while 52 per cent of depressed people have high homocysteine. When homocysteine is high it results in your losing the ability to keep brain chemicals in balance. You consequently start feeling disconnected. This can result in depression and confusion. Check yourself out on the indicators below:

- Depression
- Poor concentration and memory
- Chronic tiredness
- Headaches or migraine
- Sleeping problems
- Joint or muscle aches or arthritis
- Deteriorating eyesight
- Family history of heart disease
- Family history of schizophrenia or Alzheimer's disease
- Frequent alcohol, coffee or cigarettes

If you score five or more, you may have a high homocysteine level. You can test your homocysteine level using a simple home test kit (see Resources, page 527). The solution is to up your intake of vitamins B6, B12 and folic acid, plus Omega 3 fats.

In summary

The easiest way to find out if there's a possibility that one or more of these imbalances is contributing to your problems is by completing the mental health questionnaire on the website www.mentalhealthproject.com. It gives you a print-out, which you can copy and give to your doctor, and advises you on what to do to eliminate these common causes of mental health problems using the principles of optimum nutrition. Alternatively, come and visit our Brain Bio Centre in London (see Resources, page 524) where we specialise in optimum nutrition for mental health problems and can arrange all the tests recommended in this chapter.

Dig deeper by reading my book *Optimum Nutrition for the Mind*.

Part 5

Nutrition for All Ages

39.

Birthrights and Wrongs

We are all older than we like to think. From a health perspective, the nine months spent in the womb and the months before conception are the most critical periods of our lives. Scientists are increasingly discovering that a mother's health and nutrition during pre-conception and pregnancy have a profound effect on the health of the infant, and that patterns of disease in adulthood can be traced to infant nutrition. Optimum nutrition increases fertility, the health of a pregnancy and the chances of having a healthy baby with strong resilience to disease.

Maximising fertility

One in every four couples suffers from some degree of infertility. For some, this means having fewer children than they want; for many, it means no children at all. And even for couples who are fertile, getting pregnant is not the easy matter that it is commonly thought to be. The average length of time taken to get pregnant is six months, although eighteen months is not uncommon. But unless fertility tests show otherwise, failure to conceive within eighteen months does not necessarily mean that you are completely infertile.

While it's well known that a woman's fertility decreases with age, did you know that a man's does too? A couple's chances of conceiving within six months of trying decrease by 2 per cent for every year the man is over twenty-four, regardless of how young his partner is. And if she's in her thirties, then she'll take twice as long to conceive as a woman in her twenties. Yet, despite these statistics, research has shown that if both partners are in good health and receiving optimum levels of all the right nutrients, the effect of their age on their chances of conceiving and having a successful pregnancy can be reduced.

Fertility and the speed of conception depend on many factors, some psychological, some physical and some nutritional. Conception rate is very high during holiday periods, for example, since stress – a major factor in infertility – is reduced. Knowing how to time intercourse to coincide with ovulation (the release of the female egg to be fertilised by the sperm) greatly increases the chances of conception. Also, your nutrition and especially your vitamin status play a crucial role.

Vitamins for fertility

The male partner is responsible in about a third of infertility cases. (It should be stressed that infertility has nothing to do with sexual virility, which is usually not affected.) The usual test for infertility in a man involves a sperm count – the higher the sperm count, the greater the fertility. One study has shown that extra vitamin C increased sperm count as well as sperm mobility.[1] Likewise, vitamin E or essential fat deficiency has been found to induce sterility in both sexes by causing damage to the reproductive tissues. Unfortunately, however, simply taking vitamin E will not reverse the condition if you are sterile.

The high rate of infertility among diabetics may provide us with a clue. Diabetics are frequently low in vitamin A, which is essential for making the male sex hormones. Vitamin A is dependent on the release of zinc from the liver. Of all the nutrients known to affect male fertility, zinc is perhaps the best researched. Signs of zinc deficiency include late sexual maturation, small sex organs and infertility. With adequate supplements of zinc these problems can be corrected.

Dr Carl Pfeiffer, Director of the Princeton Biocenter, one of the first research groups to identify the importance of zinc, also found a high degree of impotence and infertility in male patients who suffer from zinc deficiency. 'With adequate dosage of vitamin B6 and zinc,' he wrote, 'the sexual ability of the male should return in one or two months' time.' In view of the fact that the average dietary intake of zinc is half the RDA, the effects of zinc on fertility may be quite substantial and widespread. Zinc is found in high concentrations in male sex glands and in the sperm itself, where it is needed to make the outer layer and the tail.

Pre-conceptual care

The best odds for a healthy offspring are achieved when both partners prepare for pregnancy. It takes three months for sperm to mature, while the egg or ovum takes a month. If, during these pre-conceptual months, each partner pursues optimum nutrition, minimises his or her intake of antinutrients, especially alcohol, and stays healthy, the chances of a healthy conception are high, especially if the couple abstain from sex during the non-fertile phases of the month.

One in three conceptions is spontaneously aborted during the first three months of pregnancy. This risk is reduced when both partners are optimally nourished and healthy. A common cause of miscarriage is a lack of progesterone, which is needed to maintain the pregnancy in the early weeks. This can be a result of oestrogen dominance (see Chapter 25).

Homocysteine is a new health marker that's been making headlines for its association with more than 100 different health conditions including infertility and pregnancy complications. One study, which looked at nearly 6,000 women, found that those with high homocysteine levels were up to 100 per cent more likely to have suffered problems with their pregnancies or had babies with birth defects. It's now easy to have your homocysteine tested and if a high level is found, this can be reduced to a healthy level in around three months with the right nutritional supplements. It's well worth checking your homocysteine level before trying to conceive, and lowering your score, if it's above 6, by supplementing folic acid, B12, B6 and TMG (see Chapter 16).

Anyone considering IVF (where a woman's egg and her partner's sperm are fertilised outside her body and then impregnated in the womb) should cover all these 'optimum nutrition' bases first. While IVF has an average success rate of 21.8 per cent (and that's among the 'cream of the crop' who are selected for this expensive treatment), the holistic approach – where both partners are given an optimum nutrition 'MOT' and any underlying health problems resolved – has a success rate of more than 78 per cent, according to the pre-conceptual care organisation Foresight, who followed up the pregnancies of 1,076 couples, 779 of which resulted in a live birth.

Vitamins for a healthy pregnancy

Optimum nutrition can greatly improve your chances of having a healthy pregnancy. Even the slightest deficiencies during pregnancy can have serious effects on the health of the offspring, and the idea that birth defects are often caused by nutritional imbalances in the mother is rapidly gaining wider acceptance. So far, slight deficiencies of vitamins B1, B2 and B6, folic acid, zinc, iron, calcium and magnesium have all been linked to birth abnormalities. So too have excesses of toxic metals, especially lead, cadmium and copper.

Severe deficiencies of any vitamin will cause birth abnormalities, since a vitamin is by definition necessary for maintaining normal growth. A healthy pregnancy will of course depend on a greater supply than normal of all these nutrients, since accommodating the needs of a growing foetus as well as her own puts extra demands on the expectant mother.

Spina bifida

As many as 5 per cent of births show some developmental defect, many of which affect the central nervous system. Spina bifida, a condition in which the spinal chord does not develop properly, has been strongly linked to a lack of folic acid and probably of other nutrients too in the mother's diet. A survey of 23,000 women found that those who supplemented their diet during the first six weeks of pregnancy had a 75 per cent lower incidence of neural tube defects than those who did not.[2] The incidence of this condition is far higher when mothers have had a nutritionally poor diet for the first three months of pregnancy. One study found that dietary counselling alone lowered the rate of spina bifida in babies born to mothers at risk, but that the administration of extra folic acid, on its own or in a multivitamin, resulted in a much lower number of babies with neural tube defects. Since the optimum daily allowance (ODA) for folic acid intake is 800mcg per day, with a good diet providing 400mcg per day, a supplement of at least 400mcg per day is recommended for women intending to become pregnant.

Morning sickness

During the first three months of pregnancy all the organs of the baby's body are completely formed, so during this period optimum nutrition is extremely important. Yet at this time many women experience continual sickness and do not feel like eating healthily. Misnamed 'morning sickness', this condition has been accepted as normal during the first three months of pregnancy and is probably due to increases in a hormone called HCG. Women with poor diets are particularly at risk.

During pregnancy the need for vitamins B6 and B12, folic acid, iron and zinc increases; supplements of these usually stop even the worst cases of pregnancy sickness. Eating small, frequent amounts of fruit or complex carbohydrates like nuts, seeds or whole grains often helps. However, the best approach is to ensure optimum nutrition well before pregnancy. At

ION we followed up four women on optimum programmes before and during pregnancy – the average number of days on which nausea or sickness was reported was two. Yet for some women nausea continues throughout pregnancy!

Pre-eclamptic toxaemia

Another common complication of pregnancy is pre-eclamptic toxaemia, characterised by an increase in blood pressure, oedema (swelling) and excessive protein in the urine. Many theories abound as to why this occurs, but once more, optimum nutrition is a vital factor. One of my clients who had had pre-eclamptic toxaemia during her first pregnancy improved her diet and added nutritional supplements: her second pregnancy was entirely healthy.

Think zinc

Getting through pregnancy without developing any stretch marks isn't just down to luck – it's related to a woman's nutritional status. So for smooth, elastic skin, boost zinc levels by eating nuts, fish, peas and egg yolks and supplementing 15mg a day, and ensure a good daily source of vitamins C and E.

Food cravings in pregnancy are usually a sign of mineral deficiencies. When a mother-to-be boosts levels of zinc, for example, cravings usually disappear, while replenishing iron can remove cravings for strange, sometimes harmful, substances such as chalk or coal.

Vitamin and mineral supplements

For the mother, optimum nutrition before and during pregnancy ensures a healthier pregnancy with fewer complications, resulting in a healthier and heavier baby. Your daily supplement programme should include 400mcg of folic acid, 20mcg of vitamin B12, 50mg of vitamin B6, 15mg of zinc, 300mg of calcium, 200mg of magnesium and 12mg of iron. Do not take more than 3,000mcg of vitamin A, and have a hair-mineral analysis carried out to check for excesses of copper, lead or cadmium.

Essential fats

Also essential during pregnancy are essential fats, especially the Omega 3 fat DHA, and choline.

Research shows that getting a good supply of choline during pregnancy helps restructure a baby's developing brain for improved performance (it also improves memory in adults). To boost levels, eat lots of free-range eggs (the Columbus brand, available in most good supermarkets, is an especially rich source) and sprinkle lecithin granules (available from health food shops) on your cereal every morning. It is also well worth supplementing the essential Omega 3 and 6 fats GLA, EPA and DHA as well as eating fish. However, large fish such as swordfish, marlin and tuna contain higher levels of mercury than salmon and sardines, which have very little by comparison and still provided plenty of Omega 3 (see also pages 61–2).

Boosters after birth

Optimum nutrition is doubly important after birth, when the mother has to continue nourishing herself and her child. The stress of motherhood and the sleepless nights, coupled with extra nutritional needs, often make the first few months hard work. Breastfeeding (see also below) is not just best for a baby, it's also beneficial for the mother. It burns up 500 calories a day (making getting back in shape easier), stimulates the uterus to contract to its pre-birth size, reduces the mother's risk of developing breast cancer in later life and saves around £450 in formula and bottles in the first year. Any nutrients you supplement also get delivered straight to your baby, as well as giving your energy a boost. So, continue supplementing the recommended levels for pregnancy. Also make sure you have good support and a good supply of easy-to-prepare nutritious foods, especially during the first few weeks.

Post-natal depression

It is not uncommon for mothers to experience depression immediately after the birth. No doubt there is a psychological component to consider: now you have a baby – a big responsibility. However, many researchers believe that post-natal depression is brought on by hormonal and chemical changes that can be stopped with good nutrition.

One possibility is an excess of copper. The levels of copper tend to rise during pregnancy, while zinc levels tend to fall because the baby requires more. In most women the zinc content in breast milk declines rapidly as the infant uses up the mother's reserves. With a World Health Organization estimated requirement of 25mg a day, and an average intake of 7.5mg a day, yet no medical advice to increase zinc-rich foods or take supplements, zinc deficiency in mothers after giving birth is commonplace. Depression is a classic symptom, which can be corrected by supplementation with zinc and vitamin B6. According to Dr Carl Pfeiffer, who helped establish the importance of zinc for brain function, 'We have never seen post-natal depression or psychosis in any of our patients treated with zinc and B6.'

Another potential cause is lack of Omega 3 fats. Eating oily fish, and supplementing fish oils and zinc and B-complex formula, can ensure that a new mother doesn't develop post-natal depression.

The importance of breastfeeding

While breastfeeding does not guarantee optimum nutrition for the baby there is little doubt that breast is best, especially when the mother is optimally nourished. The balance of nutrients in breast milk in an optimally nourished woman is far superior to that in formula milks. One key factor is the high levels of essential fatty acids necessary for intellectual development. In fact, the discovery that breast-fed babies later achieved better intellectual performance than bottle-fed babies led to the realisation of the importance of giving infants high levels of essential fatty acids.

One other great disadvantage of bottle feeding is the milk itself. The consumption of cow's milk is strongly discouraged in infants before they are at least six months old. This is because their digestive and immune systems are too immature to deal with this complex protein – the result is often allergy. The recent discovery that child-onset diabetes results from the immune system's becoming allergic to a protein in cow's milk and beef, and then cross-reacting with a virtually identical protein in the pancreas, resulting in the destruction of pancreatic tissue, has led many paediatricians not only to caution against giving infants cow's milk before the age of six months, but also to advise mothers to keep off beef and milk for as long as they are breastfeeding. If this finding proves correct, a simple sacrifice could eliminate child-onset diabetes (see Chapter 8 for a fuller discussion).

Weaning – when and what?

Once a child can no longer sleep through the night without a feed, or is developing teeth, this is a good sign that it could be time to wean them on to solid foods – usually when they are around six months old. An infant's chewing on a piece of cucumber or carrot also helps to encourage other teeth to come through. Since the longest time between meals should be dinner to breakfast, introducing some solid food for dinner may help the child to sleep through the night.

Healthy babies, like healthy adults, need food that is fresh, unprocessed, additive-free, sugar-free (which includes sucrose, glucose, dextrose, maltose and fructose), salt-free and low in fat. In other words, they should be given food that is close to how it is found in nature. The baby will eventually be eating the food that you eat (which is, of course, completely healthy if you are following the recommendations in this book) and so will need to get used to eating this way right from the start. Below are a number of suggestions on how to eat healthily without using lots of packaged baby foods.

To be fair, packaged baby foods are improving all the time; they no longer contain artificial additives, and some are sugar-free. However, the idea that a baby needs fibre or should not have sugar on his puréed roast beef dinner has not yet filtered through to all baby-food manufacturers. As in the case of adult food, if you are going to use the occasional prepared food, read the label. If it contains cereal it should be wholemeal and unrefined; it should not contain any of the sugars listed above, modified starch, hydrogenated fat, hydrolysed vegetable protein or any ingredient that you do not understand.

Fibre for babies

Some mothers will not give their baby a high-fibre diet as it 'goes straight through them'. What they often mean is that they are getting three dirty nappies a day and cannot be bothered to change them that often. Frankly I would rather change three dirty nappies a day for a year or two than nurse an older person through the horrors of bowel cancer when the 'baby' is grown up. As in the case of an adult, a healthy infant bowel should be emptying itself two to three times a day. Much of the food will come out as recognisable lentils or grape skins, owing to the fact that a baby cannot chew foods properly.

Preventing allergies

If there's a family history of allergies or related conditions such as eczema or asthma, then it's possible to reduce the chances of passing these from mother to baby by 50 per cent simply by taking a 'probiotic' supplement during pregnancy. Biotic means life, and a probiotic encourages friendly bacteria to thrive in the digestive tract. Modern living means that many people's digestive bacteria are compromised by stress, a diet high in refined carbohydrates, antibiotics and steroid drugs such as the contraceptive Pill – and these contribute to digestive problems, allergies, eczema and asthma.

At the start of weaning, give your baby food that is very easily digested and unlikely to cause an allergic reaction. Cooked, puréed vegetables and fruit are a good start. If a fruit or vegetable can be given raw, leave it like that, for example bananas, avocados, very ripe William pears or paw-

paws. The later you introduce a food, the less likelihood there is of its pro-ducing an allergic reaction. So if you suspect that your child may react allergically (if there is, for instance, a family history of allergy) or you just want to be absolutely certain that your child does not have any allergies, introduce potential allergens as late as you can. Below is a list of foods and food groups in increasing order of being likely to give an allergic reaction. Start by giving the foods at the top and, as each one is cleared, move down the list.

- Vegetables

- Fruit (except oranges)

- Nuts and seeds

- Pulses and beans

- Rice

- Meat

- Oats, barley and rye

- Oranges

- Wheat

- Milk products

- Eggs

Introduce one or two foods each day and make a note of which ones you have given and any possible reaction, which may be anything from mild to severe eczema, excessive sleepiness, a runny nose or colic to an ear infection, excessive thirst, over-activity or asthmatic breathing. If you notice a reaction, withdraw that food and carry on with new foods once the reaction has died down. You can double-check your observations a few months later: the reaction may disappear as the digestive system matures. The last four foods should not be introduced until your baby is nine or ten months old; this also applies to any foods that either parent is known to have a reaction to.

Baby-food purées

Your partly weaned baby will still be getting plenty of nourishment from breast milk, and you may well find that you are breastfeeding as much as before. This is quite all right – in fact mothers should ideally breastfeed a lot right up until the baby is a year old. Assuming your baby is getting most of his or her protein, fat and carbohydrate from breast milk, you would do best to feed him or her plenty of vitamin- and mineral-rich vegetables and fruit. Simply cook a combination of vegetables or fruit (there is no need to add sugar) and purée them. Here are some good combinations:

- Carrots alone

- Cauliflower and turnip

- Carrots, spinach and cauliflower

- Broad beans and cauliflower or carrot, plus a very little celery

- Jerusalem artichokes and carrot

- Peeled courgettes (the skins can be bitter) and fennel

- Leek and potato

- Swede, turnip and potato

Do experiment. To save time and effort, not to mention disappointment when your baby rejects your lovingly prepared purées, you can freeze these mixtures. Start by using ice-cube trays for the tiniest amounts (you can also express breast milk and freeze it in sterilised ice-cube trays to mix with purées and make them taste more like what your baby is used to) and progress to small jars and yoghurt pots with lids.

You can slowly add other ingredients to these purées. Try red split lentils, cooked bean sprouts, well-cooked brown rice, black-eyed beans and other pulses, milk, cheese, yoghurt or soya milk. Breakfast can consist of more puréed vegetables – babies do not have to have sweet breakfast cereals or fruit, which only encourage a sweet tooth. As you introduce more cereals into the diet, you can cook brown rice flour as you would semolina and add puréed fruit for a lovely breakfast. An easier alternative is to pour some boiling water on to three teaspoons of fine oatmeal and leave this to stand for a few minutes. Puréed fruit, mashed banana, yoghurt, or expressed breast or rice milk may be added. Millet flakes, which can be bought in health food shops, can be prepared in the same way as oatmeal. As the child gets older, porridge oats may be used in place of oatmeal and the banana can be sliced instead of mashed.

Dig deeper by reading my book *Optimum Nutrition Before, During and After Pregnancy* co-authored with Susannah Lawson.

chapter 40

Superkids – Nourishing the Next Generation

What you feed your child to a large extent determines their health and dietary habits for life. As a parent, the time you spend nourishing your child properly may be the greatest contribution you can make to their development. In today's snack culture, in which children and adults are bombarded with advertisements for junk food, you have to be strong to help your child develop good eating habits. But it is worth it.

Developing good habits

The taste for sugar is acquired through eating sweeter and sweeter foods. It can also be lost, usually with some resistance, by gradually reducing the level of sweetness in foods and drinks. This means replacing sweetened drinks with fruit juice, diluted half and half with water. Among the fruit juices, apple contains the slowest-releasing sugars, while grape juice contains the fastest-releasing ones. So apple juice is preferable. Few children drink enough water. You can encourage your child to drink water by putting it on the table at mealtimes, and when they are thirsty give them water for the first glass and diluted juice for the second.

Do not give sweets, sweetened foods, cola and other sweetened drinks as treats. If you do, these drinks become associated with something good, and later in life your offspring may choose to treat themselves all the time. Instead give fresh orange or pineapple juice, diluted with fizzy water. Cola drinks are especially bad because most contain caffeine, an addictive drug. It is quite amazing, given that you have to be an adult to smoke and drink alcohol, that caffeine can be freely added to drinks advertised to children who cannot even read.

Very few breakfast cereals are truly sugar-free. Food manufacturers help children to develop a sweet tooth at an early age: most processed cereals contain fast-releasing sugars and have added sugar. Instead of giving your children such cereals, provide them with a choice of oats, sugar-free cornflakes or other such unsweetened wholegrain cereals, and encourage them to sweeten their cereal with fruit such as a sliced banana, apple or pear, some berries or perhaps a few raisins.

The best snacks are fruit (especially berries), so make sure you always have a mountain of fresh, appealing fruit for your children to nibble on at their discretion. Send them to school with fruit rather than money to buy sweets. Sure, when they are older and have pocket money they will buy sweets and get them at parties. But if sweets, sweetened drinks and foods are not part of their day-to-day diet they are unlikely to crave them or develop an addiction.

Another good habit to develop in your children is eating vegetables, including raw ones, with each meal. The trick here is to find ways of preparing vegetables so that they taste good. Too many vegetables are cooked to death and taste bland. Raw organic carrots, peas, parsnip chips (made by steam frying in diluted soy sauce), and mashed and jacket-baked potatoes are naturally quite sweet and favourites with children. Serving something raw with each meal, even if it is just a few leaves of watercress, grated red cabbage, tomato or carrot, develops the taste for salad foods.

While there are many ways of making healthy desserts, if a child always ends a meal this way they acquire a habit for life. Instead, restrict healthy desserts as a treat and give the child as much of the main course as he or she wants. If my children are still hungry at the end of a meal they help themselves to fruit.

Allergies start young

Children are like the canaries once used to check whether coalmines were safe from poisonous gases: they are very sensitive and react readily to substances. This is the first stage of the stress response (see page 183). By paying attention you can find out what does not suit your child. Many children react adversely to food additives, sugar, dairy products, peanuts, wheat, detergents, house-dust mites or exhaust fumes. Some react to eggs, oranges and other gluten grains like oats. Watch out for the following symptoms:

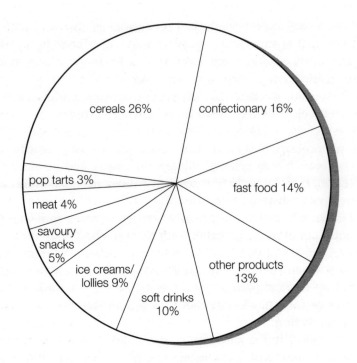

Sugar and spice and all things nice

Face Rings around the eyes, 'black' eyes, facial puffiness, constant sniffling, frequent colds, excessive mucus production, frequent earache, tonsillitis

Skin Itches, rashes, eczema, puffiness or water retention

Digestive Colic, vomiting, diarrhoea, stomach ache, wind

Mental Hyperactivity, poor concentration, being over-emotional, sleeplessness, bedwetting

Respiratory Coughing, frequent sore throats, swollen tongue or throat, asthma, respiratory infections

All these are the classic signs of allergy. The good news is that children rapidly respond once the offending substances are removed. Try removing suspected foods or environmental allergens for ten days and see if the child improves. If the allergic reactions are severe it is best to carry out what is known as an elimination/challenge investigation under the supervision of a qualified health professional. Also make sure that the child's diet is not becoming too restrictive.

Optimum nutrition, plus judicious use of supplements, can greatly decrease potential to react allergically provided the offending items are removed. Often, after a couple of months, a child can tolerate a food that previously offended, perhaps eating it only every four days to prevent the body from 'remembering' the food and learning to react allergically again. For more on allergies read Chapter 34.

Kid life crisis

Childhood should be a happy thing – a time to learn, to play and to have fun. Yet the trends show that something rather sinister is happening to many children. Learning difficulties, attention deficit hyperactivity disorder (ADHD), autism, depression and even suicide rate are rapidly increasing. More and more children are having more and more problems learning, behaving appropriately and socialising.

According to a survey by London's City University a quarter of all children 'often' or 'always' feel stressed. In the US there are now eight million children on Ritalin, a habit-forming amphetamine with many similar properties to cocaine. That's 10 per cent of all boys between the ages of six and fourteen! Alcohol abuse is up too, with one in six eleven-year-old girls drinking every week. In both the US and the UK incidence of hyperactivity is rapidly on the increase.

Diagnoses of autism more than tripled between 1987 and 1999.[3] UK figures range from three times to ten times more cases in the last decade. While autism used to occur primarily 'from birth', or at least was detected within the first six months, over the past ten years there has been a dramatic increase in 'late-onset' autism, most frequently diagnosed in the second year of life. This strongly suggests that something new is triggering this epidemic. Possible culprits include diet, vaccinations and digestive disorders, including Crohn's disease and coeliac disease, both of which are also very much more common in children than they used to be.

To understand these problems I'd like to propose that we are looking at a spectrum of problems, from learning difficulties at one end, including dyslexia and dyspraxia, to autism at the other. Somewhere in the middle of this spectrum we can put so-called attention deficit hyperactivity disorder. This condition doesn't really exist as a disease entity in the same way that diabetes or depression does. It's more of a catch-all category into which children with a variety of problems get put and then are far too often prescribed a drug like Ritalin.

Symptoms such as poor co-ordination, inability to concentrate, mood swings, inappropriate emotional reactions, fatigue, depression, digestive problems, writing and reading difficulties, poor eye-to-hand co-ordination and other visual perception problems, in varying degrees, are the hallmark of too many children. What all these have in common is the brain.

The brain drain

The brain is the most vulnerable organ of the body. Optimum nutrition during foetal development has a profound effect on the brain, learning and behaviour. Yet many of the most important nutrients for brain development, such as essential fats and fat-soluble vitamins and zinc, are commonly missing in the average twenty-first-century junk-food diet. These nutrients are also essential for digestive health. They have been replaced by high-sugar foods, highly processed fat, refined wheat and dairy products.

Essential fats and ADHD

Many children with ADHD have known symptoms of essential fatty acid (EFA) deficiency such as excessive thirst, dry skin, eczema and asthma. It is also interesting that males, who have a much higher EFA requirement than females, are more commonly affected: four out of five ADHD sufferers are boys. Researchers have theorised that ADHD children may be deficient in essential fatty acids not just because they have inadequate dietary intake (though this is not uncommon), but rather because their need is higher, because they absorb them poorly or because they don't convert them well into prostaglandins that help the brain communicate.[4]

Research at Oxford University has proven the value of these essential fats in a 'double-blind' trial involving forty-one children aged eight to twelve years with ADHD symptoms and specific learning difficulties. Those children receiving extra essential fats in supplements were both behaving and learning better within twelve weeks.[5]

Vitamins and minerals and ADHD

It is of interest, then, that EFA conversion to prostaglandins can be inhibited by most of the foods that cause symptoms in children with ADHD such as wheat and dairy products. Conversion is also hindered by deficiencies of the various vitamins and minerals needed for the enzymes that power the conversions, including vitamins B3 (niacin), B6 and C, biotin, zinc and magnesium. Zinc deficiency is common in children with learning difficulties.

Autism: the case for vitamin A

Paediatrician Dr Mary Megson from Richmond, Virginia, believes that many autistic-spectrum children are lacking in vitamin A. Otherwise known as retinol, vitamin A is essential for vision. It is also needed for building healthy cells in the gut and in the brain. There is no real doubt that something funny is going on in the digestive tracts of many of these children. Could this be related to vitamin A deficiency, she wondered?

The best sources of vitamin A are breast milk, organ meats, milk fat, fish and cod liver oil, none of which is prevalent in our modern diets. Instead, we have formula milk, fortified food and multivitamins, many of which contain altered forms of retinol such as retinyl palmitate, which doesn't work as well as the fish- or animal-derived retinol. What would happen, wondered Dr Megson, if these children weren't getting enough natural vitamin A?[6] Not only would this affect the integrity of the digestive tract, potentially leading to allergies, but also it would affect the development of their brains and disturb vision. Both brain differences and visual defects have been detected in autistic children. The visual defects, she deduced, were an important clue because lack of vitamin A would mean poor black and white vision, a symptom often seen in the relatives of autistic kids.

If you were seeing without black and white, what you'd lose is shadow. Without shadow you'd lose 3D and, as a consequence, you couldn't tell people's expressions so well. This might explain why autistic children tend not to look straight at you. They look to the side. Long thought to be a sign of poor socialisation, this may in fact be the best way they can see people's expressions because there are more black and white light receptors at the edge of the visual field than in the middle!

Of course, the proof is in the pudding, and Dr Mary Megson has, simply by giving cod liver oil containing natural, unadulterated vitamin A, reported rapid and dramatic improvements in autism, often within a week of the subjects' starting cod liver oil.[7]

Toxic foods

Sugar

A diet high in refined carbohydrates is not good for anyone, and many parents believe than eating sweets promotes hyperactivity and aggression in their children. Many studies do consistently report that hyperactive children have higher sugar consumption than other children,[8] and reducing dietary sugar has been found to halve disciplinary actions in young offenders.[9]

A study of 265 hyperactive children found that more than three-quarters displayed abnormal glucose tolerance.[10] Glucose is the main fuel for the brain and body, and when blood glucose levels fluctuate wildly all day on a rollercoaster ride of refined carbohydrates, stimulants, sweets, chocolate, fizzy drinks, juices and little or no fibre to slow the glucose absorption, it is not surprising that levels of activity, concentration, focus and behaviour will also fluctuate wildly, as is seen in children with ADHD. The calming effect sometimes observed after sugar consumption may well be the initial normalisation of blood sugar from a hypoglycemic state during which the brain and cognitive functions controlling behaviour were starved of fuel.

Wheat and milk

Not only is breast milk best for essential fats and vitamin A; breastfeeding up to the age of at least four months is essential to limit a child's chances of developing sensitivity to milk.

In addition to these likely deficiencies, the most significant contributing factor in autism appears to be undesirable foods and chemicals that often reach the brain via the bloodstream because of faulty digestion and absorption. The most common offending foods are wheat, high in gluten, and dairy products containing casein. These proteins are difficult to digest and, especially if introduced too early in life, may result in an allergy. Fragments of these proteins, called peptides, can mimic chemicals in the brain called endorphins, so are often referred to as 'exorphins'. These exporphin peptides have damaging opioid-like effects in the brain, leading to many of the symptoms found in children with behavioural problems. Researchers at the Autism Research Unit at Sunderland University have found increased levels of these peptides in the blood and urine of children with autism.[11]

To understand how these common foods can be so harmful to sensitive individuals we need to look at how they get into the body via the gut. Opioid peptides are derived from the incomplete digestion of proteins, particularly food containing gluten and casein. One such peptide (IAG), derived from gluten in wheat, is detected in 80 per cent of autistic people.[12] So the first problem is the poor digestion of proteins, which is what happens if you are zinc-deficient. But even then, these partially digested protein fragments shouldn't enter the bloodstream. So how do they? Vitamin A and essential-fat deficiency is certainly one culprit, but there may be more.

Improving children's behaviour and mental performance

To test the effect of all these factors together I designed a one-week experiment. Working with ITV's *This Morning* we selected a class of thirty children aged six to seven years in a London primary school and identified twelve children who were most disruptive and had learning difficulties.

For one week the children and their parents were asked to not eat or drink foods containing added sugar or additives. The children were also asked to eat more fish and put seeds on their morning cereal. Seeds and fish are good sources of essential fats. In addition, they were given an Optio, a fruit-juice drink with added vitamins.

Four out of the twelve children showed a dramatic improvement in behaviour, concentration, reading and writing. Reece was one of these children; at the beginning of the week he had real problems concentrating, sitting still, reading and writing. By the end of the week he had gone through a Jekyll and Hyde transformation. Below are examples of a writing test he was given at the beginning and end of the week. Not only did he latterly write one and a half pages, compared with four lines, but also his handwriting improved dramatically. His mother, who was sceptical about the trial, said, 'I thought that nothing could calm this child down. We'd seen a psychologist but they didn't help. He was very fidgety, he was hard to get into bed, hyperactive and constantly on the go and with occasional tantrums. Now he's a completely different child. He's a lot calmer and he wants to do more at school. In two weeks his reading has gone up a level. He doesn't get so over-excited and he's much nicer to be with. We are definitely going to stick with the diet.'

Of course, not everything can be blamed on diet and nutritional deficiencies. As for adults, modern living is also proving stressful for children. Too many children are pressured to perform in a century where the motto is 'succeed and achieve'. Perhaps living out their parents' dissatisfactions they go from school, to piano, to extra coaching, with no time left to do nothing or to play. Combine these psychological pressures with poor diet and too many children go over the edge into mental health problems. Some want to go further. Childline receive 1,500 calls each year from suicidal children. More than ever, our children need love, support and optimum nutrition.

Supplements for children

The best time to start supplementing a child's diet is as soon as they are no longer being breast-fed (during breastfeeding, it's the mother who needs supplements). I recommend that you start supplementing your child's diet when they begin to rely more on solid food rather than breast milk as their main source of nutrients. This is usually around the age of six to nine months. The ideal daily supplement programme, from weaning to the age of eleven, is shown in the following chart.

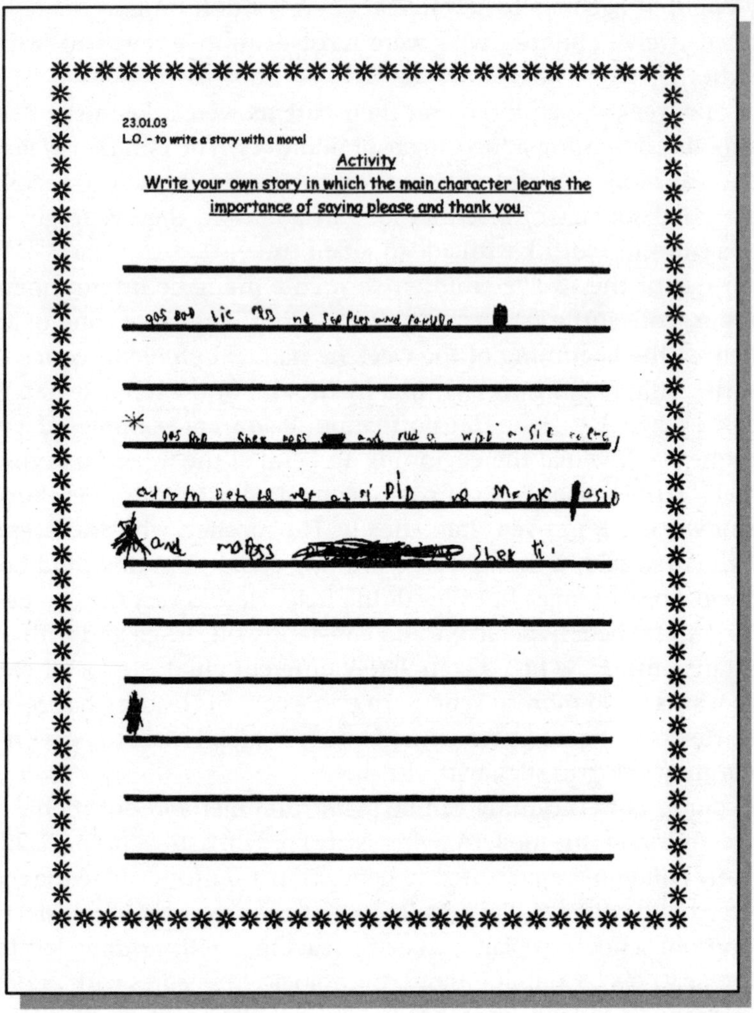

23.01.03
L.O. - to write a story with a moral

Activity

Write your own story in which the main character learns the importance of saying please and thank you.

Reece's handwriting before

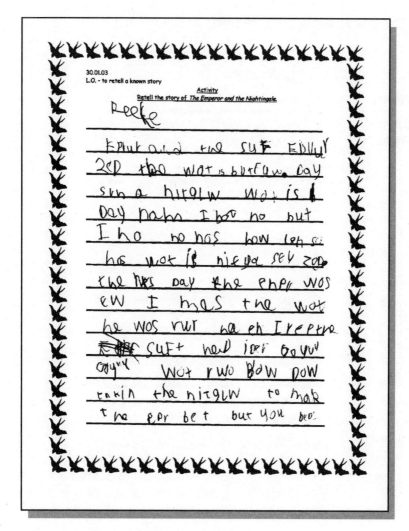

and after one week of optimum nutrition

■ The ideal daily supplement programme

		Age					
Nutrient	Less than 1	1	2	3–4	5–6	7–8	9–11
Vitamins							
A (retinol)	500mcg	600	700	800	1,000	1,500	2,000
D	1mcg	1.25	1.5	1.75	2.25	2.5	2.5
E	13mg	13	17	20	23	30	40
C	100mg	100	200	300	400	500	600
B1 (thiamine)	5mg	5	6	8	12	16	20
B2 (riboflavin)	5mg	5	6	8	12	16	20
B3 (niacin)	7mg	10	14	16	18	20	22
B5 (pantothenic acid)	10mg	10	15	20	25	30	35
B6 (pyridoxine)	5mg	5	7	10	12	16	20
B12	5mcg	6	7	8	9	10	10
Folic Acid	100mcg	100	120	140	160	180	200
Biotin	30mcg	40	50	60	70	80	90
Minerals							
Calcium	150mg	160	170	180	190	200	210
Magnesium	50mg	60	70	80	90	100	110
Iron	4mg	5	6	7	8	9	10
Zinc	4mg	5	6	7	8	9	10
Manganese	300mcg	300	350	400	500	700	1,000
Iodine	50mcg	75	100	125	150	175	200
Chromium	15mcg	17	20	23	25	27	30
Selenium	10mcg	15	20	25	28	30	35
EFAs							
GLA	50mg	65	80	95	110	135	150
EPA	100mg	150	200	250	300	350	400
DHA	100mg	125	150	175	200	225	250

Choosing the right supplements

Many companies formulate single multivitamin and mineral supplements that incorporate all the necessary nutrients especially for children (see Resources, page 532). The chart provided above gives you a guideline as to the levels of nutrients to look for. You can choose chewable (crushable in the early stages) or liquid formulas, depending on your (or your child's) preferences.

You should ideally give your child their supplement with breakfast, but certainly not last thing at night as the B vitamins can have a mild stimulatory effect. Children also tend to be more susceptible to vitamin toxicity than adults, and while the doses listed are well within any potentially toxic limits for even the most sensitive child, don't be tempted to give more than the recommended levels unless under the direction and supervision of a nutritional therapist.

Essential fats to boost IQ

As long as your child is eating oily fish three times a week and a daily portion of seeds, they should be getting a good level of essential fats to help their brains develop and boost IQ. However, if they don't eat fish or seeds every day, I recommend that you supplement their diet with an essential fatty acid (EFA) formula. Look for one that contains both GLA (Omega 6) and DHA and EPA (Omega 3), which are the most important Omega 3 fats for development (see Resources, page 530). The above chart gives you the rough quantities to aim for in a supplement, assuming the child is receiving the same again from seeds and the occasional fish.

chapter 41

Puberty, PMS, the Menopause and the Andropause

The transition from child to adult is no less easy biologically than psychologically. At puberty the body undergoes rapid changes focused on sexual development that require optimal nutrition to avoid 'side effects'. These include acne and obesity, and eating, mental and behavioural problems. These are common indications that the person is not adapting as well as possible to the changes.

Both girls and boys need relatively more vitamins A, D and B6, biotin, zinc, calcium, magnesium and essential fatty acids during puberty. In an assessment of nutritional needs (see page 402), these nutrients are upped between the ages of fourteen and sixteen. Once a child reaches fourteen their nutritional needs are essentially the same as those of adults, with a greater emphasis on these nutrients, plus an ongoing need for adequate protein because adolescents are still growing.

Of these nutrients, zinc and magnesium are most often found to be lacking. Zinc is needed for sexual maturation by both sexes, but boys need more. The relative decline in the growth rate of boys during adolescence is probably partly due to sub-optimal intake of zinc – what zinc they do have is taken for sexual maturation in preference to growth. Growth problems, 'growing pains' and acne are all possible indications of a lack of zinc.

The teenage years are also associated with increasing 'food freedom' and it is important that teenagers learn to nourish themselves. If they are not given nutrition education from school or their parents they opt for food that tastes good, rather than food that does them good. The link between food and good skin and physical and mental strength needs to be emphasised, since these are all desired qualities. The key habits to encourage are:

- Eating seeds, perhaps a tablespoon of ground seeds on cereal – these are very rich in zinc, magnesium and essential fatty acids

- Eating fruit in preference to sweets and fatty, sugary snacks

- Always having some vegetables with a meal; most schools have no idea how to make vegetables enticing and teenagers often develop an aversion to them during their school years

- Eating real meals rather than refuelling on the move

Beating PMS through diet

Pre-menstrual problems, termed pre-menstrual syndrome (PMS), were until relatively recently accepted as a woman's lot. Yet these symptoms – which include depression, tension, headaches, breast tenderness, water retention, bloating, low energy and irritability – are in most cases avoidable. Classically, they occur in the week preceding menstruation, though a small percentage of women have the symptoms from the middle of the cycle, coinciding with ovulation. Since pre-menstrual problems are a result of hormonal changes, hormone treatment has been used to correct them. But the use of such drug treatment must be seriously questioned, as it disrupts the body's chemistry and has been associated with increased risk of cancer.

The effectiveness of vitamin B6 has been proved in some studies to help 70 per cent of pre-menstrual sufferers.[13] But researchers soon found that B6 with zinc, which is needed to convert B6 into its active form, was more effective. Dr Guy Abrahams, a researcher in California, then discovered that magnesium was especially effective at reducing the symptom of breast tenderness and swelling.[14]

More recently, research has focused on the role of gamma linolenic acid (GLA), an essential fatty acid found in evening primrose and borage oils. GLA's 60 per cent success rate is almost certainly due to its role in making prostaglandins.[15]

We now know that vitamin B6, zinc and magnesium are also required to make prostaglandins and, perhaps for this reason, have been shown to help pre-menstrual tension (PMT) sufferers. These nutrients alone can easily halve symptoms, as we found out in a trial at ION. In this trial of PMT sufferers, in which both patients and their doctors rated their improvement for each pre-menstrual health problem, there was a substantial improvement of 55–85 per cent. On average, within three months a woman on a supplement programme of this kind could expect a 66 per cent improvement in each problem.

In some kinds of PMS, hormonal changes disturb blood sugar control and bring on sugar and stimulant changes, as well as symptoms of tiredness and irritation. Following a strict no-sugar, no-stimulant diet, while eating complex carbohydrates or fruit, little and often, can make all the difference. Diet, coupled with supplements, can often relieve symptoms of PMS all together.

In a small percentage of women, PMS indicates a more pronounced hormonal imbalance that cannot be corrected by diet and supplements alone. Such an imbalance is usually due to oestrogen dominance (see page 219) and a relative lack of progesterone. This condition can be brought on by a period of time on the Pill and needs testing and correcting by a qualified nutrition consultant or doctor.

The pros and cons of contraception

As a source of contraception, the Pill has too many health drawbacks. In my opinion the best method of contraception for any couple is knowing when ovulation occurs through observing temperature and vaginal mucus changes (for more details read the book *Natural Family Planning*[16]). Once a woman is in tune with her cycle she will very often have feelings and sensations that mark ovulation, and test kits can also now be bought. Once the time of ovulation is known, there is no chance of conception from three days after ovulation until seven days before the next ovulation. That is half the cycle dealt with. At other times non-invasive barrier methods such as condoms or caps can be used, or even abstinence practised.

The Chinese say that too much sex depletes vital energy, particularly in a man. We know that a man can lose up to 3mg of zinc per ejaculation. With an average daily intake of only 7.5mg, a man having sex three times a day has certainly blown it as far as zinc is concerned! This is one reason why it is better for a man to abstain in the days leading up to conception.

The only trouble with using ovulation times as a means of contraception is that sub-optimum nutrition often leads to irregular periods. Also, if there is an underlying hormone imbalance such as oestrogen dominance, it may take a while to establish a regular, healthy cycle. In such cases it is especially important to avoid synthetic hormones, which are more often than not the cause of the imbalance in the first place.

Menopausal symptoms – what works?

For many women it is not the fear of osteoporosis, breast cancer or heart disease that is most concerning about the menopause, but how to cope with the debilitating symptoms that affect their daily lives – most commonly hot flushes, fatigue, headaches, irritability, insomnia, and depression.

The usual remedy prescribed by doctors is HRT, but that is now being actively discouraged owing to the proven increased risk of breast cancer (see page 282). So, what works without the risk?

Exercise

According to a study of Swedish women conducted by Lund University, the more vigorous physical exercise you do the less likely you are to suffer from hot flushes.

Blood sugar control

Recent research at the University of Texas at Austin has proven what nutritionists have known all along: if you have 'disglycemia', which means that your blood sugar level goes up and down like a yo-yo, you are much more likely to experience fatigue, irritability, depression and hot flushes than if you don't. The best way to control this is to eat low-glycemic-load carbohydrates with protein. The system explained in my book *The Holford Diet* makes this way of eating highly practical.

Vitamins C and E

Vitamin C actually helps your hormones to work, so when levels are low, 1 or 2 grams of vitamin C a day smoothes the edges. Choose a supplement that contains berry extracts, rich in bioflavonoids, as there's evidence that these help too. Vitamin E is another all-round hormonal helper. A daily intake of 600mg helps vaginal dryness but takes at least a month to work.

Essential fats

Research isn't great on the therapeutic effect of essential fats on menopausal symptoms, but they are so essential for balancing hormones and mood that I recommend eating seeds (flax, sesame, sunflower, pumpkin) daily and supplementing some EPA (300mg), DHA (200mg) and GLA (100mg).

Soya, isoflavones and red clover

Four trials have now shown that isoflavones, which are especially rich in soya and red clover, approximately halve the incidence and severity of hot flushes. Two placebo-controlled studies did not find this effect, at least at a level of statistical significance, but did find that the higher the excretion of isoflavones the lower the incidence of hot flushes, suggesting that a high intake of isoflavones, from diet or supplements, is effective. Soya, tofu and isoflavones have also been shown to be cancer-protective, unlike oestrogen HRT. My advice is to eat some tofu regularly, meaning at least every other day. You probably need 50 grams a day for an effect. Again, don't expect immediate results. Supplements containing isoflavone extracts may help, but the research to date isn't conclusive. They are worth trying if all else fails.

Black cohosh

Most promising are the results with the herb black cohosh, which helps hot flushes, sweating, insomnia and anxiety. Also encouraging is new research that shows that black cohosh doesn't have a downside – it doesn't increase cancer risk and it isn't anti-oestrogenic. The usual recommended daily amount is 50mg, although much larger amounts, up to 500mg, are more effective. It also helps raise serotonin, relieving depression.

St John's wort

The combination of black cohosh and St John wort (300mg a day) is particularly effective for women who experience depression, irritability and fatigue. St John's wort, renowned for its anti-depressant effects, has been demonstrated to relieve other menopausal symptoms, including headaches, palpitations, lack of concentration and decreased libido. A medical trial in Germany found that 80 per cent of women felt that their symptoms had gone or substantially improved after taking St John's wort for twelve weeks.

Dong quai

The other 'hot' herb for hot flushes is dong quai, botanically called *Angelica sinensis*. One placebo-controlled experiment giving dong quai plus camomile to fifty-five post-menopausal women who complained of hot flushes and refused hormonal therapy found that they experienced a big reduction, of almost 80 per cent, in hot flushes. These results became apparent after one month. Try 600mg a day.

Progesterone cream

Menopausal symptoms are caused just as much by a fall-off in progesterone as by a drop in oestrogen. Once a woman stops ovulating, progesterone levels plummet. While HRT preparations have all used man-made, progesterone-like chemicals called progestins, which have undesirable side effects including increased cancer risk, body-identical progesterone, often called 'natural progesterone', reduces cancer risk and works very well for menopausal symptoms.

A recent trial in the US, published in the *Journal of Obstetrics and Gynaecology*, found that progesterone cream significantly relieved or arrested symptoms in 83 per cent of women, compared with 19 per cent of women on placebo. To find out more contact the Natural Progesterone Information Service (see Resources, page 525).

Combined remedies

Combinations of all these herbs, nutrients and diet and lifestyle changes should yield the best results. One recent study gave a combination of panax ginseng, black cohosh, soya, and green tea extracts in the morning and black cohosh, soya, kava, hops, and valerian extracts in the evening. By the end of the second week, the number of hot flushes was reduced by 47 per cent.[17] By the way, acupuncture and yoga have also both been proven to help.

Synthetic or natural HRT?

The conventional view is that menopausal symptoms are brought about by a lack of oestrogen. There is little doubt that the cessation of menstruation is due to declining levels of oestrogen, which are needed to trigger ovulation. For this reason oestrogen HRT is given. However, as soon as a woman starts having cycles without ovulation, often many years before her periods stop, no progesterone is produced (this is because the progesterone is produced in the sac that is left after the ovum is released). While oestrogen levels decline – they do not stop – progesterone production drops to zero. The continued relative excess of oestrogen compared over progesterone, coupled with progesterone deficiency, may prove to be the major cause of menopausal symptoms.

Both oestrogen HRT and natural progesterone augmentation (given as a small amount of skin cream twice a day) can stop symptoms. However, conventional HRT suits few women and 70 per cent stop within a year of starting it, usually because of unpleasant symptoms or a lack of results. While oestrogen and synthetic progestin HRT is strongly linked to increased risk of breast cancer and is no longer being recommended to women for osteoporosis prevention, natural progesterone is anti-cancer (see page 282) and four times more effective at reversing osteoporosis (see page 224). It is best to get professional advice, including tests, to correct hormone imbalances. However, the combination of diet, supplements and, when needed, small amounts of natural progesterone, can transform a woman's experience of the menopause.

Andropause – the male menopause

Men too can suffer from menopausal symptoms later in life. The symptoms of the male menopause, known as the andropause, are very similar to those of the female menopause – fatigue, depression, irritability, rapid ageing, aches and pains, sweating, flushing and decreased sexual performance.

Having successfully treated thousands of ailing men, Dr Malcolm Carruthers, world authority on testosterone and author of *The Testosterone Revolution*, is convinced that the andropause is real and connected to decreasing levels of free testosterone, the male sex hormone (see page 282).

Exactly why free-testosterone levels decline is a bit of a mystery; however, a number of contributors may be involved. These include stress, too much alcohol and overheating of the testes. More insidious, however, are the effects of increasing xenoestrogens, chemicals in the environment with actions similar to those of the female hormone oestrogen, which have recently been found to be anti-androgenic, blocking the action of testosterone.

Xenoestrogens are found in everything from pesticides to plastic. 'Perhaps future generations of archaeologists,' says Carruthers, 'will come across a thick stratum of plastic bags, marking the demise of *homo plasticus* or "plastic bag man" who was neutered by the by-products of the consumer society.' According to recent research, the pesticide DDT breaks down into a substance (DDE) that has little oestrogenic activity, but fifteen times the anti-androgen effect of DDT. Residues of these chemicals, long since banned, are still found in the food chain. To what extent the average intake of pesticide residues is contributing to decreasing levels of testosterone is unknown.

Testosterone is made in the body from cholesterol. Very low-cholesterol diets can lower testosterone levels, but antioxidant nutrients such as vitamin E help to protect valuable cholesterol from being damaged. Testosterone can also be made from DHEA, a natural hormone produced by the adrenal glands, which is available over the counter in the US. For those suspected of suffering from the andropause I recommend following the general optimum nutrition principles in this book, testing for testosterone deficiency and only then, if necessary, correcting with testosterone implants or creams.

chapter 42.

Preventing the Problems of Old Age

The best way to stay healthy in old age is to prevent disease before it starts. Many animals, after all, stay healthy throughout their lives. In the Western world it is barely even legal to die of old age: most death certificates require a cause, a disease. I firmly believe that it is possible to lead an active life without years of poor health and unnecessary suffering. Certainly three of the 'grandfathers' of optimum nutrition, Linus Pauling, Roger Williams and Carl Pfeiffer, all lived to a ripe old age.

The trick, of course, is to prevent heart disease and cancer by following the advice in Chapters 23 and 32. Both Pauling and Pfeiffer were convinced that, through optimum nutrition, you could add at least ten years of healthy living. Williams said, 'Well-rounded nutrition, including generous amounts of vitamins C and E, can contribute materially to extending lifespan of those who are already middle-aged. The greatest hope of increasing lifespan can be offered if nutrition – from the time of pre-natal development to old age – is continuously of the highest quality.' Pfeiffer took 10 grams of vitamin C a day towards the end of his life, while Pauling took 16 grams. There is certainly a good case for taking a gram of vitamin C (1,000mg) and 75mg of vitamin E for every decade of life. So an eighty-year-old may benefit most from 8 grams of vitamin C and 600mg of vitamin E.

Improving digestion and absorption

The production of stomach acid and enzymes often declines with age. Stomach acid production depends on zinc, so it is important to ensure that your zinc intake is adequate. A lack of zinc also reduces people's sense of taste and smell, leading to a liking for salt, sauces and strong-tasting food like cheese and meat. Zinc-deficient people often go off fruit and vegetables. Improving zinc nutrition, rather than overcooking vegetables and adding lots of strongly flavoured sauces, can improve your health considerably, including relieving constipation.

The lack of stomach acid and enzymes also leads to poor absorption of nutrients from food into the body. If you have digestive problems or are sixty-plus, to assist nutrient absorption it is worth trying a digestive enzyme supplement containing a small amount of betaine hydrochloride (stomach acid). Betaine is another name for trimethylglycine (TMG), which lowers homocysteine (see Chapter 16). This can improve the absorption of both vitamin and minerals.

Studies on the elderly clearly demonstrate that key nutrients such as vitamins B12 and folic acid are poorly absorbed. For example, while the RDA for vitamin B12 is a measly 1mcg and the average dietary intake is more like 6mcg, a recent study found that 10mcg of B12 is ineffective in restoring B12 status in those with low or borderline serum B12, a hallmark of the elderly, while 50mcg per day is effective in both restoring B12 status and lowering homocysteine levels.[18] It is also worth paying a little extra for the most easily absorbed mineral formulas (see Chapter 48).

Combating arthritis, aches and pains

One of the greatest causes of suffering in old age is aching joints and arthritis. One is often led to believe there is nothing that can be done except to take painkillers, which more often than not speed up the progression of the disease. This is completely untrue. There are many proven ways to reduce pain and inflammation without drugs, outlined in Chapter 26 and discussed fully in my book *Say No to Arthritis*, even when degeneration is severe.

Fred is a case in point. He had seen many specialists and tried all the conventional treatments. Then he tried the optimum nutrition approach. 'I used to have constant pain in my knees and joints, could not play golf or walk more than ten minutes without resting my legs. Since following Patrick's advice my discomfort has decreased 95–100 per cent. It is a different life when you can travel and play golf every day. I never would have believed my pain could be reduced by such a large degree, and no return no matter how much activity in a day or week.' Key strategies for reducing pain and inflammation are:

- Identify and avoid allergens.

- Supplement niacin (up to 500mg a day) and pantothenic acid (500mg a day).

- Supplement antioxidants.

- Supplement anti-inflammatory nutrients and herbs such as Omega 3 fats and boswellia.

- Supplement bone-building nutrients, including minerals and glucosamine.

- Good, all-round optimum nutrition.

Sometimes aches and pains occur in the muscles and not the joints. This is not arthritis and may be due to one of two conditions. The first is fibromyalgia, which is characterised by a number of tender points in specific muscles. This is now thought to be due to a problem in the energy metabolism of the muscle cells, and not to inflammation. Anti-inflammatory agents may therefore not help, although painkillers can suppress the symptoms. A particular form of magnesium, magnesium malate, is proving very effective at relieving fibromyalgia, together with a supportive diet plus supplements. Stress, which uses up magnesium, makes this condition worse. Polymyalgia, characterised by early-morning stiffness, often in the shoulders and hips, is more often brought on when the body's detoxification systems are overloaded. This means that the liver, kidneys, brain and all the cells, including muscle cells, cannot deal with the garbage produced by digestion and daily living. Different systems of the body can be affected.

Some people experience chronic fatigue, others bodily aches as in polymyalgia. Yet others find that their nervous system is affected, bringing on premature senility or multiple sclerosis-type symptoms, or else the immune system starts misbehaving, resulting in infections, allergies, inflammation and auto-immune diseases like rheumatoid arthritis. Polymyalgia, being an inflammatory condition, usually responds to antioxidant supplementation and liver detoxification. The conventional treatment is the drug prednisolone.

Avoiding the drug cycle

Most people in this scenario end up on the drug cycle, perhaps starting with painkillers or steroids, then moving on to antibiotics when infections set in. The drugs treat the symptom but not the cause – in fact they usually aggravate the cause by irritating the gut and making the intestinal wall more leaky, which is what non-steroidal anti-inflammatory drugs and antibiotics do. This means that more garbage gets into the body, further overloading detoxification pathways. Many drugs, such as paracetamol, are toxins in their own right and severely tax the liver. The result is ever-increasing over-load on body systems, leading to more serious diseases and infections.

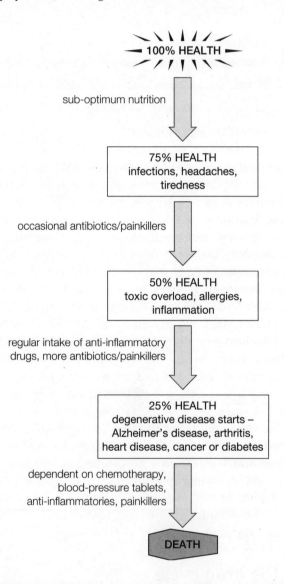

The drug dilemma. Many conventional medical drugs (such as painkillers or anti-inflammatory drugs) suppress the body's normal responses to underlying contributors. They act like toxins in the body and can contribute to decline in health and/or dependence. Then you need another drug to counteract the symptoms! It's a downward spiral.

Preventing dementia and Alzheimer's

It is very likely that age-related memory decline and Alzheimer's disease are the net consequences of inflammation and overstretching the body's ability to detoxify. This is good news because it means that Alzheimer's disease should be preventable and possibly even reversible in the early stages.[19]

Alzheimer's disease and dementia have similar causes and associated risk factors to other common degenerative disease, including cardiovascular disease and diabetes, both of which are largely preventable by optimum nutrition. The central mechanism for degeneration of brain cells is inflammation and oxidation. Increased intake of antioxidant vitamins E and C, and Omega 3 fats EPA and DHA, reduces risk. Lowering levels of the stress hormone cortisol and homocysteine levels, the latter by improving folate and vitamin B12 and B6 intake, also decreases risk. Reducing excessive exposure to aluminium, mercury and copper, which exacerbate oxidation, may also reduce risk.

Once brain-cell degeneration occurs, levels of the brain's memory molecule, acetylcholine, start to decline. In addition, there is growing evidence that precursor nutrients phosphatidyl choline, phosphatidyl serine and DMAE may also improve cognitive function, possibly by helping brain-cell generation or by helping to make more acetylcholine.

A combined dietary and lifestyle approach, together with nutrient supplementation, offers an effective strategy for prevention and early-stage reversal of age-related cognitive decline. If you'd like to know more about this approach read my book *Optimum Nutrition for the Mind*.

Treat the cause and not the symptom

The way out is to treat the cause and not the symptom, as well as ensuring optimum brain nutrition including the smart nutrients discussed in Chapter 28, which help to maximise memory.

A combination of poor diet, alcohol, drugs and infections often leads to problems in later life. Thanks to recent biochemical advances, simple urine tests can now reveal whether the sensitive balance of beneficial bacteria in the gut has been disrupted (known as dysbiosis), to what extent the gut wall has become permeable (this is a primary underlying cause of toxic overload) and exactly which pathways in the liver are overloaded. Each pathway depends on a sequence of enzymes, themselves dependent on nutrients. A nutrition consultant can devise a specific diet and supplement programme using specific vitamins, minerals, amino acids and fatty acids designed to decrease the toxic load on the body and restore the body's detoxification potential. The results are often spectacular.

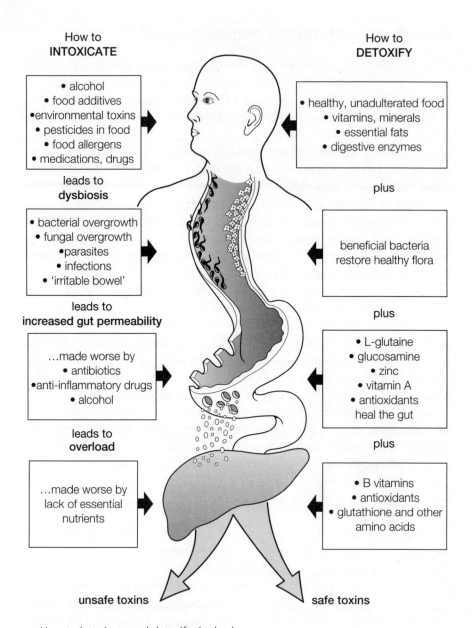

How to
INTOXICATE

How to
DETOXIFY

- alcohol
- food additives
- environmental toxins
- pesticides in food
- food allergens
- medications, drugs

- healthy, unadulterated food
- vitamins, minerals
- essential fats
- digestive enzymes

leads to
dysbiosis

plus

- bacterial overgrowth
- fungal overgrowth
- parasites
- infections
- 'irritable bowel'

beneficial bacteria
restore healthy flora

leads to
increased gut permeability

plus

...made worse by
- antibiotics
- anti-inflammatory drugs
- alcohol

- L-glutaine
- glucosamine
- zinc
- vitamin A
- antioxidants
heal the gut

leads to
overload

plus

...made worse by
lack of essential
nutrients

- B vitamins
- antioxidants
- glutathione and other
amino acids

unsafe toxins

safe toxins

How to intoxicate and detoxify the body

This is especially important since it is often decreased liver detoxification potential, exacerbated by poor nutrient status and exposure to oxidants and other anti-nutrients, that leads to the system failure called death.

Like the salmon, I believe that fully healthy humans should have enough reserves to make it to the end of their lives without a debilitating loss of either mental or physical function, and to experience finally a fairly rapid and painless system shut-down. What happens next is the ultimate adventure. I am intrigued about the growing evidence suggesting that the pineal gland releases a neurotransmitter-like substance, dimethyl tryptamine that, if injected, often produces profound experiences that exactly parallel the now thousands of well-reported near-death experiences.[20] However, discussing whether or not there is life after death is not the purpose of this book. Here, I am more concerned with whether or not there is life before death!

Part 6

Your Personal Nutrition Programme

chapter) **43.**

Working Out Your Optimum Nutrition

How healthy do you want to be? If you want to realise your full potential, mentally and physically, finding out your optimum nutritional requirements is essential. But if your needs are unique, how do you find these out? Since 1980 I have been developing and refining a precise system for analysing people's nutrient needs, based on assessing the major factors that influence individual requirements. This system has been tried and tested on over 100,000 people and is now used by nutritional therapists all over the world.

Hundreds of thousands of people have benefited from this system, so I know what sorts of results to expect. They include:

- Greater mental alertness

- Improved memory

- More physical energy

- Better weight control

- Reduced cholesterol levels

- Reversal of disease

If you'd like to hear in their own words how people's health has changed as a result of their working out and following their own personal health programme using this system, visit my website www.patrickholford.com.

Although many people with diagnosed illnesses have been helped while on a personal health programme, such a programme is not designed to treat illness so much as to prevent it. **If you suffer from a recognised medical condition, please check that this programme is compatible with any treatment you may already be receiving.**

Chapters 44 and 45 present a simplified version of the system, based on the Optimum Nutrition Questionnaire. A more comprehensive way to work out exactly what you need is available on www.patrickholford.com using the My Nutrition on-line questionnaire (see Resources, page 525). This works out how healthy you are right now and what you need to change, with specific diet and supplement recommendations, to achieve 100 per cent health. It provides a useful assessment of what you need for optimum health and is a great place to start. I recommend it for everyone. It is not, however, the same as having a personal assessment of your nutritional needs carried out by a nutritional therapist. This is, of course, highly preferable and essential for anyone who is currently unwell or suffering from a diagnosed disease. Nutritional therapists can also run the necessary biochemical tests to help you get well. Details of how to find a qualified nutrition consultant are given in Resources (see page 525).

Factors that affect your nutritional needs

At least eight factors affect your optimum nutritional requirements. Age, sex and amount of exercise are easily covered. But the effects of pollution, stress, your past health history, your genetic legacy and, of course, the nutrients (and anti-nutrients) supplied in your diet are not so straightforward to work out. But all these details and more must be taken into account. There are four basic ways to go about it:

- Diet analysis
- Biochemical analysis
- Symptom analysis
- Lifestyle analysis

Diet analysis

This may seem the obvious place to start: finding out what goes in should reveal what is missing. But unfortunately a breakdown of foods eaten over, say, a week, cannot take into account the variations in nutrient content in the food, your individual needs, or how well a nutrient is used when, and if, it is absorbed. I have seen many people who had superficially 'perfect' diets, but still showed signs of vitamin deficiency. For a high proportion of them the problem was poor absorption. These variables make some diet analyses carried out on a computer less helpful than might be expected.

Where diet analysis comes in useful is in assessing foods that are known to affect our nutrient needs, such as sugar, salt, coffee, tea, alcohol, food additives and preservatives. Other factors, such as intake of fats, carbohydrates, protein and calories, can also be determined from an analysis of your diet.

Biochemical analysis

Tests such as hair-mineral analysis or vitamin blood tests give indisputable information about your biochemical status and help a nutrition consultant to know the actual nutritional state of your body. But not all these tests provide useful information to help you build up your nutrition programme. To be accurate, any vitamin or mineral test must reflect the ability of the nutrient to function in the body. For example, iron is a vital constituent of red blood cells; it helps to carry oxygen throughout the body. By measuring the iron status in your cells it is possible to get a good measure of your iron needs.

On the other hand, vitamin B6 has no similar direct function to perform in the blood – it is used in other chemical reactions, for example the production of the brain chemical serotonin or in methylation reactions, hence lowering homocysteine levels. Therefore simply measuring vitamin B6 in the blood doesn't really tell you if you've got enough for your B6 enzymes to work properly. Testing something like your homocysteine level is much more useful. If you've got enough vitamins B6, B12 and folic acid then your homocysteine level will be low. If it's high you know you need more of one or more of these nutrients. We call this a 'functional' test because it actually measures whether a particular aspect of your body's biochemistry is functioning properly.

Because each nutrient has a different function in the body, we cannot say that blood tests are better than urine tests, or that analysis of mineral levels in the hair provides more accurate information than blood levels. For each nutrient there are different tests, depending on what we want to find out. For instance, for zinc deficiency there are over a dozen tests which involve blood, urine, hair, sweat and even taste.

To make an extensive series of tests would be expensive. My best three value-for-money tests are homocysteine and food-intolerance tests and hair-mineral analysis, which reveals a person's mineral status. From a small sample of hair the levels of calcium, magnesium, zinc, chromium, selenium and manganese can be discovered, although the results need careful interpretation. Hair-mineral analysis also provides useful information about lead, cadmium, arsenic, aluminium and copper, all of which are toxic in excess. Hair-mineral analysis can sometimes pinpoint problems of absorption, or reasons for high blood pressure or frequent infections.

Homocysteine is also good for measuring your B vitamin status. If you have a high score and follow my recommendations for supplementing B vitamins and the homocysteine-lowering diet guidelines in Chapter 16, it normally takes eight weeks to bring your homocysteine level to normal. Valda, aged seventy-three, is a case in point. She had had high blood pressure for thirty years, as well as arthritis. Her homocysteine level was very high, at 42.9. The optimal level is below 6. She followed my recommendations and within eight weeks her homocysteine had dropped by 88 per cent, to 5.1, and her blood pressure had become virtually normal, at 130/80. Her arthritis had improved and she felt much better in herself.

There are also good tests for measuring your antioxidant status, one of which is glutathione peroxidase. For example, I ran this inexpensive blood test on two volunteers in 'average' health, then put one, Janette, on an RDA-based multivitamin and gave the other, Leone, what I take daily, which is a pack of two multivitamin and mineral tablets, 2 grams of vitamin C and an essential fat supplement. Janette's initial glutathione peroxidase score was 59. The 'normal' range is 65–90, although it's better to be closer to 90. After a month her score rose by 10 points to 69, at the low end of the normal range, which is OK, but not ideal. She said she didn't feel any different. Leone started off with a score of 64; after a month of supplementation her score rose by 22 points to 86, which is just about optimum. She said, 'I didn't feel as tired as usual. And while everyone in the office went down with flu, I was fine. My skin also seemed to positively glow.'

These are the kinds of tests a nutritional therapist might want to run to work out your optimum diet and supplement programme.

Symptom analysis

Deficiency symptom analysis is the most underestimated method of working out nutritional needs. It is based on over 200 signs and symptoms that have been found in cases of slight vitamin or mineral deficiency. For example, mouth ulcers are associated with vitamin A deficiency, muscle cramps with magnesium deficiency. For many of these symptoms, the mechanism is understood. Magnesium, for instance, is required for muscles to relax. Symptoms such as these can be early warning signs of deficiency which show us that our bodies are not working perfectly. However, while deficiency in vitamins C, B3 or B5 would all result in reduced energy because they are involved in energy production, being low in energy does not necessarily mean that you are deficient. Perhaps you are just working too hard or sleeping badly. If, however, you have a cluster of symptoms, all associated with vitamin B3 deficiency, you are much more likely to be in need of more vitamin B3 to reach optimum health.

The advantage of deficiency symptom analysis is that health is being measured directly. Results are not dependent on whether you eat oranges which are high in vitamin C, or on whether you absorb and utilise food well, as dietary analysis is. Some people have criticised this method because it relies on subjective information from the person concerned – yet the large majority of medical diagnoses are based on subjective information from the patient. If you want to find out how someone feels, isn't it obvious to ask? I always ask my clients why they think they are ill. More often than not they are right.

Lifestyle analysis

These three methods of analysis, if properly applied, should define what you need right now to be optimally nourished, but it is good to check that your needs for your particular lifestyle are adequately covered. For example, if you smoke and drink alcohol frequently your nutritional needs will be higher than if you don't. If you are pregnant, live in a city, have a high-stress occupation suffer from allergies, your ideal needs may be affected.

Lifestyle analysis is the fourth piece of the jigsaw puzzle that helps a nutritionist know what you need. The next two chapters tell you how to analyse your diet, your symptoms of deficiency and your lifestyle in order to work out your own personal health programme.

chapter 44

Your Optimum Diet

Before foods can give us vitality, hundreds of chemical reactions must take place, involving twenty-eight vitamins and minerals. These micro-nutrients are the real keys that unlock the potential energy in our food.

Your vitality depends upon a careful balance of at least fifty nutrients. They include sources of energy, measured in calories, which may come from carbohydrates, fats or proteins; thirteen known vitamins; fifteen minerals; twenty-four amino acids (which we get when proteins are digested); and two essential fatty acids. Even though the requirement for some minerals, like selenium, is less than a millionth of our requirement for protein, it is no less important. In fact, one-third of all chemical reactions in our bodies are dependent on tiny quantities of minerals, and even more on vitamins. Without just one of any of these nutrients, vitality, energy and ideal weight are just not possible.

Fortunately, deficiency in protein, fat or carbohydrate is very rare. Unfortunately, deficiency in vitamins, minerals and essential fats is not, despite popular belief. Many nutritionists believe that as few as one in ten people receives sufficient vitamins, minerals and essential fats from their diet for optimum health.

As much as two-thirds of the average calorie intake consists of fat, sugar and refined flour. The calories in sugar are called 'empty' because they provide no nutrients, and those are often hidden in processed foods and snacks. If a quarter of your diet by weight, and two-thirds by calories, consists of such dismembered foods, there is little room left to get the levels you need of all the essential nutrients.

Wheat has twenty-five nutrients removed in the refining process that turns it into white flour, yet only four (iron and vitamins B1, B2 and B3) are replaced. On average, 87 per cent of the essential minerals zinc, chromium and manganese is lost. Processed meats like hamburgers and sausages are no better: the use of inferior meat high in fat lowers the nutrient content. Eggs, fish and chicken are nutrient-rich sources of protein, but protein deficiency is rarely a problem.

Vegetables, fruit, nuts, seeds, beans and grains are full of vitality, being whole foods. Many are 'seed' foods, so they have to contain everything that the plant needs to grow, including zinc. Broccoli, carrots, peas and sweet potatoes are rich in antioxidants. Peppers, broccoli and fruit are rich in vitamin C and other phytonutrients. Seeds and nuts are rich in essential fats. Beans and grains provide both protein and complex carbohydrate. Foods such as these should make up at least half, if not all, of your diet.

The perfect diet pyramid below gives you the kind of balance of foods to aim for in your diet.

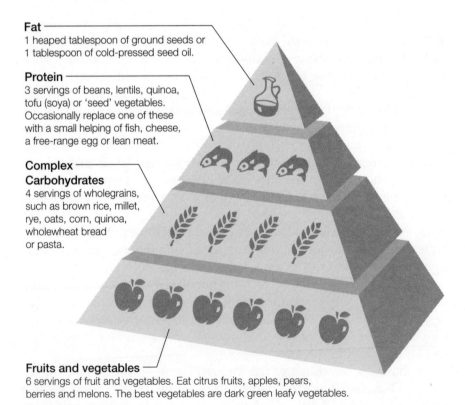

Fat
1 heaped tablespoon of ground seeds or
1 tablespoon of cold-pressed seed oil.

Protein
3 servings of beans, lentils, quinoa,
tofu (soya) or 'seed' vegetables.
Occasionally replace one of these
with a small helping of fish, cheese,
a free-range egg or lean meat.

Complex Carbohydrates
4 servings of wholegrains,
such as brown rice, millet,
rye, oats, corn, quinoa,
wholewheat bread
or pasta.

Fruits and vegetables
6 servings of fruit and vegetables. Eat citrus fruits, apples, pears,
berries and melons. The best vegetables are dark green leafy vegetables.

The perfect diet pyramid

Check out your diet

Many people would like to believe that as long as they take their vitamin supplements they can keep eating all the 'bad' foods that they love. But you cannot rely on diet, supplements or exercise alone to keep you healthy. All three are essential.

■ Diet check questionnaire

Score one point for each 'yes' answer. Maximum score is 20.

☐ Do you add sugar to food or drink almost every day?

☐ Do you eat foods with added sugars almost every day?

☐ Do you use salt in your food?

☐ Do you drink more than one cup of coffee most days?

☐ Do you drink more than three cups of tea most days?

☐ Do you smoke more than five cigarettes a day?

☐ Do you take recreational drugs such as cannabis?

☐ Do you drink more than 10oz (28g) of alcohol (one glass of wine, 1 pint or 600ml of beer, or one measure of spirits) a day?

☐ Do you eat fried food more than twice a week?

☐ Do you eat processed 'fast food' more than twice a week?

☐ Do you eat red meat more than twice a week?

☐ Do you often eat foods containing additives and preservatives?

☐ Do you eat chocolate or sweets more than twice a week?

☐ Does less than a third of your diet consist of raw fruit and vegetables?

☐ Do you drink less than ½ pint (300ml) of plain water each day?

☐ Do you normally eat white rice, flour or bread rather than whole grain?

☐ Do you drink more than 3 pints (1.7 litres) of milk a week?

☐ Do you eat more than three slices of bread a day, on average?

◯ Are there some foods you feel 'addicted' to?

◯ Do you eat oily fish less than twice a week and/or seeds less than daily?

0–4 You are obviously a health-conscious individual and your minor indiscretions are unlikely to affect your health. Provided you supplement your diet with the right vitamins and minerals you can look forward to a long and healthy life.

5–9 You are on the right track, but must be a little stricter with yourself. Rather than giving up your bad habits, set yourself easy experiments. For instance, for one month go without two or three of the foods or drinks you know are not good for you. See how you feel. Some you may decide to have occasionally, while others you may find you go off. But be strict for one month – your cravings will only be short-term withdrawal symptoms. Aim to have your score below 5 within three months.

10–14 Your diet is not good and you will need to make some changes to be able to reach optimum health. But take it a step at a time. You should aim to have your score down to 5 within six months. Start by following the advice in this chapter, backed up by the advice in Part 2. You will find that some of your bad dietary habits will change for the better as you discover tasty alternatives. The bad habits that remain should be dealt with one at a time. Remember that sugar, salt, coffee and chocolate are all addictive foods. Your cravings for them will dramatically decrease or go away altogether after one month without them.

15–20 There is no way you can continue to eat like this and remain in good health. You are consuming far too great a quantity of fat, refined foods and artificial stimulants. Follow the advice in Part 2 very carefully and make gradual and permanent changes to your lifestyle. For instance, take two questions to which you answered 'yes' and make changes so that one month later you could answer 'no' (one example would be to stop eating sugar and drinking coffee in the first month). Keep doing this until your score is 5 or less. You may feel worse for the first two weeks, but within a month you will begin to feel the positive effects of healthy eating.

Eating for vitality

One secret of longer and healthier life is to eat foods high in vitamin and mineral vitality, but this is not the only criterion for judging a food. Good food should also be low in fat, salt and fast-releasing sugars, high in fibre and alkaline-forming. Non-animal sources of protein are desirable. Such a diet will also be low in calories, but then you will not have to count them because your body will become increasingly efficient and not crave extra food. A craving for food when you have already eaten enough calories is often a craving for more nutrients, so foods providing 'empty' calories are strictly to be avoided.

Top ten diet tips

Here are ten top tips for transforming your diet for better health:

1. Eat 1 heaped tablespoon per day of ground seeds or 1 tablespoon of cold-pressed seed oil.

2. Eat 2 servings of beans, lentils, quinoa, tofu (soya), or 'seed' vegetables per day.

3. Eat 3 pieces per day of fresh fruit such as apples, pears, bananas, berries, melon or citrus fruit.

4. Eat 4 servings per day of whole grains such as rice, millet, rye, oats, wholewheat, corn, quinoa as cereal, breads or pasta.

5. Eat 5 servings per day of dark green, leafy and root vegetables such as watercress, carrots, sweet potatoes, broccoli, spinach, green beans, peas and peppers.

6. Each day, drink at least 6 glasses of water, diluted juices, herbal or fruit teas.

7. Eat whole, organic, raw food as often as you can.

8. Supplement a high-strength multivitamin and mineral, 1,000mg of vitamin C and essential Omega 3 and 6 fats every day.

9. Avoid fried, burnt, or browned food, hydrogenated fat and excess animal fat.

10. Avoid any form of sugar, and white, refined or processed food with chemical additives, and minimise your intake of alcohol, coffee and tea. Limit your alcohol intake to one alcoholic drink a day.

Dig deeper by reading my book *The Optimum Nutrition Cookbook* co-authored with Judy Ridgway, which is full of delicious 'optimum nutrition' recipes.

45.

Your Optimum Supplement Programme

Your personal nutritional needs can be calculated by looking at your lifestyle and identifying signs and symptoms associated with various deficiencies. In the sections that follow, answer the questions as best you can, then for each nutrient work out your score out of ten. If you score five or more the chances are that you do not have the optimal intake of that nutrient, given your current needs. The second part of this chapter shows you how to turn these scores into your optimum supplement programme. You can also do this by having an on-line My Nutrition assessment (see page 525) which will calculate your own personal diet and supplement programme.

Optimum Nutrition Questionnaire

■ Symptom Analysis

For each symptom that you experience often, Score **1** point. Many symptoms occur more than once, because they can be the result of many nutrient deficiencies. If you experience any of the symptoms in **bold** type, score **2** points. The maximum score for each nutrient is 10 points. **Put your score for each nutrient in the box.**

Vitamin Profile

VITAMIN A

____ **Mouth ulcers**
____ Poor night vision
____ Acne
____ **Frequent colds or infections**
____ Dry flaky skin
____ Dandruff
____ Thrush or cystitis
____ Diarrhoea

☐ *Your score*

VITAMIN D

____ **Arthritis or osteoporosis**
____ Backache
____ Tooth decay
____ Hair loss
____ **Muscle twitching or spasms**
____ **Joint pain or stiffness**
____ Weak bones

☐ *Your score*

VITAMIN E

____ Lack of sex drive
____ **Exhaustion after light exercise**
____ **Easy bruising**
____ Slow wound-healing
____ Varicose veins
____ Poor skin elasticity
____ Loss of muscle tone
____ Infertility

☐ *Your score*

VITAMIN B2

____ **Bloodshot, burning or gritty eyes**
____ **Sensitivity to bright lights**
____ Sore tongue
____ Cataracts
____ Dull or oily hair
____ Eczema or dermatitis
____ Split nails
____ Cracked lips

☐ *Your score*

VITAMIN C
____ **Frequent colds**
____ Lack of energy
____ **Frequent infections**
____ Bleeding or tender gums
____ Easy bruising
____ Nosebleeds
____ Slow wound-healing
____ Red pimples on skin
____ Bleeding or tender gums
____ Acne

▢ *Your score*

VITAMIN B1
____ Tender muscles
____ Eye pains
____ Irritability
____ Poor concentration
____ 'Prickly' legs
____ Poor memory
____ Stomach pains
____ Constipation
____ Tingling hands
____ Rapid heartbeat

▢ *Your score*

VITAMIN B6
____ **Infrequent dream recall**
____ **Water retention**
____ Tingling hands
____ Depression or nervousness
____ Irritability
____ Muscle tremors, cramps or spasms
____ **Lack of energy**

▢ *Your score*

VITAMIN B3 (NIACIN)
____ Lack of energy
____ Diarrhoea
____ Insomnia
____ Headaches or migraines
____ Poor memory
____ Anxiety or tension
____ Depression
____ Irritability

▢ *Your score*

VITAMIN B5
____ Muscle tremors, cramps or spasms
____ Apathy
____ Poor concentration
____ **Burning feet or tender heels**
____ Nausea or vomiting
____ Lack of energy
____ Exhaustion after light exercise
____ Anxiety or tension
____ Teeth-grinding

▢ *Your score*

FOLIC ACID
____ Eczema
____ Cracked lips
____ Prematurely greying hair
____ Anxiety or tension
____ Poor memory
____ **Lack of energy**
____ Depression
____ Poor appetite
____ Stomach pains

▢ *Your score*

VITAMIN B12

____ Poor hair condition
____ Eczema or dermatitis
____ Mouth over-sensitive to heat or cold
____ Irritability
____ Anxiety or tension
____ **Lack of energy**
____ Constipation
____ Tender or sore muscles
____ Pale skin

☐ *Your score*

BIOTIN

____ **Dermatitis or dry skin**
____ **Poor hair condition**
____ **Prematurely greying hair**
____ **Tender or sore muscles**
____ **Poor appetite or nausea**

☐ *Your score*

Mineral Profile

CALCIUM

____ **Muscle cramps, tremors or spasms**
____ **Insomnia or nervousness**
____ **Joint pain or arthritis**
____ **Tooth decay**
____ **High blood pressure**

☐ *Your score*

IRON

____ **Pale skin**
____ **Sore tongue**
____ **Fatigue or listlessness**
____ **Loss of appetite or nausea**
____ **Heavy periods or blood loss**

☐ *Your score*

MAGNESIUM

____ **Muscle cramps, tremors or spasms**
____ Muscle weakness
____ Insomnia, nervousness or hyperactivity
____ High blood pressure
____ Irregular or rapid heartbeat
____ Constipation
____ Fits or convulsions
____ Breast tenderness or water retention
____ Depression or confusion

☐ *Your score*

MANGANESE

____ **Muscle twitches**
____ **Childhood 'growing pains'**
____ **Dizziness or poor sense of balance**
____ **Fits or convulsions**
____ **Sore knees**

☐ *Your score*

ZINC

____ Decline in sense of taste or smell
____ White marks on more than two fingernails
____ Frequent infections
____ Stretch marks
____ Acne or greasy skin

◯ *Your score*

CHROMIUM

____ Excessive or cold sweats
____ Dizziness or irritability after six hours without food
____ Need for frequent meals
____ Cold hands
____ Need for excessive sleep or drowsiness during the day

◯ *Your score*

SELENIUM

____ Family history of cancer
____ Signs of premature ageing
____ Cataracts
____ High blood pressure

◯ *Your score*

Essential Fatty Acid Profile

OMEGA 3/OMEGA 6

____ **Dry skin or eczema**
____ Dry hair or dandruff
____ Inflammatory health problems, e.g. arthritis
____ Excessive thirst or sweating
____ PMS or breast pain
____ Water retention
____ Frequent infections
____ Poor memory or learning difficulties
____ High blood pressure or high blood lipids

◯ *Your score*

Now put all your individual scores into the appropriate spaces in the second column of the chart on page 402 (the column headed Symptom Score).

■ Lifestyle Analysis

The following checks allow you to adjust your nutrient needs according to aspects of your health and lifestyle. Again, answer the questions as best you can and work out your score. In most checks the maximum score is 10, scoring **1** point for each 'yes' answer unless otherwise specified. **If you score 5 or more in any category, you will need to add the points shown in the chart on page 402 to your individual nutrient scores.** The easiest way to do this is to circle all the numbers in the corresponding columns on page 402. For example, if you scored more than 5 on the energy check, you would circle all the numbers in the energy column on page 402. Some checks are either **'yes'** or **'no'**. If you answer 'yes', circle the numbers in the relevant columns on page 402.

Energy Check

____ Do you need more than eight hours' sleep a night?

____ Are you rarely wide awake and raring to go within twenty minutes of rising?

____ Do you need something to get you going in the morning, like a cup of tea or coffee or a cigarette?

____ Do you have tea, coffee, sugar-containing foods or drinks, or smoke cigarettes, at regular intervals during the day?

____ Do you often feel drowsy or sleepy during the day, or after meals?

____ Do you get dizzy or irritable if you have not eaten for six hours?

____ Do you avoid exercise because you do not have the energy?

____ Do you sweat a lot during the night or day or get excessively thirsty?

____ Do you sometimes lose concentration or does your mind go blank?

____ Is your energy less now than it used to be?

◯ *Your score*

Stress Check

____ Do you feel guilty when relaxing?

____ Do you have a persistent need for recognition or achievement?

____ Are you unclear about your goals in life?

____ Are you especially competitive?

____ Do you work harder than most people?

____ Do you easily get angry?

____ Do you often do two or three tasks simultaneously?

____ Do you get impatient if people or things hold you up?

___ Do you have difficulty getting to sleep, sleep restlessly or wake up with your mind racing?

⬜ *Your score*

Exercise Check

Score 2 points for each 'yes' answer

___ Do you take exercise that noticeably raises your heartbeat for at least twenty minutes more than three times a week?
___ Does your job involve lots of walking, lifting or any other vigorous activity?
___ Do you regularly play a sport (football, squash, etc.)?
___ Do you have any physically tiring hobbies (gardening, carpentry, etc.)?
___ Are you in serious training for an athletic event?
___ Do you consider yourself fit?

⬜ *Your score*

Immune Check

___ Do you get more than three colds a year?
___ Do you find it hard to shift an infection (cold or otherwise)?
___ Are you prone to thrush or cystitis?
___ Do you generally take antibiotics twice or more each year?
___ Have you had a major personal loss in the last year?
___ Is there any history of cancer in your family?
___ Have you ever had any growths or lumps removed or biopsied?
___ Do you have an inflammatory disease such as eczema, asthma or arthritis?
___ Do you suffer from hay fever?
___ Do you suffer from allergy problems?

⬜ *Your score*

Pollution Check

___ Do you live in a city or by a busy road?
___ Do you spend more than two hours a week in heavy traffic?
___ Do you exercise (do your job, cycle, play sports) by busy roads?

___ Do you smoke more than five cigarettes a day?

___ Do you live or work in a smoky atmosphere?

___ Do you buy foods exposed to exhaust fumes from busy roads?

___ Do you generally eat non-organic produce?

___ Do you drink more than 1 unit of alcohol a day (one glass of wine, 1 pint or 600ml of beer, or one measure of spirits)?

___ Do you spend a considerable amount of time in front of a TV or computer screen?

___ Do you usually drink unfiltered tap water?

Your score

Cardiovascular Check

___ Is your blood pressure above 140/90?

___ Is your pulse rate after fifteen minutes' rest above 75?

___ Are you more than 14lb (7kg) over your ideal weight?

___ Do you smoke more than five cigarettes a day?

___ Do you do less than two hours of vigorous exercise (one hour if you are over fifty) a week?

___ Do you eat more than one tablespoon of sugar each day?

___ Do you eat meat more than five times a week?

___ Do you usually add salt to your food?

___ Do you have more than two alcoholic drinks (or units of alcohol) a day?

___ Is there a history of heart disease or diabetes in your family?

Your score

Female Health Check

Do you regularly suffer from pre-menstrual syndrome?   *Yes / No*

Are you pregnant or trying to get pregnant?   *Yes / No*

Are you breastfeeding?   *Yes / No*

Do you have menopausal symptoms or are you post-menopausal?   *Yes / No*

Age Check

Are you under 11?   *Yes / No*
Are you 11–16?   *Yes / No*
Are you over 50?   *Yes / No*

Now put all your individual scores into the appropriate spaces in the second column, headed Symptom Score, of the chart on page 402.

How to work out your optimum nutrient needs

From the Symptom Analysis section of the Optimum Nutrition Question-naire you will have arrived at your basic score for each nutrient, which then needs to be adjusted depending on your answers to the Lifestyle Analysis questions. To do this, add all the numbers you have circled to your symptom score. Do this for each row, entering each total in the first column on page 403, headed Your Total Score. The higher your score for any given nutrient, the greater your need for that nutrient.

Once you have arrived at your score for each nutrient you can work out your supplement needs by looking at the column that corresponds to your score in the chart on page 403. For example, if your vitamin C score was 6, your estimated ideal supplementary intake of this vitamin is 1,600mg per day. Now work out your own supplemental levels for each nutrient.

If you score 0–4 on any nutrient I still recommend you to supplement it on a basic level, which can easily be achieved with a good daily multi-vitamin supplement. Remember: these levels are your supplementary needs, not your overall needs including what you should get from your diet. I have assumed that you have improved your diet – or will do so – so that it provides a basic intake of these nutrients. You will not get the same results from adding supplements to a poor diet.

For example, the ideal daily intake of calcium is 800 to 1,200mg (if needs are high, as for pregnant women or elderly people). The average intake is around 900mg. If you have a dairy-free diet, but eat seeds, you should still be able to achieve at least 800mg. So, if you have no symp-toms or lifestyle factors that increase your need, you don't need to supplement extra. If, on the other hand, you are pregnant, your supple-mental requirement is 1,200 – 800 = 400mg. This is why the range given for supplementation on page 483 goes from zero up to 400mg.

Levels of minerals other than those in the chart are generally sufficient in most people's diets and can be increased through dietary changes.

Potassium, which balances sodium (salt), is best supplied by eating plenty of raw fruit and vegetables. Phosphorus deficiency is exceedingly rare, and the mineral is contained in almost all supplements as calcium phosphate. Iodine deficiency is also extremely rare. Copper is frequently over-supplied in our diets and can be toxic. A wholefood diet almost always contains enough copper.

Scores for children

For children under the age of fourteen, there is a simple method for adjusting the nutrient-need figures (which are based on adult requirements). Take the weight of the child in pounds and divide by 100. (Alternatively, take the weight of the child in kilograms and divide by 50.) Now multiply their (adult) supplemental levels by the number you have worked out to give the child's actual supplemental level. For example, if a child weights 50lb, and we divide that by 100, we get 0.5. If the child scored 6 for vitamin C, giving a supplemental level of 2,000mg, we would multiply by 0.5 and get 1,000mg. This is the child's approximate optimal intake of vitamin C.

Alternatively, use the guide to optimal supplement intakes for children up to the age of eleven on page 364. From fourteen onwards, adult levels can be given.

Planning your ideal supplement programme

In case you are wondering, it is not necessary to take thirty different supplements every day! Your needs can be compressed into four or five different supplements, each combining the nutrients above. The most common combinations are a multivitamin (containing vitamins A, B, C, D and E) and a multimineral for all the minerals. Vitamin C is usually taken separately, since the basic optimum requirement of 1,000mg (1g) makes quite a large tablet without the addition of any more nutrients.

Choosing the right formula is an art in itself. Chapter 46 helps you through the maze by showing you how to decipher the small print and read between the lines, while Chapter 47 explains how to devise a simple daily routine of vitamin supplements. Alternatively you can walk into your local health food store, show the product adviser your calculations of your personal requirements and ask him or her to suggest a supplement programme that meets your needs.

NUTRIENTS	SYMPTOM SCORE	ENERGY	STRESS	EXERCISE	IMMUNE	POLLUTION	CARDIOVASCULAR	PREGNANT/FEEDING	PMS	MENOPAUSE	AGE 14-16	AGE OVER 50
A (beta-carotene)						2	1				1	
D								1		1	1	1
E					1	1	1	1		1		
C		1	2	1	1	2	1					
B1		1	2	1								
B2		1	2	1								
B3		2	2	1			1					
B5		1	2	1								
B6		1	2	1	1			1	2		1	
B12								2				
Folic acid								2				
Biotin								1			1	
Omega 3/Omega 6 Fats									2	2	1	1
Calcium		1			1	1	2		2	1	1	1
Magnesium		1	1	1	1					2		1
Iron												
Zinc		1	1			2	2		2	2	1	1
Manganese												
Selenium						1	1	1				1
Chromium		2	1									1

| YOUR TOTAL SCORE | Nutrient | SCORE | | | | WHAT YOU NEED |
		0–4	5–6	7–8	9 or more	
	A	1000	2000	2500	3000	mcg
	D	3	4	5	5	mcg
	E	150	200	300	400	mg
	C	800	1600	2000	2800	mg
	B1	15	25	35	45	mg
	B2	15	25	35	45	mg
	B3	25	30	40	50	mg
	B5	30	50	100	130	mg
	B6	45	60	75	95	mg
	Folic acid	200	350	500	600	mcg
	B12	10	20	30	40	mcg
	Biotin	30	60	120	180	mcg
	GLA	110	150	200	260	mg
	EPA/DHA	250	500	700	1050	mg
	Cal	0	200	300	400	mg
	Iron	5	7	9	15	mg
	Mag	50	100	200	250	mg
	Zinc	5	10	15	20	mg
	Sel	25	75	100	150	mcg
	Chro	25	50	100	200	mcg
	Man	1	3	6	9	mg

chapter 46

Everything You Need to Know about Supplements

Not all supplements are the same. Analysis of a wide variety of multi-vitamin tablets to find out how much it would cost to get the basic optimum vitamin requirements produced a range between 30p and over £5 a day! And with so many supplements available, all promising perfect health, it is easy to get confused. For instance, if you are looking for a simple multivitamin preparation to meet the basic optimum requirements, you have at least twenty products to choose from. This chapter explains what to look for in a good supplement.

Reading the label

Labelling laws vary from country to country, but many of the principles are the same. However, since the laws keep changing, many manufacturers are as confused as the public. Below is a typical label with advice on how to interpret the small print.

On this label the dosages are easy to understand, the chemical names for the different vitamins are given and the fillers (for example calcium phosphate) are listed. Directions for when and how to take the tablets are given. These are the things to go for when you are buying supplements: do not be misled by an attractive-looking label or a very cheap price, but do not pay too much either!

Unfortunately, however, not all supplements are true to their labels, so it is not always best to buy the cheapest. Reputable vitamin companies should give you a list of all the ingredients on the label.

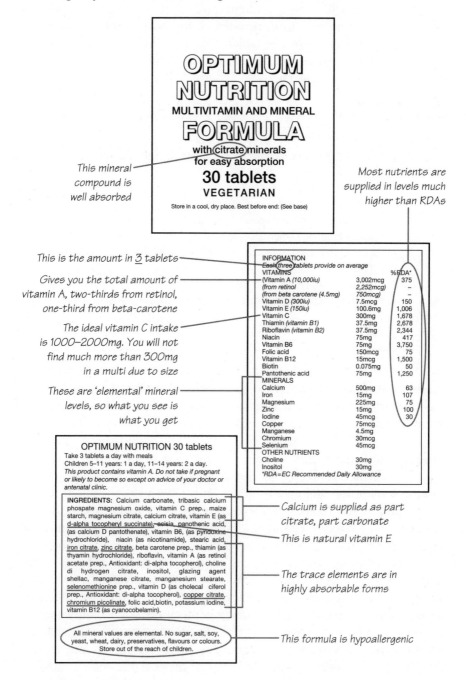

This mineral compound is well absorbed

Most nutrients are supplied in levels much higher than RDAs

This is the amount in 3 tablets

Gives you the total amount of vitamin A, two-thirds from retinol, one-third from beta-carotene

The ideal vitamin C intake is 1000–2000mg. You will not find much more than 300mg in a multi due to size

These are 'elemental' mineral levels, so what you see is what you get

OPTIMUM NUTRITION

MULTIVITAMIN AND MINERAL

FORMULA

with citrate minerals for easy absorption

30 tablets

VEGETARIAN

Store in a cool, dry place. Best before end: (See base)

INFORMATION

Each three tablets provide on average

VITAMINS		%RDA*
(Vitamin A (10,000iu)	3,002mcg	375
(from retinol	2,252mcg)	–
(from beta carotene (4.5mg)	750mcg)	–
Vitamin D (300iu)	7.5mcg	150
Vitamin E (150iu)	100.6mg	1,006
Vitamin C	300mg	1,678
Thiamin (vitamin B1)	37.5mg	2,678
Riboflavin (vitamin B2)	37.5mg	2,344
Niacin	75mg	417
Vitamin B6	75mg	3,750
Folic acid	150mcg	75
Vitamin B12	15mcg	1,500
Biotin	0.075mg	50
Pantothenic acid	75mg	1,250
MINERALS		
Calcium	500mg	63
Iron	15mg	107
Magnesium	225mg	75
Zinc	15mg	100
Iodine	45mcg	30
Copper	75mcg	
Manganese	4.5mg	
Chromium	30mcg	
Selenium	45mcg	
OTHER NUTRIENTS		
Choline	30mg	
Inositol	30mg	

*RDA=EC Recommended Daily Allowance

OPTIMUM NUTRITION 30 tablets

Take 3 tablets a day with meals
Children 5–11 years: 1 a day, 11–14 years: 2 a day.
This product contains vitamin A. Do not take if pregnant or likely to become so except on advice of your doctor or antenatal clinic.

INGREDIENTS: Calcium carbonate, tribasic calcium phospate magnesium oxide, vitamin C prep., maize starch, magnesium citrate, calcium citrate, vitamin E (as d-alpha tocopheryl succinate), acisia panothenic acid, (as calcium D pantothenate), vitamin B6, (as pyridoxine hydrochloride), niacin (as nicotinamide), stearic acid, iron citrate, zinc citrate, beta carotene prep., thiamin (as thyamin hydrochloride), riboflavin, vitamin A (as retinol acetate prep.), Antioxidant: di-alpha tocopherol), choline di hydrogen citrate, inositol, glazing agent shellac, manganese citrate, manganesium stearate, selenomethionine prep., vitamin D (as cholecal ciferol prep., Antioxidant: di-alpha tocopherol), copper citrate, chromium picolinate, folic acid,biotin, potassium iodine, vitamin B12 (as cyanocobelamin).

All mineral values are elemental. No sugar, salt, soy, yeast, wheat, dairy, preservatives, flavours or colours. Store out of the reach of children.

Calcium is supplied as part citrate, part carbonate

This is natural vitamin E

The trace elements are in highly absorbable forms

This formula is hypoallergenic

Reading the supplement label

Vitamin names and their amounts

For most supplements the ingredients have to be listed in order of weight, starting with the ingredient present in the greatest quantity. This is often confusing, since included in this list are the non-nutrient additives needed to make the tablet. Often the chemical name of the nutrient is used instead of the common vitamin code (for example ergocalciferol for vitamin D).

Vitamin	Chemical name(s)
A	retinol, retinyl palmitate, or betacarotene
B1	thiamine, thiamine hydrochloride, thiamine mononitrate
B2	riboflavin
B3	niacin, niacinamide
B5	pantothenic acid, calcium pantothenate
B6	pyridoxine, pyridoxal-5-phosphate, pyridoxine hydrochloride
B12	cyanocobalamine, methylcobalamine
C	ascorbic add, calcium ascorbate, magnesium ascorbate, sodium ascorbate
D	ergocalciferol, cholecalciferol
E	d(l) alpha tocopherol, tocopheryl acetate, tocopheryl succinate
Biotin	biotin
Folic acid	folate

When you have identified which nutrient is which, look at the amount provided by each daily dose. Some supplements state this in terms of two tablets ('Each two tablets provide . . .', since the supplement is designed to be taken twice a day. The amount supplied will be given in milligrams (mg) or micrograms (mcg or μg). Most countries have now switched to 'μg' as the symbol for micrograms, which are thousandths of a milligram.

Vitamin A measurements are a little tricky. This is because betacarotene is not actually vitamin A but can be turned into vitamin A by the body. So, to indicate the equivalent effect of a certain amount of betacarotene compared with vitamin A (retinol), a unit called a 'μgRE' is used. This stands for 'micrograms of Retinol Equivalent'. What it is saying is that this amount of betacarotene has the equivalent effect of so many μg of retinol. In fact, 6mcg of betacarotene is equivalent in potency to 1mcg of retinol, and is therefore written as 1mcgRE of betacarotene. If a supplement contains both vitamin A and betacarotene, add the two amounts of μgRE to arrive at the total vitamin A dose provided.

Elemental minerals

Minerals in multivitamin and mineral tablets often omit the 'elemental' value of the compound, stating only the amount of the mineral compound. For instance, 100mg of zinc amino acid chelate will provide only 10mg of zinc and 90mg of the amino acid to which it is chelated (attached). What you want to know is the amount of the actual mineral, in this example 10mg. This is called the 'elemental value'. Most reputable manufacturers make your life easy by stating something like 'zinc amino acid chelate (providing 5mg zinc) 50mg' or 'zinc (as amino acid chelate) 5mg', both of which mean you are getting 5mg of elemental or actual zinc. Otherwise you may have to contact the manufacturer for more detailed information. Most good companies declare this information either on the label or in literature that comes with the product.

Supplement labels are also required to show the percentage of the RDA that is met by the product. But for the purposes of achieving optimum nutrition this is largely irrelevant, since the amounts needed are often many times higher than the RDA.

Fillers, binders, lubricants and coatings

Supplements often contain other ingredients which are necessary in their manufacture. While capsules do not really need to have anything added, tablets usually do to enable the ingredients to stick together to form a tablet. Tablets start off as powders, and to get the bulk right 'fillers' are added. 'Binders' are added to give the mixture the right consistency, and lubricants are also used. Only when this is done can the mixture be turned into small, uneven granules, which are then pressed into tablets under considerable force. Granulating allows the mixture to lock together, forming a solid mass. The tablet may then be covered with a 'protein coating' to protect it from deterioration and make it easier to swallow.

Unfortunately, many tablets also have artificial colouring and flavouring added, as well as a sugar coating. For instance, many vitamin C tablets are coloured orange and made to taste sweet, since we associate vitamin C with oranges! Vitamin C is naturally almost white and certainly is not sweet – nor should your supplement be. As a rule of thumb, buy only supplements that declare their fillers and binders (sometimes also called 'excipients'). Companies with integrity are usually only too happy to display this information. The following fillers and binders are perfectly acceptable, and some even add further nutritious properties to the tablet:

Dicalcium phosphate   A natural filler providing calcium and phosphate

Cellulose   A natural binder consisting of plant fibre

Alginic acid/sodium alginate   A natural binder from seaweed

Gum acacia/gum arabic   A natural vegetable gum

Calcium stearate or magnesium stearate   A natural lubricant (usually from animal source)

Silica   A natural lubricant

Zein   A corn protein for coating the tablet

Brazil wax   A natural coating derived from palm trees

Stearate, which is the chemical name for saturated fat, is used as a lubricant. The cheapest comes from animal sources, although non-animal stearates are available. If you are a strict vegan or vegetarian you may want to check this with the supplement company. If a product is labelled 'suitable for vegans' it cannot legally contain any ingredients sourced from animals.

Most large tablets are coated. This makes them shiny, smooth and easier to swallow. It is not so necessary with small tablets. If a tablet is chalky or rough on the outside, it is not coated. Coating, depending on the substance used, can also protect the ingredients, increasing their shelf-life. Avoid sugar-coated, artificially coloured supplements. Natural colours, for example from berry extracts, are fine.

Very occasionally a manufacturer over-coats a batch of tablets and, particularly in people with a shortage of stomach acid, this can inhibit the tablet's disintegration. Most reliable companies check the disintegration time of each batch to rule out this possibility, so it is a rare problem.

Free from sugar, gluten, animal products, etc.

Many of the better supplements will declare that the product is free from sugar and gluten. If you are allergic to milk or yeast, do check that the tablets are also free from lactose (milk sugar) and yeast. B vitamins can be derived from yeast, so you need to be careful. If in doubt, contact the company and ask for an independent 'assay' of the ingredients: good companies will supply this information.

Sometimes glucose, fructose or dextrose is used to sweeten a tablet and yet the packaging still declares 'no sugar'. These products are best avoided. A small amount of fructose is the least evil if you are having difficulty enticing a child to take vitamins. Any other preservatives or flavouring agents should be avoided unless they are natural. Pineapple essence, for instance, is a natural additive.

If you are vegan or vegetarian, choose supplements that state they are suitable for vegans or vegetarians. Retinol (vitamin A) can be derived from an animal source, synthesised or derived from a vegetable source such as retinyl palmitate. Vitamin D can be synthesised, or derived from sheep's wool or from a vegetable source. Companies do not have to state the source of the nutrients, just their chemical form.

Advisory statements

Some supplements are required by law to carry 'advisory notices'. In my view these cautions are, in most cases, exceedingly overcautious. For example, vitamin B6 supplements containing above 10mg have to say that 'long-term intakes may lead to mild tingling and numbness'. I know of not one single case where this has actually happened, although it will happen at higher doses, above 500mg. If you are particularly concerned by such warnings on labels read Chapter 49, which gives you a realistic upper limit for nutrients, based on the latest science.

47.

Building Your Own Supplement Programme

So now you know how to read the labels and find out if a particular supplement contains what you need. Here's how to turn your nutrient needs into a supplement programme.

Theoretically, at one extreme you could take just one mega-mega-multivitamin and mineral that has everything you could possibly need in it. The trouble is that it would be enormous, impossible to swallow and no doubt give you a lot more than you need of some nutrients. The other extreme is to take one supplement for each nutrient, exactly matching your requirements – but you'd end up with handfuls of pills.

Instead, nutritionists use 'formulas' – combinations of vitamins and minerals – which when combined appropriately more or less reach your needs. In a typical supplement programme you might end up with four supplements to take. These formulas are like building blocks. The essential building blocks are shown in the 'supplement jigsaw' below.

1. Start with a high-potency multivitamin and mineral

The starting point of any supplement programme is a high-potency multivitamin and multimineral. Your daily supplement should provide the following nutrients:

Multivitamin

A good multivitamin should contain at least 1,500mcg of A, 5mcg of D, 100mg of E, 250mg of C, 25mg each of B1, B2, B3, B5 and B6, 10mcg of B12, and 50mcg of folic acid and biotin.

Multimineral

This should provide at least 150mg of calcium, 75mg of magnesium, 10mg of iron, 10mg of zinc, 2.5mg of manganese, 20mcg of chromium, 25mcg of selenium and, ideally, some molybdenum, vanadium and boron.

Multivitamin and mineral

You simply can't fit all of the above vitamins and minerals into one tablet. Good quality, combined multivitamin and mineral formulas recommend two or more tablets a day to meet these kinds of levels. The bulkiest nutrients are vitamin C, calcium and magnesium. These are often insufficiently supplied in multivitamin and mineral formulas – and vitamin C is best taken separately anyway, simply because you'll never get 1,000mg (the ideal daily dose) into a multi.

2. Add extra vitamin C and other immune-boosting nutrients

Vitamin C

This is worth taking separately because the amount you need won't fit in a multivitamin. The supplement should provide around 1,000mg of vitamin C. Some vitamin C formulas also provide other key immune-boosting nutrients such as bioflavonoids or anthocyanidins, zinc and cat's claw.

3. Add extra antioxidant nutrients

The evidence is now very conclusive that an optimal intake of antioxidant nutrients slows down the ageing process and prevents a variety of diseases. For this reason it is well worth supplementing extra antioxidant nutrients – on top of those in a good multivitamin – to ensure you are achieving the best possible ageing protection. This is especially important the older you are, and if you live in a polluted city or have frequent strong sun exposure. The kinds of nutrients that are provided in an antioxidant supplement are vitamins A, C, E and betacarotene, zinc and selenium, possibly iron, copper and manganese, the amino acids glutathione or cysteine, plus phytonutrients such as bilberry extract, pycnogenol and grape seed extract. These plant chemicals, rich in bioflavonoids and anthocyanidins, are also often supplied in more comprehensive vitamin C formulas.

4. Are you getting enough fat?

There are two ways of meeting your essential-fat requirements: one is from diet, by eating a heaped tablespoon of ground seeds every day, having a tablespoon of special cold-pressed seed oils and/or eating fish three times a week; the other is to supplement concentrated oils. For Omega 3 this means either flax seed oil capsules or the more concentrated fish oil capsules providing EPA and DHA. For Omega 6 this means supplementing a source of GLA such as evening primrose oil or borage oil. Even better is a combination of all three – EPA, DHA and GLA.

These are the basic building blocks of a good supplement programme. I take these every day. Then, there are optional extras – from nutrients that support your brain and your mood and give you an energy boost when you need it, to natural relaxants or hormone-balancers.

Bone mineral complexes

If the above formulas still leave you short on calcium and magnesium, or if you are pregnant, breastfeeding, post-menopausal or elderly, you may meet your needs by adding a complex of minerals including calcium, magnesium, vitamin D, boron and a little zinc, vitamin C or silica. These help to build healthy bones.

Brain-food formulas

I also supplement a complex of brain-friendly nutrients which includes phosphatidyl choline, phosphatidyl serine, DMAE, pyroglutamate, ginkgo biloba, plus extra B vitamins. Together with Omega 3 fats, these give me optimum nutrition for the mind.

You will also find supplements that help support hormonal health, mood, energy and relaxation. My book *Natural Highs* explains how to use nutrients and herbs to keep you calm and connected.

Individual nutrients

Sometimes even the above formulas may still leave you short on specific nutrients. Shortfalls are commonly found in vitamin B3 (niacin), vitamin B5 (pantothenate), vitamin B6 (pyridoxine), zinc and chromium. If you need both vitamin B3 and chromium, take chromium polynicotinate, which is a complex of the two. If you need extra B3, remember that ordinary niacin makes you blush, so look for niacinamide or 'no-flush niacin'. If you need vitamin B6 and zinc you can often find them in one tablet. A list of recommended supplement companies whose products meet these levels of vitamin and mineral intake is given on page 533.

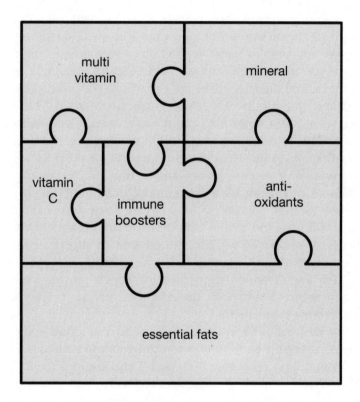

Your ideal supplement programme

How to turn your nutrient needs into a simple supplement programme

From your scores in the questionnaire on page 403 you will have worked out your optimum daily nutrient needs. If you scored less than 5 on each vitamin and mineral your needs will be easily covered by this programme:

Supplement	Daily dose (tablets)
Multivitamin/mineral	2
Vitamin C 1,000mg	1
Essential Omega 3 and 6	1

If you scored 5 or more for vitamins A, D or E, you will probably need to double the multivitamin. A score of 7 or more on vitamin E will warrant a separate vitamin E supplement or perhaps an antioxidant complex that contains vitamin E. If you scored 7 or more on at least two B vitamins your best bet is to take a B-complex tablet in addition to your multivitamin per day. However, if you scored high only on B6, for example, adding a B6 supplement of the desired strength will be more practical. The same applies to vitamin C. If your optimum level is 2,000mg, take two vitamin C tablets a day.

If you scored 5 or more for at least two minerals, you will probably meet your needs by doubling your multimineral intake. However, if only calcium and magnesium were deficient, these can be provided together in a 'bone formula'. If you are particularly in need of chromium you may also require extra vitamin B3; some manufacturers combine the two. The same is true for zinc and B6, so look out for these combined nutrients since they will save you money and decrease the number of tablets you need to take. If you have a weak immune system or are exposed to a lot of pollution you may need more vitamins A, C and E, and zinc and selenium. These are all antioxidant nutrients which protect the immune system and help you deal with the effects of pollution. They are often combined in one supplement.

In three months' time, reassess your needs. You'll find you need less and may end up on a basic supplement programme such as a multivitamin, vitamin C and an essential Omega 3 and 6 supplement. This is a good basic supplement programme for everybody.

Supplements – when to take them

Now that you have worked out what to take, you will want to know when to take it. This depends not only on what is technically best, but also on your lifestyle. If taking supplements twice a day means that you would forget the second lot, you are probably best advised to take them all at once! After all, nature supplies them all in one go, with a meal. Here are the 'ten commandments' of supplement-taking:

1. Take vitamins and minerals fifteen minutes before or after a meal, or during it.

2. Take most of your supplements with your first meal of the day.

3. Don't take B vitamins late at night if you have difficulty sleeping.

4. Take extra minerals, especially calcium and magnesium, in the evening – they help you sleep.

5. If you are taking two or more B-complex or vitamin C tablets, take one at each meal.

6. Do not take individual B vitamins unless you are also taking a general B complex, perhaps in a multivitamin.

7. Do not take individual minerals unless you are also taking a general multimineral.

8. If you are anaemic (iron-deficient), take extra iron with vitamin C.

9. Always take at least ten times as much zinc as copper. If you know you are copper-deficient, take copper only with ten times as much zinc, for example 0.5mg copper to 5mg zinc.

10. Take amino acid supplements on an empty stomach or with a carbo-hydrate food, for example a piece of fruit.

Most of all, always take your supplements. Irregular supplementation doesn't work. There are two supplement-taking strategies that I have found to work for most people. Take most supplements in the morning and a few in the evening, so that you do not have to take any to work. Or, if your supplement programme consists of say, three multivitamins, three vitamin Cs and three antioxidants, put all three in a sachet and take one of each with each meal. Some supplement companies supply small plastic bags so you can 'bag up' your daily supplements. Others have supplement packs that you can buy that already contain the supplements you need (see Resources, page 533).

Are there any side effects?

The side effects of optimum nutrition are increased energy, mental alert-ness and a greater resistance to disease. In fact, a survey of supplement-takers found that 79 per cent noticed a definite improvement in energy, 66 per cent felt more emotionally balanced, 60 per cent had better memory and mental alertness, skin condition had improved in 55 per cent of peo-ple and, overall, 61 per cent had noticed a definite improvement in their well-being. As long as you stick to the levels given in this book and do not take toxic levels (explained in Chapter 49), the only side effects are beneficial.

A small number of people do, however, experience slight symptoms on starting a supplement programme. This may be because they take too many supplements with too little food, or perhaps because a supplement contains something that does not agree with them, for example yeast. These problems are usually solved by stopping the supplements, then taking one only for four days, then adding another for the next four days, and so on until all the supplements have been taken. This will usually reveal whether a supplement is causing a problem. More often than not, the problem simply goes away.

Sometimes people feel worse before they feel better. Imagine your body coping with the onslaught of pollution, poor diet, toxins and stimulants, and then suddenly getting a wonderful diet and all the supplements it needs. This can lead to the process called detoxification, in which the body cleanses itself. This is not a bad thing, and usually subsides within a month. However, if you have inexplicable symptoms, see a nutritional therapist.

What health improvements to expect

Vitamins and minerals are not drugs, so you should not expect an overnight improvement in your health. Most people experience a definite improvement within three months – the shortest length of time that you should experiment with a supplement programme. The earliest noticeable changes are increased energy, mental alertness and emotional stability, and better skin condition. Most people notice these improvements in the first thirty days. Your health will continue to improve as long as you are following the right programme. If you do not experience any improvement in three months, it is best to see a nutritional therapist.

When should you reassess your needs?

Certainly at the beginning your needs will change, and a reassessment every three months is sensible. Your nutrient needs should decrease as you get healthier. Remember, you need optimum nutrition most when you are stressed. So when emergencies arise, or you are working especially hard, make doubly sure that you eat well and take your supplements every day.

chapter 48

Choosing the Best Supplements

While the golden rule of any supplement programme is to work out the right doses and take them regularly, there are many other issues to consider when choosing supplements. Is it better to have natural rather than synthetic nutrients? Are capsules better than tablets? Are certain forms of minerals better absorbed? Are there good and bad combinations? What if you are on medication – are there any situations when you should not take supplements?

Capsules versus tablets

Capsules always used to be made of gelatine, which is an animal product and therefore not suitable for strict vegetarians. However, thanks to technological advances there are now capsules made from vegetable cellulose. The advantage of tablets is that, through compression, you can get more nutrients into them. The disadvantage is the need for fillers and binders. Some people think capsules allow for better nutrient absorption; however, provided the tablet is properly made there is little difference, even if you have poor digestion. Most vitamins, including the oil-based ones, can be provided in tablet form. For instance, natural vitamin E comes in two forms: d-alpha tocopherol acetate (oil) and d-alpha tocopherol succinate (powder). They are equally potent.

Natural versus synthetic

A great deal of nonsense has been said and written about the advantages of natural vitamins. First of all, many products that claim to be natural are simply not. By law, a certain percentage of a product must be natural before the product can be declared 'natural' on its label. The percentage varies from country to country. Through careful wording some supplements are made to sound natural when they are not. For instance, 'vitamin C with rosehips' invariably means synthetic vitamin C with added rosehips, although it is often confused with vitamin C from rosehips. So which is better?

By definition, a synthetic vitamin must contain all the properties of the vitamin found in nature. If it does not, the chemists have not done their job properly. This is the case with vitamin E. Natural d-alpha tocopherol succinate is 36 per cent more potent than the synthetic vitamin E called dl-alpha tocopherol (in this case the 'l' dictates the chemical difference). So natural vitamin E, usually derived from wheat germ or soya oil, is better.

However, synthetic vitamin C (ascorbic acid) has the same biological potency as the natural substance, according to Dr Linus Pauling, although advanced scientific techniques have shown visible differences between the two. No one has yet shown that natural vitamin C is more potent or more beneficial to take. Indeed, most vitamin C is synthesised from a 'natural' sugar such as dextrose; two chemical reactions later you have ascorbic acid. This is little different from the chemical reactions that take place in animals, which convert sugar to vitamin C. Vitamin C derived from, say, acerola cherries – the most concentrated source – is also considerably bulkier and more expensive. Acerola is only 20 per cent vitamin C, so a 1,000mg tablet would be five times as large as a normal tablet and would cost you ten times as much!

It is true that vitamins derived from natural sources may contain unknown elements that increase their potency. Vitamin E or d-alpha tocopherol is found with beta, gamma and delta tocopherol, and the inclusion of these with a measured amount of d-alpha tocopherol may be of benefit. Vitamin C is found in nature together with the bioflavonoids, active nutrients that appear to increase its potency, particularly its capacity for strengthening tiny blood vessels. Good sources of bioflavonoids are berries and citrus fruit, so the addition of citrus bioflavonoids or berry extracts to vitamin C tablets is one step closer to nature.

It is possible that yeast and rice bran, which are excellent sources of B vitamins, also contain unknown beneficial ingredients, so these vitamins are best supplied with yeast or rice bran. Brewer's yeast tablets or powder are far less efficient ways of taking B vitamins than B-complex vitamin supplements with a little added yeast – one would have to eat pounds of yeast tablets to get optimum levels of B vitamins. However, some people are allergic to yeast, and if you react badly to any supplements it could be yeast that is the problem. For this reason many supplements are yeast-free.

There are many other potentially helpful substances that may be provided with nutrients in a complex. Included here are substances called coenzymes, which help to convert the nutrient into its active form. Vitamin B6 needs to be converted from pyridoxine to pyridoxal-5-phosphate before it becomes active in the body. This process requires zinc and magnesium, which are now included in a number of B6 supplements. Supplements of pyridoxal-5-phosphate are also available, and should, theoretically, be more usable. Time will tell how much of an advantage these innovations will prove. But the key point is to make sure you get enough of each of the essential nutrients.

Vitamin and mineral absorption

Vitamins and particularly minerals come in different forms which affect their absorption and availability. Apart from the form of the nutrient, there are dietary and lifestyle factors that help or hinder their availability to the body.

■ Water-soluble nutrients

Vitamin or mineral	Best form to take	When best absorption	What helps absorption	What hinders absorption
B1	thiamine	alone or with meals	B complex, manganese	alcohol, stress, antibiotics
B2	riboflavin	alone or with meals	B complex	alcohol, tobacco, stress, antibiotics
B3	nicotinic acid, nicotinamide	alone or with meals	B complex	alcohol, stress, antibiotics
B5	calcium pantothenate	alone or with meals	biotin, folic acid, B complex	antibiotics, stress
B6	pyridoxine hydrochloride phosphate	alone or with meals	zinc, magnesium, B complex	alcohol, antibiotics, stress
B12	methylcobalamin	alone or with meals	calcium, B complex	alcohol, intestinal parasites, stress, antibiotics
C	ascorbic acid, calcium ascorbate	away from meals	hydrochloric acid in stomach	heavy meals
Folic acid		alone or with meals	C, B complex	alcohol, stress, antibiotics

Biotin	alone or with meals	B complex	avidin (in raw egg whites), stress, antibiotics

Fat-soluble vitamins

A	retinol, betacarotene	take with foods containing fats or oils	zinc, E, C	lack of bile
E	D-alpha tocopherol	take with foods containing fats or oils	selenium, C	lack of bile, ferric forms of iron, oxidised fats
D	ergocalciferol, cholecalciferol	take with foods containing fats or oils	calcium, phosphorous, E, C	lack of bile

Minerals

Vitamin or mineral	When best to take	What helps absorption	What hinders absorption
Calcium (Ca)	with protein food	magnesium, D, hydrochloric acid in stomach	Tea, coffee, smoking
Magnesium (Mg)	with protein food	calcium, B6, D, hydrochloric acid in stomach	Alcohol, tea, coffee, smoking
Iron (Fe)	with food	C, hydrochloric acid in stomach	oxalic acid, tea, coffee, smoking
Zinc (Zn)	on an empty stomach, p.m.	B6, C, hydrochloric acid in stomach	phytic acid, lead, copper, calcium, tea, coffee
Manganese (Mn)	with protein food	C, hydrochloric acid in stomach	high-dosage zinc, tea, coffee, smoking
Selenium (Se)	on an empty stomach	E, hydrochloric acid in stomach	coffee, mercury, tea, smoking
Chromium (Cr)	with protein food	B3, hydrochloric acid in stomach	tea, coffee, smoking

Mineral bioavailability

Most of the minerals essential for health are supplied from food to the body as a compound bound to a larger (food) molecule. This binding is known as chelation, from the Greek word *chele*, meaning a claw. Some form of chelation is important, since most essential minerals in their 'raw' state have a slight electrical positive charge. The gut wall is slightly negatively charged, so once separated from food through the process of digestion these unbound minerals would become loosely bound to the gut wall. Instead of being absorbed, these minerals would easily become bound to undesirable substances like the phytic acid in bran, the tannic acid in tea, oxalic acid and so on – these acids would remove the mineral from the body.

Bioavailability of a mineral, which is defined as the proportion that can be utilised, depends on many factors, including the amount of 'enhancers' and 'inhibitors' present, such as phytates, other minerals and vitamins, as well as the acidity of the digestive environment. Most minerals are absorbed in the duodenum, the first part of the small intestine, assisted by the presence of stomach acid.

Minerals are bound, or chelated, to different compounds to help their absorption. Amino acid-chelated minerals are bound to amino acids, examples of which are chromium picolinate, and selenocysteine or zinc amino acid chelate. These are well absorbed, as are other 'organic' compounds including citrates, gluconates and aspartates. Inorganic compounds such as carbonates, sulphates and oxides are less well absorbed.

For some minerals the extra cost of amino acid-chelated minerals outweighs the advantage. For example, magnesium amino acid chelate is only twice as well absorbed as magnesium carbonate, an inexpensive source of magnesium. Iron amino acid chelate, on the other hand, is four times better absorbed, making the price differential worth it. Generally speaking, the following forms are most readily available to the body, listed in decreasing order of their bioavailability (i.e. the very best first).

Calcium   Amino acid chelate, ascorbate, citrate, gluconate, carbonate

Magnesium   Amino acid chelate, ascorbate, citrate, gluconate, carbonate

Iron   Amino acid chelate, ascorbate, citrate, gluconate, sulphate, oxide

Zinc   Picolinate, amino acid chelate, ascorbate, citrate, gluconate, sulphate

Manganese   Amino acid chelate, ascorbate, citrate, gluconate

Selenium   Selenocysteine or selenomethionine, sodium selenite

Chromium   Picolinate, polynicotinate, ascorbate, gluconate

What about sustained release?

Some vitamins are called prolonged, sustained or time released, implying that the ingredients are not all made available for absorption in one go. This can be useful when taking large amounts of water-soluble vitamins such as B complex or vitamin C. However, absorption depends also on the person and the dosage. Some people are able to absorb and use 1,000mg of vitamin C taken in one dose; taking it in sustained-release form would provide little benefit. However, if you take three 1,000mg tablets a day, sustained release would allow you to take them all in one go. Since sustained-release vitamins are more expensive, you have to weigh up the pros and cons. And there is no point in having a sustained-release fat-soluble vitamin, such as A, D or E, as these can be stored in the body.

The best sustained-release products are capsules containing tiny 'beads', each containing the desired nutrients, which dissolve at different rates and so release the nutrients over time. This method, however, consumes a lot of space, so the dose is not usually very high, making the necessity for sustained release less relevant.

What about food form?

A critical question is 'do vitamins and minerals in food work better than those in supplements?' Some companies sell 'food-form' vitamins and minerals and claim they absorb better into the body. These food-form supplements are made by feeding nutrients to yeast, having the yeast ferment and incorporate the nutrient into its food matrix, then killing off the yeast by a combination of heat and enzymes from pineapple and papaya. This ensures there are no yeast cells left and hence no adverse effects for those sensitive to yeast.

While the research to date, which has looked at the ability of supplements to raise body levels, appears to be positive, there is still much to be done to find out what exactly makes food-form nutrients more bioavailable and also to prove the extent to which they work better in promoting health. The answer is bound to be as complex as nature herself.

In nature, nutrients are bound in a complex way to peptides, proteins, glycoproteins and so on. When we eat, the high acid content of the stomach, plus enzymes, breaks down these bonds to liberate the nutrients. The nutrients then have to be reassembled into forms that can be transported and used by the body. It looks as if the complex way food incorporates nutrients, which is what the food-form process mimics, allows the nutrients to be more easily released, transported and used.

Given that we have evolved over millions of years to use the nutrients available to us in foods it certainly makes good sense to provide nutrients in supplements in a form a close as possible to that found in nature. That said, a nutrient in the form found in food may not in all cases be better for you than that in a supplement. Taking folic acid supplements, for example, has been well proven to be twice as effective in raising blood levels of folic acid and lowering homocysteine as eating the equivalent amount of folate in food.

Good and bad combinations

The general rule is to take supplements with food. This is primarily because the presence of stomach acid helps many minerals to be absorbed, and because the fat-soluble vitamins are carried by the fats or oils present in most meals. Nutrients do, however, compete for absorption. For example, if you want to absorb a large amount of a specific amino acid such as lysine (good for the arteries and for preventing herpes), more will be absorbed if you take it on an empty stomach or with non-protein foods such as a piece of fruit. Similarly, a tiny mineral like selenium will be absorbed better on its own than as part of a multimineral.

However, no one wants to end up taking each supplement separately. So unless you have a specific need or deficiency and want to maximise absorption by taking the nutrient on its own, spread your nutrients out through the day and take them with meals as nature intended.

There is, however, always one exception. If you want to take the alkaline-forming 'ascorbate' type of vitamin C in quite large doses (3 grams or more a day), take it away from meals to avoid neutralising the acidity in your stomach. If you ever experience a burning sensation after taking vitamin C as ascorbic acid (a weak acid), you may have some gastrointestinal irritation or even an ulcer. See your doctor and have this possibility checked out. While vitamin C helps to heal wounds, the acid form can aggravate an existing problem and should be avoided.

Drug-nutrient interactions: difficulties and dangers

There are very few dangerous drug-nutrient interactions. However, there are many drugs that interfere with the action of nutrients, increasing your need.

- Aspirin increases the need for vitamin C.

- The birth-control Pill and HRT increase the need for B6, B12, folic acid and zinc.

- Antibiotics increase the need for B vitamins and beneficial bacteria.

- Paracetamol increases the need for antioxidants.

Here are details of some potentially dangerous combinations that must be avoided:

- Warfarin (a blood-thinning drug), aspirin, vitamin E and high-EPA/DHA fish oils all thin the blood, and the combined effect would be too much. It is better to reduce the drugs and increase the nutrients, but first check with your doctor.

- When taking MAOI anti-depressants (such as Nardil or Parstelin) you must avoid yeast (including supplements), alcohol and certain specific foods.

- Some anti-convulsants are anti-folate, creating an increased need for folic acid, yet supplementation can impair the action of the drug. Specialist advice from your doctor and nutrition consultant is recommended. Epileptics should be careful about supplementing the brain nutrient DMAE.

- In cases of vitamin B12 deficiency, supplementing folic acid can reduce the symptoms while the underlying deficiency gets worse. Therefore it is best to supplement both nutrients, preferably as part of a B complex.

Dos and don'ts of supplement-taking

Very few problems occur with vitamin supplements, but it is sensible to be aware of the following:

- Vitamin A (retinol) in doses in excess of 2,500mcg should not be taken by pregnant women or women trying to conceive. Check that the total provided by all your supplements (e.g. a multivitamin, antioxidant complex, etc.) does not exceed this level.

- Betacarotene in excess makes your skin go very yellow. If you have excessively yellowing skin, check your betacarotene intake from food and supplements. This is quite different from jaundice or hepatitis, in which the whites of your eyes go yellow. Also, don't supplement betacarotene on its own if you are a smoker. Take it as part of an all-round antioxidant complex.

- Vitamin B2 (riboflavin) makes your urine bright yellow. This is normal.

- Vitamin B3 in the form of niacin, usually in doses of 100mg or more, can make you flush and go red, hot and itchy for up to thirty minutes.

This is normal and is not an allergy. While the nutrient is beneficial, if you do not like this side effect, take less or else take half the dose twice a day. Your flushing potential will reduce with regular supplementation. (Alternatively, buy the 'no-flush' type of niacin.)

- Vitamin C has a laxative effect in very high doses, normally above 5 grams a day. A small number of people are very sensitive even at 1 gram a day, while others can tolerate 10 grams a day. The ideal level is the 'bowel-tolerance' level, so adjust your intake accordingly.

- Copper is an essential mineral but it is toxic. Do not take supplements containing copper unless they contain at least ten to fifteen times as much zinc. So, for example, if there is 1mg of copper, make sure there is 10–15mg of zinc. This will prevent copper accumulation. Conversely, zinc is an antagonist of copper so don't take large amounts of zinc without adding a little copper.

Value for money

For a supplement to be good value it must be well made, well formulated and well priced. The quality of manufacture is hard to assess unless you have an advanced chemistry laboratory in your back room! However, there are four simple tests you can do:

1. Is the stated number of tablets actually in the bottle? (When we tested one manufacturer's product at ION we found an average of ninety-five tablets instead of a hundred.)

2. Is the tablet coated all round and therefore easy to swallow? (Uncoated or badly coated tablets can break up or taste unpleasant.)

3. Does the label tell you everything you need to know? (The better the company, the more information it will want to give you.)

4. Does the company emphasise its quality control and, if asked, can it supply you with independent analyses of its products?

If you are buying fish oil supplements make sure the company emphasises the purity of its fish oils. Good products are free from residues of mercury or PCBs and other undesirable pollutants found in fish. Less expensive supplements often come out badly on independent analysis.

chapter 49

Vitamins and Minerals – How Much Is Safe?

Just how safe are supplements? What happens if you take more vitamins or minerals than you need? How much is too much? These are common concerns, fuelled by media reports linking vitamin C with kidney stones and warnings against vitamin A in pregnancy. How much is fact and how much is fiction?

The optimal intake of a nutrient varies considerably for each individual, depending on their age, sex, health and numerous other factors. It is therefore to be expected that the level that would induce signs of toxicity also varies considerably. When certain illnesses are present, a person's need for a vitamin can increase dramatically: vitamin C is the prime example, when you are fighting an infection. In this chapter I have erred on the side of caution by listing the levels of nutrients that may induce toxicity in a small percentage of people, if taken both over a short period (up to one month) and over a long period (three months to three years), indicating which symptoms persist and which go away once the high level is reduced.

It is important to realise that just about everything is toxic if the dose is high enough. In 1990 a man died as a result of drinking 10 litres of water in two hours. So the critical question is: how much more of the substance than is normally consumed do you need to consume to reach toxic levels? In other words, what is the safety margin?

The safety of vitamins

The general conclusion from a survey we conducted at the Institute for Optimum Nutrition of the results of over one hundred research papers in scientific journals is that for the majority of vitamins, with the exception of A and D, levels one hundred times greater than the RDA are likely to be safe for long-term ingestion.[1] Two recent comprehensive reviews broadly support this position.[2]

In practical terms, this means that the chances of having a toxic reaction to even the higher-dose supplements available in health food shops is extremely unlikely unless you take considerably more tablets than recommended. This is consistent with the public health record of deaths attributed to nutritional supplements. To date, no one has been reported as dying as a result of a vitamin supplement. Very rarely there are deaths due to children's swallowing handfuls of their mother's sugar-coated iron supplements. Compare this with deaths attributed to prescribed drugs. These were the conclusions of a survey of hospitalised patients, published in the *Journal of the American Medical Association*: 'We estimate that in 1994 overall 2,216,000 hospitalised patients had serious Adverse Drug Reactions and 106,000 had fatal Adverse Drug Reactions, making these reactions between the fourth and sixth leading cause of death.'[3] Similar findings have also been reported in Britain.[4]

In the table below you can see that you are more than 100,000 times more likely to die from a highly preventable medical injury, including prescribed drugs, than you are from a dietary supplement. Death, however, is a rather severe yardstick. What about toxicity or adverse effects? These too are extremely uncommon as a result of nutritional supplements. In nearly twenty years of practice, teaching and writing I have yet to come across a single case of actual toxicity.

Vitamin A

Vitamin A comes in two forms: the animal form, retinol, which is stored in the body; and the vegetable form, betacarotene, which is converted into retinol unless body levels are already high. Betacarotene is therefore not considered toxic, with the exceptions that excessive intake can cause a reversible yellowing of the skin, and that there is possibly an increased cancer risk, only for smokers, if it is supplemented on its own.

There have been a number of incidences of adverse reactions to retinol, usually from intakes of 150,000mcg or more over a considerable length of time. The symptoms include peeling and redness of the skin, disturbed hair growth, lack of appetite, and vomiting. According to Dr John Marks,

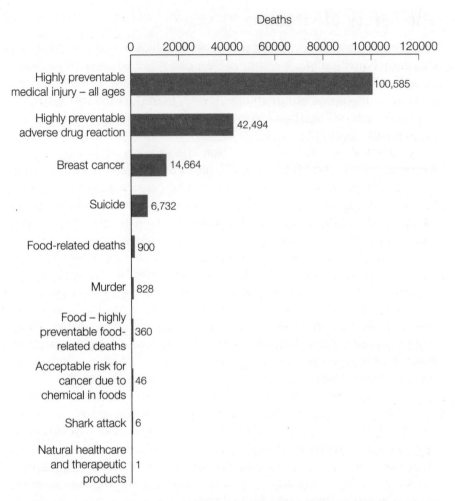

Relative risk of death from dietary supplements versus medical treatment. This assessment of risk, from Australia, shows that if the risk of dying from a natural or dietary supplement is 1, your risk of dying from a shark attack is 6, of being murdered 828, and of dying from a highly preventable medical injury, including an adverse drug reaction, more than 100,000 times higher![5]

medical director at Girton College, Cambridge, 'toxic reactions have been extremely rare below 30,000ius (10,000mcg) ... daily administration in adults up to about 50,000ius (17,000mcg) would appear to be safe'. This is consistent with estimates of the intake of 15,000mcg of vitamin A that our ancestors would have eaten in a more tropical environment, although a large part of this would have come from betacarotene.

A number of cases of toxicity and birth defects have been reported for a synthetic relative of vitamin A, isocretinoin, sold as the drug

Roaccutane. These effects have been wrongly extended to natural vitamin A. Five cases of birth defects have been reported in babies born to women taking large amounts of retinol (75,000–150,000mcg per day); however, no clear cause-and-effect relationship has ever been established in any of these cases.

One study published in 1995 found a possible association: in a group of 22,747 women, 121 gave birth to children with the kind of defect associated with, among other things, vitamin A toxicity. Of these 121, two of the cases could have been attributable to supplementing in excess of 3,300mcg of vitamin A in the form of retinol. In view of the possibility that large amounts of retinol could induce birth defects, it is wise for women of childbearing age to take no more than 3,300mcg of retinol in supplemental form. (Other studies have shown that women who supplement their diet with multivitamins including vitamin A, usually at a level of 2,500–7,500mcg, have a lower incidence of defects in their babies.)

The same caution as for retinol does not apply to betacarotene. This has, however, been shown to slightly increase the risk of lung cancer and colon cancer if given in isolation to smokers. My advice here is to stop smoking and, if you haven't, supplement betacarotene only as part of a multivitamin or antioxidant complex. Betacarotene in food reduces the risk of cancer even for smokers.

Vitamin D

Of all the vitamins, D is the most likely to cause toxic reactions. It encourages calcium absorption, and excessive intake can lead to calcification of soft tissue. However, the levels that create this effect are certainly in excess of 3,000mcg and probably more like 15,000mcg. A daily intake not exceeding 6,600mcg for adults and 330mcg for children is generally considered safe.

Vitamin E

Vitamin E has been well researched for toxicity. A review of 216 trials of high-dose vitamin E in 10,000 people showed that daily doses of 2,000mg for up to eleven years and 35,000mg for a few months had no detrimental effect. However, adverse reactions have occasionally been reported at lower levels of 1,300mg, especially in children, possibly due to an allergic reaction to the source of the vitamin E.

Vitamin E appears to increase the anti-clotting effects of the drug Warfarin, and therefore high levels are not recommended for those on Warfarin. High levels are also best avoided by people suffering from rheumatic fever. Some old reports that vitamin E should not be taken in supplement form by women with breast cancer are inaccurate: it is highly beneficial to do so. A daily intake of up to 1,000mg is considered safe.

Vitamin C

Vitamin C is water-soluble and therefore excess is readily excreted from the body. RDAs vary considerably from country to country. A general consensus based on up-to-date research is that 100mg a day represents a good basic intake; the optimal intake is probably between 1,000 and 3,000mg a day.

A number of studies have investigated the effects of vitamin C on specific diseases, using over 10,000mg a day. The recommendation of these high levels has attracted controversy and allegations that vitamin C can cause kidney-stone formation, interferes with B12 absorption, and causes a 'rebound scurvy' when supplementation is stopped. All these allegations have been shown to be without substance. The only drawback to taking large amounts of vitamin C is that it can have a laxative effect. Generally, supplementing up to 5,000mg of vitamin C a day can be considered safe.

Vitamin B

The B vitamins are water-soluble and excess is readily excreted from the body in the urine, so they are generally of very low toxicity. Thiamin (B1), riboflavin (B2), pantothenic acid (B5), B12 and biotin show no sign of toxicity at levels of at least 100 times the US RDA. Vitamin B3 in the form of niacin causes blushing at levels of 75mg or more; this is part of its natural action and therefore is not generally considered to be a toxic effect.

According to Dr John Marks at Girton College, Cambridge, 'doses of 200mg to 10g daily have been used therapeutically to lower blood cholesterol levels under medical control for periods of up to ten years or more, and though some reactions have occurred at these very high dosages, they have rapidly responded to cessation of therapy, and have often cleared even when therapy has been continued'. Levels of up to 2,000mg per day on a continuous basis are considered safe.

Vitamin B6 has been extensively tested for toxicity by a number of research groups including the US Government Food and Drug Administration, which concluded that 'in man, side effects were not encountered with daily administration of 50–200mg over periods of months'. Most of the unfounded reports of low-dose B6 causing nerve damage appear to be based on one well-documented case of a woman who increased her B6 intake from supplements of 500mg to 5,000mg over a period of two years, and developed muscle weakness and pain which were attributed to nerve damage.

One researcher, investigating seven cases of people taking 2,000–5,000mg of B6 a day for considerable lengths of time, said that 'substantial improvement occurred in all cases in the months after withdrawal of pyridoxine, usually with improvement in gait and less discomfort in the extremities, but in some patients, residual neurological discomfort remained'. In rats, daily injected doses of 600mg/kg, equivalent to 38,000mg a day in a person weighing 100 stone, caused 'peripheral neuropathy', with tingling and numbing of the hands and feet.

Deficiency of vitamin B6 induces the same symptoms. The likely explanation is that, in order to become active in the body where it helps enzymes to work, pyridoxine must be converted to pyridoxal phosphate. If the body is saturated with excessive pyridoxine this conversion does not take place: enzymes become saturated with simple pyridoxine and so do not work properly. So B6 excess may, in fact, induce what are effectively B6-deficiency symptoms. Since zinc is required for the conversion of pyridoxine to pyridoxal phosphate, taking B6 with zinc is likely to reduce its toxicity. In any event, a daily intake of up to 200mg on a continuous basis is generally considered safe.

The safety of minerals

The safety of minerals depends on three factors: the amount, the form and the balance with other minerals in the diet. First, all minerals show toxicity at exceedingly high doses. Where form is concerned, trivalent chromium, for example, is essential, while hexavalent chromium (found in neither foods nor supplements) is very toxic. And as for balance, iron supplementation can exacerbate zinc deficiency since it is a zinc antagonist. The reason for such antagonism is that the shape of the atoms of many minerals is very similar. They are really just different sizes of cogs, so if you lack one mineral but take in an excess of a similar-shaped one it can slot into the wrong enzyme, speeding it up, slowing it down or simply stopping it from working altogether.

In view of these factors, the levels given in the following pages as safe for long-term consumption presuppose that other essential minerals are also adequately supplied. Larger amounts than those stated may also be safe for short-term use, particularly for people with certain illnesses which result in an extra requirement for a mineral. Selenium requirement, for example, is thought to increase in certain types of cancer.

Calcium

The best-absorbed of calcium's many forms include calcium ascorbate, amino acid chelate, gluconate, orotate and carbonate. In normal, healthy people there is little danger of toxicity since the body excretes excessive amounts. In some cultures people consume in excess of 2g a day from their diet alone, so this amount is certainly considered safe. Calcium-deficiency disorders are treated with 3.6g per day.

Problems of excessive calcium arise from other factors, such as excessive vitamin D intake (above 25,000ius per day), or parathyroid or kidney disorders. Calcium interacts with magnesium and phosphorus, so calcium supplementation should be given only to people with adequate magnesium and phosphorus intake, or supplementing these elements. Phosphorus is rarely deficient, while magnesium deficiency is quite common. The ideal calcium: phosphorus ratio is probably 1:1. Less than 1:2 is not desirable. The ideal calcium: magnesium ratio is probably 3:2.

Magnesium

The best-absorbed of magnesium's many forms include magnesium aspartate, ascorbate, amino acid chelate, gluconate, orotate and carbonate. Toxic effects include blushing of the skin, thirst, low blood pressure, loss of reflexes and respiratory depression. Toxicity is likely to occur only in people with kidney disease who are taking magnesium supplements. For normal, healthy adults a daily intake of up to 1,000mg is considered safe. Magnesium interacts with calcium, so magnesium supplements should be given only to people with adequate calcium intake, or supplementing calcium. The ideal ratio of magnesium to calcium is probably 2:3, and in cases of magnesium deficiency 1:1.

Iron

This is one of the most frequently deficient minerals. The diets of at least 6 per cent of women in the UK contain less than the RDA. Iron comes in many different forms, the best absorbed of which include ferrous aspartate, amino acid chelate, succinate, lactate and gluconate (ferric forms are less well absorbed).

Ferrous sulphate is less toxic than ferric forms of iron. Even so, 3g of ferrous sulphate can cause death in an infant, compared with 12g for an adult. Supplements containing a significant amount of iron should be kept in a child-proof container. Iron is stored in the body and therefore toxicity can result from chronic over-intake, producing haemosiderosis, a generalised deposition of iron within body tissue, or haemochromatosis, normally a hereditary condition resulting in cirrhosis of the liver, bronze pigmentation of the skin, diabetes, arthritis and heart abnormalities.

Haemochromatosis is far more common than is realised. One in 200 people has these genetic mutations that mean they are at risk of suffering from iron overload, the symptoms of which are extreme fatigue and abdominal pain. Provided you don't have haemochromatosis, 50mg a day as a supplement is generally considered safe; however, even this is unnecessary to correct acute anaemia. A third of pregnant women show some level of iron-deficiency anaemia, which is easily corrected by supplementing up to 25mg a day.

Iron is antagonistic to many other trace minerals including zinc, which is often deficient especially among pregnant and lactating women. Therefore extra iron should not be supplemented without ensuring adequate zinc status or supplementing zinc. The normal requirement for zinc and iron is approximately equal.

Zinc

This is one of the most thoroughly researched and commonly deficient minerals. About a thousand papers are published each year indicating its value for a variety of conditions. The best-absorbed forms of zinc include zinc picolinate, amino acid chelate, citrate and gluconate. Zinc supplementation is relatively non-toxic. When it's taken in doses of 2,000mg, symptoms of nausea, vomiting, fever and severe anaemia have been reported. Small amounts of zinc, particularly in the form of zinc sulphate, can act as an irritant in the digestive tract when taken on an empty stomach. There is also some evidence that, at levels of 300mg per day, zinc may impair rather than improve immune function. It is generally considered safe to supplement up to 50mg per day.

Zinc is an iron, manganese and copper antagonist; therefore an adequate intake of these minerals is advisable if large amounts of zinc are taken over a long period. Manganese is very poorly absorbed, so it is generally advisable to supplement half as much manganese as zinc if more than 20mg of zinc a day is supplemented. The normal requirement for zinc is about ten times that of copper. Since the average intake of copper for people on a healthy diet is in the order of 2mg, those supplementing more than 20mg of zinc may be advised to add 1mg of copper for each additional 10mg of zinc. It is also best to ensure that at least 12mg of iron is supplemented when you are taking more than 20mg of zinc.

Copper

Deficiency of this mineral is quite rare, probably because we get it from drinking water as well as from unrefined foods. The best-absorbed forms of copper include copper amino acid chelate and gluconate.

Requirements are low (2mg per day), and only 5mg a day is required to correct deficiency. Toxicity does occur, mainly due to excessive intake from water that flows through copper pipes. Copper is also a strong antagonist of zinc, and for this reason it is advisable not to supplement more than 2mg or a tenth of one's intake of zinc. Copper also depletes manganese.

Manganese

No more than 2–5 per cent of dietary manganese is absorbed, so increasing your intake from food has only a slight effect on overall body levels. The better forms for absorption include amino acid chelates, gluconates and orotates. There is some evidence that vitamin C may help the absorption of manganese. In animals it is one of the least toxic of all trace elements. Toxicity has never been reported in man. A daily intake of up to 50mg is considered safe. Excessive zinc or copper intake interferes with manganese uptake.

Selenium

This trace element is required in very small amounts of 25–200mcg per day. It comes in two forms: organic, such as selenomethionine or selenocystine, sometimes in the form of selenium yeast; and inorganic, as sodium selenite. The inorganic form is more toxic, with toxicity occurring at levels of 1,000mcg or more. The organic forms show toxicity above 2,000mcg. No toxicity has been reported with either form at intakes of 750mcg. An intake of up to 500mcg for an adult is generally considered safe. In view of the relatively small difference between beneficial and detrimental intake, selenium should be kept out of reach of children.

Chromium

Of the two forms of chromium found in nature, hexavalent and trivalent, hexavalent is much more toxic. However, it is found neither in food nor in supplements, so contamination can occur only from occupational exposure. The better-absorbed forms of chromium are picolinate, amino acid chelate and polynicotinate. Trivalent chromium has a very low toxicity, partly because so little is absorbed. An intake of up to 500mcg is certainly considered safe.

You might have heard a rumour that chromium picolinate could cause DNA damage. This was based on a study in 1995 in which hamsters were given amounts of chromium several thousands of times higher than you would ever take in a supplement.[6] A further animal study in 1997 gave amounts 5,000 times higher than the 200mcg I recommend and failed to find any evidence of toxicity.[7] Since then a decade of research including more than thirty human trials has also shown no safety concerns. The fact is there is no evidence that supplementing chromium picolinate, let alone any other form of chromium, has the potential to cause cancer in either animals or humans. In the US, the National Toxicology Program investigated chromium picolinate and found no evidence of 'genotoxicity' or any other ill effects. And now, even the FSA agrees that chromium is non-toxic, even in amounts ten times higher than the average 200mcg supplement.

Part 7

A to Z of Nutritional Healing

A to Z of Nutritional Healing

While there is no substitute for individual assessment of nutrient needs, the following nutritional advice is helpful for people suffering from particular health problems. For the more serious conditions it is best to follow these programmes under the supervision of your doctor or nutrition consultant. The supplements recommended are for adults and are based on the formulas given in Chapter 47. Since dosage is crucial, it is best to get supplements close to these formulas. When individual amounts of a nutrient are given, these are the total required. Check that you are not 'doubling up' by receiving, for example, vitamin A in a multivitamin, an antioxidant and a separate supplement.

For further guidance on supplement doses stay within the ranges given in Chapter 45, using the higher amounts for conditions that are specifically helped by these nutrients, or when symptoms of deficiency are present.

All the recommendations given here are for adults. For guidance on supplemental levels for children see Chapter 40. For babies and infants I recommend you read my book *Optimum Nutrition Before, During and After Pregnancy*.

The recommendations given are aimed at helping to restore health in these conditions. They do not replace medical advice, nor should they be continued on an ongoing basis once the condition is corrected.

The basics for any supplement programme, given on page 413, are 2 x a high-strength multivitamin and mineral (you can't get optimum levels in only 1 pill), 1 gram or more of vitamin C and an essential Omega 3 and 6 supplement. You can get daily packs of these 'basics', which is a good place to start, adding any extras. The supplement directory on pages 528–33 gives some 'best fit' products that meet the recommendations given below.

Acne

This condition is most prevalent among teenagers, and the hormonal changes that take place at this age are certainly at the root of many skin problems. These changes cause the sebaceous glands to produce too much sebum and keratin, which block up the skin pores making them more likely to get infected. A diet high in saturated fat or fried food also makes pores more likely to get blocked. Vitamin A deficiency produces skin congestion through over-keratinisation of skin cells. Vitamin A and zinc deficiency leads to lowered ability to fight infection, as does lack of beneficial bacteria (through overuse of antibiotics). Optimum nutrition helps by balancing hormones as well as reducing the risk of infection. The most important nutrients are vitamins A, B complex (especially B6), C and E, zinc, niacin for skin-flushing, and vitamin E for wound-healing. Good diet and cleanliness are essential. Be careful of supplements with added iodine, which can make acne worse.

Diet advice
Follow an optimum diet and drink plenty of water. Sulphur-rich foods such as eggs, onions and garlic are also helpful. Avoid sugar, cigarettes, fried and high-fat foods. Eat plenty of fresh fruit and vegetables (high-water-content foods).

Supplements
- 2 × multivitamin and multimineral
- 2 × antioxidant complex
- 2 × vitamin C 1,000mg
- Niacin (B3) 100mg for thirty days (for flushing and cleansing the skin)
- Zinc 15mg
- Vitamin E 400mg (helps heal the skin)

Use topical vitamin A cream (see Skin-care products in Resources). Also read Chapter 27.

Alcoholism

Particularly prevalent among histadelic (high-histamine) people (see page 337), alcoholism may in part be a way of coping with the excess energy that such individuals produce. B vitamins, especially B1, B2, B3 and B6, are destroyed by alcohol, which primarily affects the liver and nervous system. Vitamins A and C help protect the liver. Glutamine heals the gut and reduces cravings. A very alkaline diet reduces the craving for alcohol. Tyrosine and adaptogens help to prevent emotional and physicals lows after stopping. Emotional problems almost always underlie alcoholism, and these, as well as the addiction – which usually also exists for sugar – must be addressed.

Diet advice

Follow the recommended diet and eat plenty of whole grains, beans and lentils. Drink plenty of water. Often, sugar addiction is substituted for dependency on alcohol, which is just another form of sugar, so sugar and stimulants are also best avoided. Eat frequent meals containing some protein foods such as nuts, seeds, fish, chicken, eggs or milk produce.

Supplements

- 3 × multivitamin and multimineral
- 2 × antioxidant complex
- 3 × vitamin C 1,000mg
- Adaptogen herbs, plus tyrosine
- Bone mineral complex (providing 500mg calcium and 300mg magnesium)
- Glutamine powder 5g twice a day in water on an empty stomach

Also read Chapters 35 and 38.

Allergies

'Allergy' is a word that often invokes connotations beyond its original meaning. An allergy is an intolerance to a particular substance. We have an intolerance to coffee, for example, if large amounts produce symptoms. Some people have more pronounced symptoms, even in reaction to simple foods like wheat or milk. Since an allergy is like an addiction, it is often the foods that one is most 'addicted' to that are suspect. If you feel that you might have allergies but do not know what they are, it is best to see a nutrition consultant or an allergy specialist who can test you and solve any underlying digestive imbalances that provoke allergies. Optimum nutrition will greatly reduce or clear up allergic reactions in most cases. Vitamin C, calcium and magnesium help to reduce the severity of allergic reactions. L-glutamine heals the gut and supports the immune system, reducing allergic potential.

Diet advice

Follow a general healthy diet. Avoid suspect foods, dairy products and grains (the most common allergens), especially wheat. After two months you may be able to reintroduce suspect foods every fourth day without having a reaction. Eventually you may be able to tolerate your allergens in small amounts on a daily basis.

Supplements
- 2 × multivitamin and multimineral
- 2 × antioxidant complex
- 4 × vitamin C 1,000mg
- Calcium/magnesium complex (providing 500mg and 300mg respectively)
- L-glutamine powder 3g a day

Also read Chapter 34.

Alzheimer's and dementia

Like many degenerative diseases, Alzheimer's stems primarily from not looking after your diet and lifestyle. The actual damage in the brain is caused by inflammation linked to too many oxidants, blood sugar problems, raised cortisol, high homocysteine and exposure to toxic metals. These include aluminium, copper and mercury. Trace amounts of mercury can cause the type of damage to nerves that is characteristic of Alzheimer's. If you are experiencing significant decline in mental function, and have a mouth full of amalgam fillings, I'd recommend you seriously consider having them replaced. One of the best predictors of dementia and Alzheimer's risk is your blood level of homocysteine. If it's high, supplementing large amounts of B6 (100mg), B12 (100mcg) and folic acid (800mcg) helps lower it.

Diet advice
Eat plenty of fresh fruit and vegetables (aim for a mix of all colours, combining blueberries, beetroot, carrots, yellow peppers and green vegetables), seeds and fish such as mackerel, salmon or tuna, rich in Omega 3 and vitamin E. Eat wholefoods, and avoid refined foods and sugar, smoking, alcohol and fried foods.

Supplements
- 2 × multivitamin and mineral
- 3 × antioxidant complex
- 4 × vitamin C 1,000mg
- 3 × brain-food formula
- 3 × Omega 3 fish oils
- Homocysteine-lowering formula, if your homocysteine score is high
- Lecithin granules (1 tablespoon)

Also read Chapters 28 and 42.

Anaemia

Anaemia can be caused by iron, B12 or folic acid deficiency. A blood test can determine if you have such deficiencies. Iron is needed in the body to make haemoglobin – a key part of blood responsible for the delivery of oxygen and other nutrients to your tissues, brain, muscles and organs. If you're low in iron you can't make enough red blood cells, hence your pale appearance, and with fewer red blood cells, your brain and body don't get the levels of oxygen and other nutrients they need. If you're low in folic acid or B12 the haemoglobin is misshapen and doesn't work properly. The result? Tiredness.

Two simple tests of your iron status involve your eyelids and fingernails. Look in the area under your lower eyelids – it should be a rich pink/red colour, not pale; press on the end of your fingernail, turning the bed white – it should come back to red quickly when you release it, not stay pale.

Diet advice

Red meat is well known as a good source of iron, but can also be rich in saturated fat. Sources that do not have a high fat content include eggs, spinach and other greens, beans, lentils, prunes, dried apricots, molasses and pumpkin seeds so eat plenty of these, as well as green vegetables and beans, which are rich in folate. Only foods of animal origin contain vitamin B12.

Supplements

- 2 × multivitamin and mineral
- Amino acid-chelated iron 10mg
- 2 × vitamin C 1,000mg

Angina and atherosclerosis

Atherosclerosis is a narrowing of the arteries due to fatty deposits. When the condition becomes more pronounced, blood pressure begins to increase. If a pronounced block occurs in the arteries that supply the heart with oxygen, then angina, experienced as chest pain on exertion, may result. Optimum nutrition is the primary method for preventing both of these conditions. Antioxidant nutrients help prevent the cellular damage that may underlie these problems. Vitamin C and lysine help to reverse atherosclerosis. Vitamin B3 (niacin) raises HDL, the cholesterol-remover. Fish oils, rich in EPA and DHA, thin the blood and reduce cholesterol.

Diet advice

Follow the dietary advice in this book strictly, avoiding sugar, salt, foods high in saturated fat, coffee and excess alcohol. Ensure there are sufficient essential fats in the diet by eating seeds. Take plenty of exercise within your capacity.

Supplements
- 2 × multivitamin and multimineral (with at least 300mg magnesium)
- 2 × antioxidant complex
- 4 × vitamin C 1,000mg
- 2 × lysine 1,000mg
- 'No-flush' niacin 500mg
- 3 × Omega 3-rich fish oils (providing EPA 1,200mg)
- Homocysteine-lowering formula, if your hymocysteine score is high
- Vitamin E 400mg

Also read Chapter 23.

Arthritis

There are two major forms of arthritis and many different causes of both. Osteoarthritis, more common in the elderly, describes a condition in which the cartilage in the joints wears away, inducing pain and stiffness mainly in weight-bearing joints. Rheumatoid arthritis affects the whole body, not just certain joints. Antioxidant nutrients, essential fats and herbs such as boswellia, curcumin and certain hop extracts reduce inflammation. B vitamins and vitamin C support the endocrine system, which controls calcium balance. Vitamin D, calcium, magnesium and boron support bone health. Glucosamine and MSM help to build healthy joints.

Diet advice
Follow the perfect diet in this book and be sure to avoid adrenal stimulants such as tea, coffee, sugar and refined carbohydrates. Drink plenty of water and herb teas. Check for allergies, and have a hair-mineral analysis done to check your mineral levels.

Supplements
- 2 × multivitamin and multimineral
- 2 × antioxidant complex
- 2 × vitamin C 1,000mg
- 2 × essential Omega 3 and 6 oil capsules
- Joint-support complex
- Bone mineral complex

Also read Chapter 26.

Asthma

This inflammatory condition affects the lungs and respiration and is characterised by difficulty in breathing and frequent coughing. Often attacks are brought on by underlying allergies, stressful events or changes in environmental conditions like the weather. Vitamin A helps protect the lining of the lungs, while vitamin C helps to deal with environmental toxins. Antioxidant nutrients and essential fats are anti-inflammatory.

Diet advice
Follow the perfect diet in this book, ensuring an adequate intake of essential oils, and see a nutrition consultant if you suspect you have allergies.

Supplements
- 2 × multivitamin and multimineral
- 2 × antioxidant complex
- 2 × vitamin C 1,000mg
- 2 × essential Omega 3 and 6 oil capsules

Also read Chapter 34.

Breast cancer

Most breast cancers are hormonally related, linked to oestrogen dominance and progesterone deficiency. Stress, excessive use of stimulants and exposure to pesticides all disrupt hormone balance. Some forms of breast cancer, however, are linked more to carcinogens. Antioxidant nutrients have been shown to decrease risk and increase survival. Use of natural progesterone has been shown to reverse the proliferation of tumour cells. See your doctor or a nutrition consultant to get your hormone levels tested and consider natural progesterone cream.

Diet advice
Follow the diet in this book, with an emphasis on foods high in antioxidants, avoiding milk and meat, beef in particular, because of their IGF hormone content, and eating organic as much as possible. Have plenty of phytoestrogen-rich foods – beans, lentils, seeds and nuts – and lots of fresh organic fruit and vegetables. Keep saturated fat very low and ensure you have adequate essential fats from seeds and their cold-pressed oils.

Supplements
- 2 × multivitamin and multimineral
- 2 × antioxidant complex

- 2 × vitamin C 1,000mg
- 2 × essential Omega 3 and 6 oil capsules

Also read Chapters 24 and 32.

Bronchitis

In this condition the tissues of the lung get inflamed. Optimum nutrition can help prevent it by strengthening the immune system and helping to maintain healthy lung tissue. Vitamins A, B complex, C and E, and the minerals selenium and zinc, all strengthen the immune system. Vitamins A and C protect lung tissue.

Diet advice
Follow the diet in this book and do not smoke. You may also find some relief from following a diet low in mucus-forming foods, such as milk and milk products. Keep saturated fat very low and ensure you have adequate essential fats from seeds and their cold-pressed oils.

Supplements
- 2 × multivitamin and multimineral
- 2 × antioxidant complex
- 2 × vitamin C 1,000mg
- 2 × essential Omega 3 and 6 oil capsules
- Vitamin E 400mg

Burns, cuts and bruises

All these conditions require skin to heal, which depends on a good supply of vitamins A, C and E, zinc and bioflavonoids. These reduce bruising, speed up healing and minimise scar tissue. Vitamin E oil can be rubbed around, but not on, cuts and burns; you can get it by piercing a vitamin E capsule. Also useful are creams rich in vitamin A, C or E in a form that can penetrate the skin, such as retinyl, ascorbyl or locopheryl palmitate.

Diet advice
Follow the diet recommended in this book. Drink plenty of water. Ensure you have adequate essential fats from seeds and their cold-pressed oils.

Supplements
- 2 × multivitamin and multimineral with 2,270mcg of both vitamin A and betacarotene
- 2 × antioxidant complex
- 2 × vitamin C complex 1,000mg with at least 150mg of bioflavonoids
- 2 × essential Omega 3 and 6 oil capsules

- Vitamin E 400mg
- Zinc 15mg

Cancer

There are many different kinds of cancer, with different causes. Most cancers are associated with exposure to or ingestion of cancer-causing agents, coupled with immune insufficiency. Often there is an association with free-radical damage of cells, which then become cancerous. Depending on the type of cancer, the first step is to eliminate cancer-stimulating agents such as smoking, a high-fat diet, HRT, excessive exposure to sunlight or pesticides, a high-meat diet, alcohol and so on. The next step is to build up the strength of the immune system with diet and supplements and to increase your intake of antioxidant nutrients.

Diet advice

Stick strictly to the diet advice in this book. Increase the amount of high-antioxidant foods you eat (see page 133). Cut out red meat and alcohol, and reduce your intake of all sources of saturated fat. A vegan-type diet is best. Also, drink plenty of water and herb tea, especially cat's claw, which is a potent immune-booster.

Supplements

- 2 × multivitamin and multimineral
- 2 × antioxidant complex
- 4 × vitamin C 1,000mg (up to 10g a day)
- 2 × essential Omega 3 and 6 oil capsules
- Vitamin A 3,000mcg a day
- Vitamin E 400mg a day
- Selenium 200mcg a day

Also read Chapters 24 and 32.

Candidiasis

The overgrowth of *Candida albicans*, a yeast-like fungus, can occur anywhere in the body, most commonly in the digestive tract or the vagina, and causes thrush or yeast infection. Mild overgrowth can be eliminated by a four-point plan: anti-fungal agents such as caprylic acid and grapefruit seed extract; supplementation of beneficial bacteria; an immune-boosting diet and supplements; and an 'anti-candida' diet (see below). It is usually best to work with a nutrition consultant, who can confirm the extent of the infection with proper tests.

Diet advice

Avoid all sources of sugar and especially fast-releasing sugars (including fruit for the first month). Also stay away from yeast-containing foods, mushrooms and fermented foods such as alcohol and vinegar. Intake of wheat is often best reduced since it irritates the gut. This means living off vegetables, grains, beans, lentils, nuts and seeds. It is worth getting a good anti-candida recipe book!

Supplements

- 2 × multivitamin and multimineral
- 2 × antioxidant complex
- 2 × vitamin C 1,000mg
- Caprylic acid 700mg twice a day
- Grapefruit seed extract 15 drops twice a day
- A probiotic supplement such as *Lactobacillus acidophilus* or *Bifidobacteria* (take separately from caprylic acid and grapefruit seed extract, perhaps before bed)

Also read Chapters 24 and 33.

Colds and flu

Exposure to viruses is unavoidable, unless you live like a hermit. However, whether you succumb to a virus depends on the strength of your immune system at the time of infection. Studies have repeatedly shown that taking a daily supplement of 1 gram of vitamin C or more reduces the incidence, severity and duration of colds. However, optimum nutrition, together with immune-boosting nutrients during cold epidemics, can produce even better results.

Diet advice

Avoid all dairy products, eggs and excessive meat or soya consumption, since these foods are mucus-forming. This is a great time to give your body a high-energy pure food diet packed with fresh fruit and vegetables and their juices. Drink cat's-claw tea three times a day to boost the immune system.

Supplements

- 2 × multivitamin and multimineral
- 2 × antioxidant complex
- 2 × vitamin C 1,000mg (4g every four hours only when infected)
- Elderberry extract (1 dessertspoon four times a day only when infected)
- Echinacea drops (10 drops, two or three times a day)

Also read Chapter 33.

Colitis

In this condition part of the large intestine is inflamed. It is often stress-induced; however, it can also be due to poor diet, poor elimination, an allergy or sub-optimum nutrition. Since there is inflammation, the first step is to reduce any aggravating foods including alcohol, coffee and wheat. These can be replaced by foods and drinks that pass easily through the digestive tract, such as steamed vegetables, rice, fish and fruit, plus digestive enzyme supplements. Essential fats rich in GLA are powerful anti-inflammatory agents. Antioxidants also help to reduce inflammation.

Diet advice
While the diet recommended in this book is a good one, the high fibre content can act as an irritant in this condition. So a diet of lightly steamed vegetables, fish and cooked grains is often preferable, with easy-to-digest fruit as snacks. Avoid all digestive irritants, which can include any food you are allergic to, wheat, alcohol, coffee and spices.

Supplements
- 2 × multivitamin and multimineral
- 2 × antioxidant complex
- 2 × essential Omega 3 and 6 oil capsules
- Vitamin C 500mg (up to 2,000mg as ascorbate, because ascorbic acid can irritate an already inflamed bowel)
- Digestive enzyme formula with each main meal

Also read Chapter 22.

Constipation

Contrary to popular belief, we should empty our bowels not once but two or three times a day. A healthy stool should break up easily and be no strain to pass. By these criteria, a large majority of people suffer from constipation. A high-fibre diet will help, as will a reduction in meat and milk products. Exercise is crucial, as it strengthens the abdominal muscles. Vitamins B1 and E help, while vitamin C may loosen the bowels. A non-irritant laxative, fructo-oligosaccharides powder, helps relieve severe constipation.

Diet advice
Follow the diet advice in this book, in particular eating high-fibre foods. Drink at least a litre (1¾ pints) of water a day, preferably between meals. Reduce your consumption of meat and milk products. Include oats and prunes in your diet, as well as linseeds, which can be ground and sprinkled on food.

Supplements
- 2 × multivitamin and multimineral
- 3 × vitamin C 1,000mg
- Digestive enzymes/probiotics with each meal

Also read Chapter 22.

Chronic fatigue

There are many causes of chronic fatigue, the most common of which is sub-optimum nutrition. Nutrients needed in energy production include vitamins C and B complex, iron and magnesium. However, more pronounced symptoms, sometimes called ME, can include extreme tiredness on exertion. These can result from the body's ability to detoxify being overloaded. Any generation of energy (exercise) or digestion (eating) produces toxins for the body to deal with. If symptoms occur after eating or exercise, see a nutrition consultant who can test your liver detoxification potential.

Diet advice
Eat little and often, choosing from slow-releasing carbohydrates and snacking on fruit. Avoid sugar and stimulants such as tea, coffee, chocolate and alcohol. In general, follow the dietary recommendations in this book.

Supplements
- 2 × multivitamin and multimineral
- 3 × vitamin C 1,000mg
- 2 × antioxidant complex

Also read Chapters 29 and 35.

Crohn's disease

Crohn's disease is an inflammatory bowel disorder that responds very well to nutritional therapy. A few factors should be considered. Sensitivity to certain foods, most commonly gluten (the protein found in wheat, oats, rye and barley) and milk, can aggravate Crohn's, so avoiding them can help. The amount of good bacteria in the gut is likely to be low, so restore the balance with a probiotic supplement such as *Lactobacillus acidophilus*. Taking some Omega 3-rich fish or flax oil, which contain Omega 3 fats, helps calm the inflammation. Certain herbs such as slippery elm or marshmallow are very soothing to the gut lining, while others such as boswellia and curcumin can reduce inflammation. The amino acid glutamine, 5 to 10 grams taken as a powder in water last thing at night, also helps to repair the gut.

Most people with Crohn's are allergic to certain foods, most commonly gluten, and also have raised homocysteine levels. It is well worth working with a nutritional therapist, who can test for these factors and help you find your perfect diet and supplement programme.

You can't avoid fibre completely and wouldn't want to. Fibre is a natural constituent of a healthy diet high in fruit, vegetables, lentils, beans and whole grains and by eating such a diet you have less risk of bowel cancer, diabetes or diverticular disease, and are unlikely to suffer from constipation. However, be really careful with *insoluble* fibre found in bran and whole grains. It's harsh on the bowel and doesn't suit a sensitive or inflamed digestive system. There are, however, many different kinds of fibre. *Soluble* fibres, found in oats, lentils, beans, fruit, vegetables and flax seeds or linseeds (which you should continue to eat plenty of), are a whole other story. Soluble fibre-rich foods contain many other nutrients as well, so are an important part of any healthy diet, including the diets of Crohn's sufferers.

Diet advice
Avoid coffee, alcohol and sugar, drink 1.5 litres of water daily and eat fresh wholefoods that are naturally high in soluble fibre, such as lentils, beans, ground seeds, fruit and lightly cooked vegetables. Have ground flax seeds or soaked flax seeds.

Supplements
- 2 × multivitamin and mineral
- Vitamin C 1,000mg (less if irritating)
- 3 × Omega 3-rich fish oils (providing EPA 1,200mg)
- L-glutamine powder 5g, twice a day

Cystitis

This is an inflammation and infection of the bladder, which causes frequent and painful urination. Vitamins C and A protect you from such infections, and vitamin C can be particularly helpful at clearing it up. So too can grapefruit seed extract. The following recommendations apply only to clear up a bout of cystitis and should not be followed on a regular basis.

Diet advice
Follow the diet in this book. Avoid all sugar. Drink 2 litres (3½ pints) of water a day.

Supplements
- 2 × multivitamin and multimineral

- Calcium ascorbate powder 10 grams in water/juice a day until clear
- 2 × vitamin A 2,270mcg
- Grapefruit seed extract 10 drops three times a day

Also read Chapter 33.

Depression

There are many nutritionally related causes of depression, the most common being sub-optimum nutrition resulting in poor mental and physical energy. Disturbed blood sugar balance can result in periods of depression. Lack of Omega 3 fats can make you depressed. If you are low in serotonin you may benefit from 5-HTP. People who produce excessive amounts of histamine are also prone to depression. Adrenal exhaustion usually brought on by stress and overuse of stimulants can result in it. Allergies too can bring on depression. A nutrition consultant can help identify any factor that can be corrected by nutrition.

Diet advice
Cut out or avoid sugar and refined foods. Cut down on stimulants – tea, coffee, chocolate, cola drinks, cigarettes and alcohol. Follow the diet in this book. Experiment for two weeks without wheat or dairy products.

Supplements
- 2 × multivitamin and mineral
- 2 × vitamin C 1,000mg
- 2 × 5-HTP 100mg
- 3 × Omega 3-rich fish oils (providing EPA 1,200mg)

Also read Chapters 28 and 38.

Dermatitis

This condition literally means 'skin inflammation', and is similar to eczema. Usually the term 'dermatitis' is used when the primary cause appears to be a contact allergy. Go through all possibilities such as metals in jewellery and watches, perfumes, cosmetics, detergents, soaps and shampoos. Where there is a contact allergy there is often a food allergy too: common culprits are dairy products and wheat. Sometimes a combination of eating an allergy-provoking food and contact with an external allergen is needed in order for symptoms to develop. Another frequently encountered factor is a lack of essential fatty acids from seeds and their oils, which in the body turn into anti-inflammatory prostaglandins. Their formation is also blocked by too much saturated fat or fried food, or a lack of certain key vitamins and minerals. The skin is also a route that the body can use to get rid of toxins. A certain kind of dermatitis, called acro-dermatitis, responds exceptionally well to zinc supplementation and is primarily caused by zinc deficiency.

Diet advice
Generally a vegan-type diet, low in saturated fat but with enough essential fats from seeds, is best. If you suspect an allergy to dairy products or wheat, test for this by avoiding these foods.

Supplements
- 2 × multivitamin and multimineral (with magnesium 300mg and zinc 15mg)
- 2 × vitamin C 1,000mg
- 2 × antioxidant complex
- 2 × essential Omega 3 and 6 oil capsules
- Vitamin E 400mg

Also read Chapter 27.

Diabetes

Both child-onset diabetes and adult-onset diabetes are conditions caused by too high blood sugar. Child-onset diabetes is thought to develop through a cross-reaction between a protein in milk and beef and a protein in the pancreas. This can occur if genetically susceptible infants are fed dairy products or beef in their first few months, before their digestive tract and immune system are fully matured. Adult-onset diabetes is usually a consequence of poor eating habits (too much sugar and stimulants), often preceded by hypoglycemia or low blood sugar. Ensuring that adrenal hormones, insulin and glucose-tolerance factor are properly produced by the liver is fundamental in dealing with all forms of glucose intolerance and diabetes. Particularly important are vitamins C, B3, B5 and B6, zinc and chromium. It is best to discuss any proposed changes in your diet with your doctor.

Diet advice
The key to a diabetic diet is to keep your blood sugar level even. This is achieved best by eating little and often, choosing foods that contain slow-releasing carbohydrates plus some protein. This means eating some nuts with fruit, 'seed' vegetables like corn, peas, green beans or whole grain, beans or lentils, which contain both slow-releasing carbohydrate and protein. Avoid all sugar and forms of concentrated sweetness, such as concentrated fruit juice, and even excesses of faster-releasing fruit such as dates and bananas, or of dried fruit. Also avoid too many adrenal stimulants such as tea, coffee, alcohol, cigarettes and salt.

Supplements

- 2 × multivitamin and multimineral
- 2 × vitamin C 1,000mg
- Chromium 200mcg
- Zinc 15mg

Also read Chapter 10.

Diverticulitis

This is a condition of the small and large intestine, in which pockets in the intestinal wall become distended and are then more likely to get infected and inflamed. The condition, probably the result of not enough fibre and exercise, is rarely seen in primitive cultures. A general vitamin programme is recommended to support the muscle tone surrounding the intestines and to maintain a strong infection-fighting system. Increased soluble fibre and regular exercise such as swimming are the key treatments.

Diet advice

Follow the recommended diet in this book, with particular reference to the high-fibre foods (see Part 9). However, if the inflammation is severe it is best to eat lightly steamed vegetables, oats (which contain soluble fibre) and ground seeds or nuts, and to stay away from added 'hard' fibres like wheat bran. It is best to soak grain like oats so as to maximise their water content; these foods provide fibre without irritating the inflamed area. Also have a cold-pressed oil blend rich in Omega 3 and Omega 6 fatty acids, as these help to calm down inflammation.

Supplements

- 2 × multivitamin and multimineral
- Vitamin E 400mg
- Vitamin C 1,000mg

Also read Chapter 22.

Ear infections

Infections of this kind are most frequently the result of an underlying allergy. An allergic reaction induces inflammation that blocks the thin tube that runs from the sinuses to the ears. Once this swells and blocks, the inner ear chamber becomes a favourite site for infection. Treatment with antibiotics quadruples the risk of another infection. This may be because antibiotics irritate the gut wall, making it more leaky, which exacerbates underlying allergies.

Diet advice

Follow the diet recommended in this book. Eat and drink plenty of fruit, vegetables and their juices. Drink plenty of water, herb teas and three cups of cat's-claw tea a day. Stay away from mucus-forming foods – dairy produce, meat and eggs. Dairy allergy is the single most common cause of ear infections.

Supplements

- 2 × multivitamin and multimineral
- 2 × antioxidant complex
- 3 × vitamin C 1,000mg
- Echinacea 10 drops twice a day
- Aloe vera a measure a day as instructed on the bottle (get the best, since the concentration of active ingredient varies a lot)
- Grapefruit seed extract 10 drops twice a day

Scale these amounts down, according to weight, for children. Give a child weighing 60lb (half an average adult), for instance, 5 drops of both echinacea and grapefruit seed extract, 500mg of vitamin C three times a day (1,500mg in total) and a children's multivitamin and multimineral and antioxidant complex.

Also read Chapter 33.

Eczema

In this unpleasant condition the skin becomes scaly and itchy; it can crack and be very sore. Dermatitis is very similar in nature and probably also in cause. The possibility of allergy must be strongly considered. Although the mechanism is unknown, optimum nutrition does usually help this condition. Vitamins A and C strengthen the skin, while vitamin E and zinc improve healing. When there is no open wound, vitamin E oil can help to heal the skin. Essential fats also help to reduce inflammation.

Diet advice

Generally a vegan-type diet, low in saturated fat and with sufficient essential fats from seeds, is best. If you suspect an allergy to dairy produce or wheat, test for it by avoiding these foods.

Supplements

- 2 × multivitamin and multimineral (with magnesium 300mg and zinc 15mg)
- 2 × vitamin C 1,000mg
- 2 × antioxidant complex

- 2 × essential Omega 3 and 6 oil capsules
- Vitamin E 400mg

Also read Chapter 27.

Fibromyalgia

Fibromyalgia is a chronic condition accompanied by many symptoms, including widespread pain and fatigue. Research indicates that the painful muscles characteristic of fibromyalgia are due to reductions in energy production and in the ability of muscles to relax. Supplementing magnesium malate has been shown to reduce pain after as little as forty-eight hours. Also supplement other key vitamins and minerals in a good multivitamin, plus 600mg of magnesium malate. Finally, reduce your stress levels, learn how to relax and increase exercise slowly.

Diet advice
Eat a healthy diet with plenty of magnesium-rich foods such as green vegetables, nuts and seeds.

Supplements
- 2 × multivitamin and mineral
- 2 × vitamin C 1,000mg
- 2 × essential Omega 3 and 6 oil capsules
- Magnesium malate 600mg

Gallstones

These are accumulations of calcium or cholesterol in the duct running from the liver to the gall bladder, which stores bile used for digesting fats. If this duct is blocked, fats cannot be properly absorbed and jaundice occurs. It is not excesses of calcium or cholesterol in the diet that are to blame, but rather how these substances are dealt with in the body. Often, gallstone victims have inherited very narrow bile ducts, increasing their risk of this condition. Lecithin helps to emulsify cholesterol, and optimum nutrition in general should help prevent such abnormalities occurring. Digestive enzyme supplements contain lipase to help digest fat.

Diet advice
Follow the diet recommended in this book, avoiding saturated fat and keeping your essential-fat intake regular, perhaps with seeds for breakfast and a dessertspoon of cold-pressed oil rich in Omega 3 and Omega 6 at lunch and dinner. Avoid meals containing large amounts of fat.

Supplements
- 2 × multivitamin and multimineral
- 2 × antioxidant complex
- 2 × vitamin C 1,000mg
- Lecithin granules (1 dessertspoon) or a lecithin capsule, with each meal
- Digestive enzyme (containing lipase) with each meal

Also read Chapter 17.

Gout

This is caused by improper metabolism of proteins, resulting in uric acid crystals being deposited in fingers, toes and joints and causing inflammation. Diets low in fat and moderate in protein help this condition, as does exercise. However, the many nutrients involved in protein metabolism, especially B6 and zinc, are also an essential part of a nutritional programme for preventing gout.

Diet advice
Follow the diet in this book, avoiding red meat and alcohol. Be sure to drink at least 1 pint (600ml) of water a day.

Supplements
- 2 × multivitamin and multimineral
- 3 × vitamin C 1,000mg
- Bone mineral complex (rich in alkaline-forming calcium and magnesium)
- Vitamin B6 50mg
- Zinc 15mg

Hair problems

There are many different kinds of hair problems, from dry or oily hair to premature hair loss, but most are linked to what you eat. Oily hair can occur with vitamin B deficiency. Dry or brittle hair is often a sign of essential-fat deficiency. Poor hair growth, or loss of colour, is a sign of zinc deficiency. Hair loss is connected with general nutritional deficiency, especially a lack of iron, vitamin B1, vitamin C or lysine (an amino acid). Some hair supplements contain all these. Massaging the scalp also helps, as does hanging upside down, including doing headstands and 'inversion' poses in yoga, which improve circulation to the scalp. The combination of optimum nutrition, stimulating scalp circulation and correcting underlying hormonal imbalances (see Chapter 25) has proved the most effective answer for hair loss. Unfortunately there is no answer yet for grey hair, nor any apparent connection with nutrition.

Diet advice
Follow the diet recommended in this book. Make sure you do not go short of essential fats and water. Avoid sugar and stimulants like tea, coffee and chocolate.

Supplements
- 2 × multivitamin and multimineral (with 10mg iron and 10mg zinc)
- 2 × essential Omega 3 and 6 oil capsules
- 2 × vitamin C 1,000mg
- Lysine 1,000mg (for hair loss only)

Hangovers

The symptoms of excess alcohol are half dehydration and half intoxication. Once the liver's ability to detoxify alcohol is exceeded the body produces a toxic substance and it is this that brings about a headache. The advice below, if followed before drinking, will reduce any 'morning after' symptoms. So will drinking masses of liquid, which dilutes the alcohol. Needless to say, drinking large amounts of alcohol is not optimum nutrition!

Diet advice
Follow the recommendations in this book. Eat pure foods that will not add to the body's toxic burden. Fruit and vegetable juices, high in antioxidants, are very beneficial, as is lots of water – 2 litres (3½ pints) in a day. Also drink cat's-claw tea.

Supplements
- 2 × multivitamin and multimineral (preferably with molybdenum)
- 6 × vitamin C 1,000mg (1 every two hours)
- 3 × antioxidant complex
- L-glutamine powder 5g in water

Hay fever

Even though allergic reactions to pollen are the identified cause of hay fever, other factors make one person more likely to sneeze than another. The incidence of hay fever has risen dramatically in cities compared with rural areas, which led to the discovery that pollutants such as exhaust fumes prime the immune system to react. During the summer the air in polluted areas contains more free radicals due to the action of sunlight on oxygen molecules, so city-dwellers breathe in more pollutants. Taking a good all-round antioxidant supplement containing vitamins A, C and E, betacarotene, selenium and zinc, plus the amino acids cysteine or glutathione, helps increase your resistance (the most effective forms of these amino acids are N-acetyl cysteine, sometimes called NAC, and 'reduced' glutathione). The amino acid methionine, in combination with calcium, is an effective anti-histamine. You need to take 500mg of l-methionine with 400mg of calcium twice a day. Vitamin C helps to control excessive histamine levels. Vitamin B6 and zinc have a role to play in balancing histamine levels and strengthening the immune system. Vitamin B5 helps reduce symptoms.

The three most common substances reacted to are pollen, wheat and milk. Although there is no proven connection, it is interesting to note that all these are originally grass products. It may be that some hay-fever sufferers become sensitised to proteins that are common to grains, grasses and possibly milk. In any event, dairy products encourage mucus production. Similarly, modern strains of wheat are high in gluten, which irritates the digestive tract and stimulates mucus production.

Diet advice
Avoid or at least limit wheat, dairy products and alcohol. Eat plenty of antioxidant-rich fruit and vegetables, plus seeds rich in selenium and zinc. Where possible, avoid exposure to pollen and traffic fumes.

Supplements
- 2 × multivitamin and multimineral (providing B6 100mg and zinc 15mg)
- 2 × antioxidant complex
- 3 × vitamin C 1,000mg

If you are really suffering, try . . .

- L-methionine 500mg twice a day
- Calcium 400mg twice a day
- Pantothenic acid 500mg twice a day

Headaches and migraines

There are many causes of headaches and migraines, ranging from blood sugar drops, dehydration and allergy to stress and tension, or a critical combination. Peaks and troughs in adrenalin and blood sugar can bring on a headache. Often headaches go away with optimum nutrition. If they persist, look carefully at the possibility of allergy. See if you can notice any correlation between the foods you eat and the incidence of headaches.

For migraine sufferers, instead of taking an aspirin, or migraine drugs that constrict the blood vessels, try taking 100–200mg of vitamin B3 in the niacin form, which is a vasodilator. Start with the smaller dose: this will often stop or reduce a migraine in the early stages. It is best to do this at home in a relaxed environment, so the customary warm blushing sensation will probably not bother you.

Diet advice
Eat little and often and avoid long periods without food, especially if you are stressed or tense. Also make sure you drink regularly. Avoid sugar and stimulants like tea, coffee and chocolate.

Supplements
- 2 × multivitamin and multimineral
- Vitamin C 1,000mg
- B3 niacin 100mg

Herpes

The herpes virus feeds off an amino acid called arginine. If you supplement lysine, an amino acid that looks like arginine, you fool the virus and effectively starve it. I recommend supplementing 1,000mg of lysine every day, away from food, to keep the virus at bay. When you have an active infection, supplement 3,000mg of lysine a day and cut right back on foods rich in arginine, which include beans, lentils, nuts and chocolate. The more stressed you are, the weaker your immune system becomes and the more chances the virus has to become active. A good way to boost your immune system is to supplement 2g of vitamin C every day. Some people also find MSM reduces an infection. It's worth trying if lysine doesn't clear things up.

Diet advice
Avoid arginine-rich foods during an attack. These include beans, lentils, nuts and chocolate.

Supplements
- 2 × multivitamin and mineral
- 2 × vitamin C 1,000mg
- Lysine 1,000mg (take 3g a day during active infection)
- MSM 1,000mg (take 3g a day during active infection)

High blood pressure

Hypertension or high blood pressure can be caused by atherosclerosis (a narrowing and thickening of the arteries), arterial tension or thicker blood. Arterial tension is controlled by the balance of calcium, magnesium and potassium in relation to sodium (salt). Stress also plays a part. Correcting this balance can lower blood pressure in thirty days. Vitamins C and E and fish oils high in EPA and DHA help to keep the blood thin. To reverse atherosclerosis, see page 206.

Diet advice
Follow the diet recommended in this book. Avoid salt and foods with added salt. Increase your intake of fruit (eat at least three pieces a day) and vegetables, which are rich in potassium. Take a tablespoon of ground seeds as a source of extra calcium and magnesium. Unless you are vegetarian, eat poached, grilled or baked tuna, salmon, herring or mackerel twice a week.

Supplements
- 2 × multivitamin and multimineral
- Antioxidant
- 2 × vitamin C 1,000mg
- Bone mineral complex (providing 500mg calcium and 300mg magnesium)
- EPA/DHA fish oils 1,200–2,400mg or eat oily fish
- Providing vitamin E 400mg

Also read Chapter 23.

HIV infection and AIDS

The main focus of current research is on antioxidant nutrients that strengthen the immune system. Leading researcher Dr Raxit Jariwalla from the Linus Pauling Institute in California has shown vitamin C's ability to suppress the HIV virus in laboratory cultures of infected cells. He found that with continuous exposure to ascorbic acid (vitamin C), in concentrations not harmful to cells, the growth of HIV in immune cells could be reduced by 99.5 per cent. Dr Jariwalla suggests that in healthy humans a daily dose of at least 10g is needed for an anti-viral effect. N-acetyl cysteine (NAC), an altered form of the amino acid cysteine that is a powerful antioxidant, has also been found to have anti-viral properties. Dr Jariwalla discovered that adding vitamin C to NAC created an eightfold increase in anti-HIV activity.

Diet advice
Eat a high-energy, wholefood organic diet packed with fresh fruit and vegetables and their juices. Eat fish rather than meat. Drink cat's-claw tea twice a day to boost the immune system.

Supplements
- 2 × multivitamin and multimineral
- 2 × antioxidant complex
- 2–10 × vitamin C 1,000mg (2g every four hours up to bowel tolerance)
- 1–4 × N-acetyl cysteine 1,000mg

Indigestion

This unpleasant state can be caused by many different factors including too much or too little hydrochloric acid production in the stomach. Excessive stomach acid or a hiatus hernia usually causes heartburn. Insufficient hydrochloric acid or digestive-enzyme deficiency usually causes a feeling of indigestion and reduced well-being after a meal. A bacterial imbalance or fungal infection in the gut can also result in these symptoms, plus bloating after a meal, because undesirable organisms multiply on feeding. Nutrition consultants can test these possibilities and identify the cause. The following advice is, however, a good starting point.

Diet advice
Follow the recommended diet in this book. Balance your diet for acid- and alkaline-forming foods (see Part 9). Avoid stomach irritants such as alcohol, coffee and chilli, concentrated proteins and any foods that you suspect you are intolerant to.

Supplements
- 2 × multivitamin and multimineral
- Vitamin C 1,000mg
- Probiotics such as *Lactobacillus acidophilus/Bifidobacteria*
- Digestive enzyme (without betaine hydrochloride if heartburn is present) with each main meal

Also read Chapter 22.

Infections

When the immune system is run down, infections occur. Many nutrients and phytonutrients help to enhance immune function. These include vitamin C, all antioxidants, and the plants echinacea, cat's claw and aloe vera. There are also many natural infection-fighters including probiotics (for bacterial infection), caprylic acid (for fungal infection), elderberry extract (for viral infection) and grapefruit seed extract for all three. Read Chapters 19 and 28 to find out which remedies are most helpful, depending on the infection. Below is a general infection-fighting programme.

Diet advice
Follow the diet recommended in this book. Eat and drink plenty of fruit, vegetables and their juices. Drink plenty of water, herb teas and three cups a day of cat's-claw tea. Stay away from mucus-forming foods – dairy produce, meat and eggs.

Supplements
- 2 × multivitamin and multimineral
- 2 × antioxidant complex
- 3 × vitamin C 1,000mg
- Echinacea 10 drops twice a day
- Aloe vera a measure a day, as instructed on the bottle (get the best since the concentration of active ingredient varies a lot)
- Grapefruit seed extract 10 drops twice a day

Also read Chapters 24 and 33.

Infertility

This unfortunate condition is more common in women than in men, although in 30 per cent of couples who have difficulty conceiving the problem is due to the man. Vitamins E and B6, selenium and zinc are important for both sexes, and vitamin C is important for men. Also important are essential fatty acids. There are, however, many causes other than nutritional deficiency, perhaps the most common being hormonal imbalances, particularly in women. These can be checked by a nutrition consultant or your doctor, from saliva samples taken at intervals over a month.

Diet advice
Follow the diet in this book. Essential fatty acids are found in cold-pressed vegetable oils, so make sure your daily diet includes a tablespoon of an oil blend to provide Omega 3 and Omega 6 fatty acids, or a heaped tablespoon of ground seeds.

Supplements
- 2 × multivitamin and multimineral (to include zinc 15mg and selenium 100mcg)
- Vitamin E 400mg
- 2 × vitamin C 1,000mg
- 2 × essential Omega 3 and 6 oil capsules

Also read Chapters 25 and 41.

Inflammation

Many health problems, including all those ending in 'itis', are inflammatory. This means that a part of the body such as a muscle or joint, the gut or respiratory tract, is inflamed. This is a sign that the body is reacting, or overreacting, to something. A tendency to overreact can arise if a person is deficient in essential fats and their supportive nutrients, vitamins B3 and B6, biotin, vitamin C, zinc and magnesium. Pantothenic acid (vitamin B5) is also needed to make cortisol, the body's anti-inflammatory hormone. Boswellic acid, found in the plant frankincense, is a natural anti-inflammatory agent which is available in the form of a cream for inflamed joints and muscles. L-glutamine helps to calm gut inflammation. Antioxidant nutrients are also intimately involved in inflammatory responses. However, there is little point in calming down an inflammation if the source of irritation remains. This may be a food allergy or an irritating substance such as alcohol.

Diet advice

Avoid immune-suppressing or potentially irritating substances such as coffee, alcohol and strong spices. Avoid suspect foods such as wheat and dairy produce for ten days to gauge your reaction to them. Otherwise, just follow the diet guidelines in this book.

Supplements

- 2 × multivitamin and multimineral (with 300mg magnesium and 15mg zinc)
- 2 × antioxidant complex
- 2 × vitamin C 1,000mg
- Pantothenic acid 500mg
- L-glutamine powder 3 grams a day
- 3 × essential Omega 3 and 6 oil capsules
- Anti-inflammatory herbal joint complexes or cream (optional)

Also read Chapter 26.

Irritable bowel syndrome

This term is used to describe intermittent diarrhoea or constipation, urgency to defecate, abdominal pain or indigestion. There are many possible contributory causes to one or more of these symptoms. They include food allergy, gut inflammation, over-excitation of the gut muscles, stress, infection and toxic overload. It is therefore best to see a nutrition consultant who can determine which factors are relevant. Essential fats and the amino acid glutamine calm gut inflammation, antioxidants help the body to detoxify and the right mineral balance helps the muscles of the gut to work properly.

Diet advice

Pursue a simple, pure diet of lightly cooked vegetables, fish, non-gluten grains (rice, millet, corn, quinoa), lentils and beans, plus ground seeds for essential fats. Avoid any suspect allergens, including wheat and dairy products, coffee, alcohol and spices, for ten days to see if this makes a difference.

Supplements

- 2 × multivitamin and multimineral
- 2 × antioxidant complex
- 2 × vitamin C 500mg
- L-glutamine powder 3 grams
- 2 × essential Omega 3 and 6 oil capsules
- Digestive enzymes with each main meal (if indigestion is a symptom)

Also read Chapter 22.

Kidney stones

Kidney stones are abnormal accumulations of mineral salts found in the kidneys, bladder or anywhere along the urinary tract, and can range in size from a grain of sand to a fingertip. There are various kinds, but 80 per cent of kidney stones are calcium oxalate stones. Excessive calcium in too alkaline urine crystallises and stones begin to form.

By far the most important thing to do to prevent kidney stones is to drink plenty of filtered or bottled water – at least 2 litres a day – to flush the kidneys and urinary tract regularly. Nutrient deficiencies can also contribute to the formation of kidney stones, especially lack of magnesium, vitamin B6, vitamin D and potassium, all of which are involved in proper calcium metabolism.

Diet advice

Green leafy vegetables, whole grains, bananas, nuts and seeds should be consumed regularly. Vitamin A, abundant in carrots, red peppers, sweet potatoes and green leafy vegetables, also benefits the urinary tract and helps inhibit the formation of stones. Avoid antacids and minimise your consumption of animal protein, as they cause the body to excrete calcium and uric acid, the key components in the two most common forms of kidney stones.

Supplements

- 2 × multivitamin and mineral
- 2 × vitamin C 1,000mg
- 2 × essential Omega 3 and 6 oil capsules

Menopausal symptoms

These include fatigue, depression, weight gain, osteoporosis, reduced sex drive, vaginal dryness and hot flushes. While optimum nutrition often helps relieve these, many women respond to small amounts of natural progesterone used as a cream. This is available on prescription from your doctor. Supplementing vitamin C with vitamin E and bioflavonoids may help reduce hot flushes. Also important for this and other symptoms, including vaginal dryness, are sufficient essential fatty acids, which make the prostaglandins that help to balance hormone levels. For prostaglandins to work, sufficient vitamin B6, zinc and magnesium are required.

Diet advice
Follow the diet recommended in this book, being careful to cut down on sources of sugar and stimulants. Have a tablespoon of a cold-pressed oil blend or a heaped tablespoon of ground seeds for essential fats, magnesium and zinc.

Supplements
- 2 × multivitamin and multimineral
- 2 × vitamin C 1,000mg with 500mg of bioflavonoids
- Vitamin E 400mg
- Bone mineral complex (including extra magnesium and zinc)
- Herbal complex with agnus castus, dong quai, black cohosh or St John's wort
- 2 × essential Omega 3 and 6 oil capsules

Also read Chapters 25 and 41.

Muscle aches and cramps

Cramps are most commonly due to calcium/magnesium imbalances and are corrected by supplementing 500mg of calcium and 300mg of magnesium. Despite popular belief, the condition is very rarely due to a lack of salt. In fact it is best to avoid added salt and to keep fluid intake high. Fruit is naturally rich in potassium and water, and contains sufficient sodium for the body's needs. Muscle aches can occur for the same reason, or when muscle cells are not able to make energy efficiently from glucose. Magnesium, particularly in the form of magnesium malate, helps here too, as do B vitamins. Aches can also occur as a result of inflammation (see page 228).

Diet advice
Follow the diet recommended in this book. Avoid salt and increase your intake of fruit (rich in potassium) and seeds (rich in calcium and magnesium). Drink plenty of water.

Supplements
- 2 × multivitamin and multimineral
- Vitamin C 1,000mg
- Bone mineral complex (to provide 500mg calcium and 300mg magnesium) or magnesium malate plus calcium

Obesity

As well as eating no more than you need, choosing foods that keep the blood sugar even, backed up by an optimal intake of nutrients that help stabilise blood sugar, will help you to lose weight by stabilising your appetite and burning fat. These nutrients include vitamins B3, B6 and C, zinc and chromium. Konjac fibre, a source of glucomannan, also helps to stabilise blood sugar levels. Also helpful is HCA, which slows down the ability of the body to turn excess fuel into body fat, and 5-HTP, which stabilises appetite. In some people, food allergies cause water retention which can contribute to obesity. If you suspect any foods, the most common being wheat and dairy products, eliminate them for ten days to test whether they are associated with your weight gain. Thyroid problems can also be a factor in obesity. If all else fails, ask your doctor to check your thyroid.

Diet advice
Follow the diet in this book, emphasising high-water-content foods such as fresh fruit and vegetables and slow-releasing carbohydrates (see Part 9). Avoid all sources of fast-releasing sugars. Experiment with fasting one day a week, or sticking to fruit only. Make aerobic exercise a regular part of your day.

Supplements
- 2 × multivitamin and multimineral
- 2 × vitamin C 1,000mg
- 2 × essential Omega 3 and 6 oil capsules
- Chromium 200mcg and HCA 750mg and 5-HTP 100mg
- Glucomannan/konjac fibre 3g (optional)

Also read Chapter 36.

Osteoporosis

In this condition the density of the bones decreases, increasing the risk of fracture and compression of the spinal vertebrae. From a nutritional perspective there are three main contributors. These are excessive protein consumption, leading to leaching of calcium from the bone to neutralise excess blood acidity; relative dominance of oestrogen to progesterone, the latter being a major trigger for bone growth; and deficiency of bone-building nutrients, which include calcium, magnesium, vitamin D, vitamin C, zinc, silica, phosphorus and boron. The use of natural progesterone cream, prescribable by your doctor, has proved four times more effective than synthetic oestrogen HRT in restoring bone density.

Diet advice

Follow the diet in this book, keeping all sources of saturated fat to a minimum because of their oestrogenic effects. Have a heaped tablespoon of ground seeds each day as a source of calcium, magnesium and zinc.

Supplement advice

- 2 × multivitamin and multimineral
- Vitamin C 1,000mg
- Bone mineral complex

Also read Chapter 26.

PMS

Pre-menstrual syndrome describes the occurrence of a cluster of symptoms including bloating, tiredness, irritability, depression, breast tenderness and headaches, occurring most commonly in the week leading up to menstruation. There are three main causes: oestrogen dominance and relative progesterone deficiency – corrected by natural progesterone and avoiding sources of oestrogen; glucose intolerance, marked by a craving for sweet foods and stimulants; and deficiency in essential fatty acids and vitamin B6, zinc and magnesium, which together create prostaglandins, which help to balance hormone levels. While the need for these is greatest just before a period is due, it is wise to take the supplements throughout the month. If dietary and supplementary intervention do not result in significant improvement, consider seeing a nutrition consultant and having your hormone balance checked.

Diet advice

Follow the diet in this book. Eat little and often before menstruation, snacking on fruit but avoiding sugar, sweets and stimulants. Ensure that your daily diet contains one tablespoon of cold-pressed vegetable oil rich in both Omega 3 and Omega 6 fatty acids.

Supplements

- 2 × multivitamin and multimineral
- 2 × vitamin B6 100mg with zinc 10mg
- Vitamin C 1,000mg

- 2 × essential Omega 3 and 6 oil capsules
- Herbal complex with agnus castus, dong quai, black cohosh or St John's wort
- Magnesium 300mg

Also read Chapter 41.

Prostate problems

The most common prostate problem is prostatitis or benign prostatic hyper-plasia, in which the prostate gland enlarges, interfering with the flow of urine. This is thought to be due to hormonal imbalances, possibly testos-terone deficiency and oestrogen dominance, affecting prostaglandins, which have an anti-inflammatory effect. Reversal can be achieved through supplementing essential fatty acids and testosterone. Also important are zinc and a herb called saw palmetto. The prostate gland is also a common site of cancer, most likely triggered by hormonal imbalances with risk-factor similarities to breast cancer.

Diet advice
Follow the diet in this book, with an emphasis on foods high in antioxi-dants, avoiding milk and meat because of their hormone content and eat-ing organic as much as possible. Keep saturated fat very low and ensure that you have adequate essential fats from seeds and their cold-pressed oils.

Supplements
- 2 × multivitamin and multimineral
- 2 × antioxidant complex
- 2 × vitamin C 1,000mg
- 2 × essential Omega 3 and 6 oil capsules
- Saw palmetto 300mg (for enlarged prostate only)

Also read Chapter 41.

Psoriasis

This is a completely different kind of skin condition from eczema or dermatitis and does not generally respond as well to nutritional inter-vention. It can occur when the body is 'toxic', perhaps owing to an overgrowth of the organism *Candida albicans*, to digestive problems leading to intoxication, or to poor liver detoxification. Otherwise con-sider the factors discussed for dermatitis and eczema (see pages 451–2 and 454–5).

Diet advice

Follow the diet recommended in this book, with an emphasis on low levels of meat and dairy products (to keep you low in saturated fat) and plenty of seeds and their oils for essential fats. If you suspect allergy to dairy products or wheat, test by avoiding these foods.

Supplements

- 2 × multivitamin and multimineral
- 2 × antioxidant complex
- Vitamin C 1,000mg
- 2 × essential Omega 3 and 6 oil capsules

Use topical vitamin A cream (see Skin-care products in Resources, page 526). Also read Chapter 27.

Schizophrenia

This severe form of mental health problem is suffered by one in a hundred people. There are many causes, the majority of which can be alleviated by nutrition. It is strongly advised that you see a nutrition consultant who can run tests to determine whether biochemical imbalances may underlie this condition. Nutrients that can help include folic acid, essential fatty acids and megadoses of niacin (B3). These do not help all sufferers, and can make certain types of the condition worse – hence the need for testing. Often there is an underlying glucose imbalance and allergies.

Diet advice

Cut out or at least avoid sugar and refined foods. Cut down on stimulants – tea, coffee, chocolate, cola drinks, cigarettes and alcohol. Follow the diet recommended in this book. Experiment for two weeks without wheat or dairy products.

Supplements

- Multivitamin
- 2 × vitamin C 1,000mg
- Multimineral with zinc, magnesium, manganese and chromium
- Extra folic acid, niacin or essential fatty acids are best tried only under supervision

Also read Chapter 38.

Sinusitis

An inflammation of the sinus and nasal passages, sinusitis often leads to sinus infections. Contributory factors are nasal irritants such as exhaust fumes, cigarettes, smoky places, dust and pollen; allergies, often to dairy products and wheat, which are mucus-forming; plus a weakened immune system. Too much alcohol, fried food or stress, lack of sleep and overeating all weaken the immune system. Vitamins A and C and zinc, among other nutrients, help boost immunity. Essential fats are also needed to control inflammation.

Diet advice
Eat lightly, but do eat – lots of essential foods such as the best organic fruit and vegetables (baby vegetables, just sprouted), plus seeds. You do need protein (from quinoa, seeds, nuts, fish, tofu, quorn and so on) but avoid mucus-forming foods such as milk, eggs and meat.

Also inhale tea tree oil or olbas oil, in the bath or by holding it under your nose (be careful not to irritate the skin too much), to stop your nasal passages from blocking. Tiger balm is good on the chest. Drink home-made ginger and cinnamon tea (five slices of fresh ginger root and one stick of cinnamon in a thermos with ½ pint of boiling water) or cat's-claw tea to boost the immune system.

Supplements
- 2 × multivitamin and multimineral
- 2 × antioxidant complex
- 2 × vitamin C 1,000mg (3g every four hours only when infected)
- 2 × vitamin A 7,400mg (2,270mcg) when infected, or a glass of carrot juice
- 2 × zinc 15mg
- Echinacea 15 drops in water three times a day

Also read Chapters 24, 33 and 34.

Sleeping problems

For some sufferers the major problem of insomnia is waking up in the middle of the night; for others it is not getting to sleep in the first place. Both can be the effect on the nervous system of poor nutrition or too much stress and anxiety. Calcium and magnesium have a tranquil-lising effect, as does vitamin B6. Tryptophan, a constituent of protein, has the strongest tranquillising effect and, if taken in doses of 1,000–3,000mg, it is highly effective for insomnia. It takes about an hour to work and remains effective for up to four hours. While tryptophan is non-addictive and has no known side effects, its regular use in not recommended – it is better to adjust your lifestyle so that no tranquillising agents are needed.

Diet advice
Follow the diet recommended in this book, avoiding all stimulants. Do not eat sugar or drink tea or coffee in the evening. Also, do not eat late. Eat seeds, nuts, root and green leafy vegetables, which are high in calcium and magnesium.

Supplements
- 2 × multivitamin and multimineral
- Vitamin B6 100mg with zinc 10mg
- Calcium 600mg and magnesium 400mg
- Vitamin C 1,000mg
- 2 5-HTP 100mg (only if absolutely necessary)

Thyroid problems

The thyroid gland, situated at the base of the throat, controls our rate of metabolism. In hyperthyroidism or overactive thyroid, symptoms such as over-activity, loss of weight and nervousness are common; in hypothyroidism or underactive thyroid, the symptoms are lack of energy, becoming overweight and goitre, in which the throat region swells. Over-stimulation of the endocrine system through living off stress and stimulants, and oestrogen dominance, are common causes of an underactive thyroid later in life. This can also be caused by a lack of iodine, although this is rare, and taking iodine in kelp is advised to help the condition. Since the thyroid gland is controlled by the pituitary and adrenal glands, the nutrients involved in hormone production and regulation for all three glands are particularly important. These are vitamins C and B complex (especially B3 and B5), manganese and zinc. Selenium also appears to have a role to play in thyroid health, as does the amino acid tyrosine from which thyroxine is made. Often, a low dose of thyroxine is required to correct this condition.

Diet advice
Avoid all stimulants and follow the diet in this book.

Supplements
- 2 × multivitamin and multimineral
- 2 × vitamin C 1,000mg
- Manganese 10mg
- Kelp with iodine and tyrosine 2,000mg (for hypothyroidism only)

Also read Chapter 25.

Ulcers

These can occur in the stomach and duodenum – the first section of the small intestine, which is not as well protected as the rest of the intestines against the acid secretions of the stomach. In prolonged stress the stomach can over-secrete acid, so stress can be a cause. Also, diets that are too acid-forming are to be avoided. Vitamin A is the primary nutrient needed to protect the lining of the duodenum. While vitamin C does help people with duodenal ulcers, not more than 500mg should be taken as it can cause irritation. If a burning sensation is experienced after taking vitamin C, the dose is too high. The most common cause of ulcers is infection with *Helicobacter pylori*. This should be tested for by your doctor and treated with a specific anti-bacterial agent. Also, check for food allergies.

Diet advice
Follow the diet recommended in this book, keeping mainly to alkaline-forming foods as listed in Part 9.

Supplements
- 2 × multivitamin and multimineral
- 2 × vitamin A 2,270mcg (retinol) short-term only and not if pregnant
- Vitamin C 500mg (as calcium ascorbate)
- Beneficial bacteria, such as *Lactobacillus acidophilus/Bifidobacteria*, after antibiotics if treated for helicobacter infection

Varicose veins

Veins carry blood returning to the heart. A varicose vein is one that has become enlarged and swollen; the condition usually occurs in the legs, where circulation is most difficult. It is unlikely that optimum nutrition can do much for veins that are already varicose; however, adequate vitamins C and E as well as other antioxidants can help to prevent further occurrences. Also, there is some evidence that a high-fibre diet can help to prevent varicose veins.

Diet advice
Follow the diet recommended in this book. Regular exercise, especially swimming, will improve the circulation. Putting your feet up and gentle leg massages are all helpful. Application of vitamin E cream is beneficial.

Supplements
- 2 × multivitamin and multimineral
- 2 × antioxidant complex
- Vitamin E 400mg
- 2 × vitamin C 1,000mg plus bioflavonoids

Part 8

Nutrient Fact File A to Z

Nutrient Fact File A to Z

What does each nutrient do? What are the symptoms of deficiency? How much should you take in from food and from supplements? How much is too much? These are the questions answered here for each key nutrient – vitamins, minerals, essential fats and other key nutrients.

RDA stands for the EU recommended daily amounts.

ODA is the average optimum daily amount for an adult. In truth there is a range of ODAs depending on the individual (see Chapter 45 to define your needs).

SUPPLEMENTARY RANGE is the difference between this range and what you are likely to get from your diet. This defines the minimum you should supplement daily, and the maximum, if your needs are very high. Supplementary ranges for babies and children, according to their age, are given in Chapter 40.

TOXICITY is the level at which adverse effects can occur.

Best food sources lists foods with the highest nutrient amount per calorie, in descending order, with the figures in parentheses being the amount *per 100g serving*. This tells you both which nutrient-rich foods to choose and how much you'll be getting in a serving.

Best supplement details the most easily absorbed and used form of this nutrient.

Helpers and **Robbers** are the factors that assist or hinder absorption or utilisation of this nutrient.

Vitamins

● Vitamin A (retinol and betacarotene)

What it does Needed for healthy skin, inside and out, protecting against infections. Antioxidant and immune-system booster. Protects against many forms of cancer. Essential for night vision.

Deficiency signs Mouth ulcers, poor night vision, acne, frequent colds or infections, dry flaky skin, dandruff, thrush or cystitis, diarrhoea.

How much?
RDA 800mcgRE
ODA 2,500mcgRE
SUPPLEMENTARY RANGE 1,000–3,000mcg retinol (if pregnant or trying to conceive do not exceed 3,000mcg retinol); 3,000–30,000mcg betacarotene
TOXICITY May occur above 8,000–30,000mcg per day long term or 300,000mcg single dose of retinal. Betacarotene above 6mcgRE a day is not advised if taken on its own by smokers.

Best food sources Beef liver (10,800mcg), veal liver (8,000mcg), carrots (8,500mcg), watercress (1,424mcg), cabbage (900mcg), squash (2,100mcg), sweet potatoes (5,170mcg), melon (1,000mcg), pumpkin (500mcg), mangoes (1,180mcg), tomatoes (350mcg), broccoli (460mcg), apricots, papayas (610mcg), tangerines (280mcg).

Best supplement Retinol (animal source), natural betacarotene and retinyl palmitate (vegetable source).

Helpers Works with zinc. Vitamin C and E help protect it. Best taken within a multi or antioxidant formula with food.

Robbers Heat, light, alcohol, coffee and smoking.

● B1 (thiamine)

What it does Essential for energy production, brain function and digestion. Helps the body make use of protein.

Deficiency signs Tender muscles, eye pains, irritability, poor concentration, prickly legs, poor memory, stomach pains, constipation, tingling hands, rapid heartbeat.

How much?
RDA 1.4mg
ODA 35mg
SUPPLEMENTARY RANGE 15–45mg
TOXICITY Not a concern.

Best food sources Watercress (0.1mg), squash (0.05mg), courgette, lamb (0.12mg), asparagus (0.11mg), mushrooms (0.1mg), peas (0.32mg), lettuce (0.07mg), peppers (0.07mg), cauliflower (0.10mg), cabbage (0.06mg), tomatoes (0.06mg), Brussels sprouts (0.10mg), beans (0.55mg).

Best supplement Thiamine.

Helpers Works with other B vitamins, magnesium and manganese. Best supplemented as part of a B complex with food.

Robbers Antibiotics, tea, coffee, stress, birth-control Pill, alcohol, alkaline agents, e.g. baking powder, sulphur dioxide (preservative), cooking and food refining/processing.

● B2 (riboflavin)

What it does Helps turn fats, sugars and protein into energy. Needed to repair and maintain healthy skin, inside and out. Helps to regulate body acidity. Important for hair, nails and eyes.

Deficiency signs Burning or gritty eyes, sensitivity to bright lights, sore tongue, cataracts, dull or oily hair, eczema or dermatitis, split nails, cracked lips.

How much?
RDA 1.6mg
ODA 35mg
SUPPLEMENTARY RANGE 15–45mg
TOXICITY No known toxicity. Loss or excess results in bright yellow-green urine.

Best food sources Mushrooms (0.4mg), watercress (0.1mg), cabbage (0.05mg), asparagus (0.12mg), broccoli (0.3mg), pumpkin (0.04mg), beansprouts (0.03mg), mackerel (0.3mg), milk (0. 19mg), bamboo shoots, tomatoes (0.04mg), wheat germ (0.25mg).

Best supplement Riboflavin.

Helpers Works with other B vitamins and selenium. Best supplemented as part of a B complex with food.

Robbers Alcohol, birth-control Pill, tea, coffee, alkaline agents, e.g. baking powder, sulphur dioxide (preservative), cooking and food refining/processing.

● B3 (niacin)

What it does Essential for energy production, brain function and the skin. Helps balance blood sugar and lower cholesterol levels. Also involved in inflammation and digestion.

Deficiency signs Lack of energy, diarrhoea, insomnia, headaches or migraines, poor memory, anxiety or tension, depression, irritability, bleeding or tender gums, acne, eczema/dermatitis.

How much?
RDA 18mg
ODA 85mg
SUPPLEMENTARY RANGE 25–50mg
TOXICITY None known below 3,000mg.

Best food sources Mushrooms (4mg), tuna (12.9mg), chicken (5.2mg), salmon (7.0mg), asparagus (1.11mg), cabbage (0.3mg), lamb (4.15mg), mackerel (5.0mg), turkey (5.5mg), tomatoes (0.7mg), courgettes and squash (0.54mg), cauliflower (0.6mg) and wholewheat (4.33mg).

Best supplement Niacin (may cause flushing) and niacinamide.

Helpers Works with other B-complex vitamins and chromium. Best taken with food.

Robbers Antibiotics, tea, coffee, birth-control Pill and alcohol.

● B5 (pantothenic acid)

What it does Involved in energy production, controls fat metabolism. Essential for brain and nerves. Helps make anti-stress hormones (steroids). Maintains healthy skin and hair.

Deficiency signs Muscle tremors or cramps, apathy, poor concentration, burning feet or tender heels, nausea or vomiting, lack of energy, exhaustion after light exercise, anxiety or tension, teeth-grinding.

How much?
RDA 6mg
ODA 100mg
SUPPLEMENTARY RANGE 30–130mg
TOXICITY None known below 100 times RDA level.

Best food sources Mushrooms (2mg), watercress (0.10mg), broccoli (0.10mg), alfalfa sprouts (0.56mg), peas (0.75mg), lentils (1.36mg), tomatoes (0.33mg), cabbage (0.21mg), celery (0.40mg), strawberries (0.34mg), eggs (1.5mg), squash (0.16mg), avocados (1.07mg), wholewheat (1.1mg).

Best supplement Pantothenic acid.

Helpers Works with other B-complex vitamins. Biotin and folic acid aid absorption. Best taken with food.

Robbers Stress, alcohol, tea, coffee. Destroyed by heat and food processing.

● B6 (pyridoxine)

What it does Essential for protein digestion and utilisation, brain function and hormone production. Helps balance sex hormones, hence use in PMS and the menopause. Natural anti-depressant and diuretic. Helps control allergic reactions.

Deficiency signs Infrequent dream recall, water retention, tingling hands, depression or nervousness, irritability, muscle tremors or cramps, lack of energy, flaky skin.

How much?
RDA 2mg
ODA 75mg
SUPPLEMENTARY RANGE 45–95mg
TOXICITY Cases of pyridoxine toxicity reported with dosages above 1,000mg – unaccompanied by a B complex to help balance the intake.

Best food sources Watercress (0.13mg), cauliflower (0.20mg), cabbage (0.16mg), peppers (0.17mg), bananas (0.51mg), squash (0.14mg), broccoli (0.21mg), asparagus (0.15mg), lentils (0.11mg), red kidney beans (0.44mg), Brussels sprouts (0.25mg), onions (0.10mg), seeds and nuts (varies).

Best supplement Pyridoxine, pyridoxal-5-phosphate only if enterically coated (as stated on the label).

Helpers Works with other B-complex vitamins, as well as zinc and magnesium. Best supplemented with food and zinc.

Robbers Alcohol, smoking, birth-control Pill, high protein intake, processed foods.

● B12 (cyanocobalamin)

What it does Needed for making use of protein. Helps the blood carry oxygen, hence essential for energy. Needed for synthesis of DNA. Essential for nerves. Deals with tobacco smoke and other toxins.

Deficiency signs Poor hair condition, eczema or dermatitis, mouth oversensitive to heat or cold, irritability, anxiety or tension, lack of energy, constipation, tender or sore muscles, pale skin.

How much?
RDA 1mcg
ODA 25mcg
SUPPLEMENTARY RANGE 10–40mcg
TOXICITY None reported with oral dose. Very rarely, an allergic reaction to injection occurs.

Best food sources Oysters (15mcg), sardines (25mcg), tuna (5mcg), lamb (trace), eggs (1.7mcg), shrimp (1mcg), cottage cheese (5mcg), milk (0.3mcg), turkey and chicken (2mcg), cheese (1.5mcg).

Best supplement Cyanocobalamin.

Helpers Works with folic acid. Best taken as B complex with food.

Robbers Alcohol, smoking, lack of stomach acid.

● Folic acid

What it does Critical during pregnancy for development of brain and nerves. Always essential for brain and nerve function. Needed for utilising protein and red blood cell formation.

Deficiency signs Anaemia, eczema, cracked lips, prematurely greying hair, anxiety or tension, poor memory, lack of energy, poor appetite, stomach pains, depression.

How much?
RDA 200mcg
ODA 800mcg
SUPPLEMENTARY RANGE 200–600mcg
TOXICITY Seldom reported, but gastrointestinal and sleep problems have occurred above 15mg.

Best food sources Wheat germ (325mcg), spinach (140mcg), peanuts (110mcg), sprouts (110mcg), asparagus (95mcg), sesame seeds (97mcg), hazelnuts (72mcg), broccoli (130mcg), cashew nuts (69mcg), cauliflower (39mcg), walnuts (66mcg), avocados (66mcg).

Best supplement Folic acid.

Helpers Works with other B-complex vitamins, especially B12. Best supplemented as part of B complex with food.

Robbers High temperature, light, food processing and birth-control Pill.

● Biotin

What it does Particularly important in childhood. Helps your body use essential fats, assisting in promoting healthy skin, hair and nerves.

Deficiency signs Dry skin, poor hair condition, prematurely greying hair, tender or sore muscles, poor appetite or nausea, eczema or dermatitis.

How much?
RDA 150mcg
ODA 225mcg
SUPPLEMENTARY RANGE 30–180mcg
TOXICITY None reported.

Best food sources Cauliflower (1.5mcg), lettuce (0.7mcg), peas (0.5mcg), tomatoes (1.5mcg), oysters (10mcg), grapefruit (1.0mcg), watermelon (4.0mcg), sweetcorn (6.0mcg), cabbage (1.1mcg), almonds (20mcg), cherries (0.4mcg), herrings (10.0mcg), milk (2.0mcg), eggs (25mcg).

Best supplement Biotin.

Helpers Works with other B vitamins, magnesium and manganese. Best supplemented as part of a B complex with food.

Robbers Raw egg white, which contains avidin (but this is not significant in cooked egg whites), fried food.

● Vitamin C (ascorbic add)

What it does Strengthens immune system – fights infections. Makes collagen, keeping bones, skin and joints firm and strong. Antioxidant, detoxifying pollutants and protecting against cancer and heart disease. Helps make anti-stress hormones, and turns food into energy.

Deficiency signs Frequent colds, lack of energy, frequent infections, bleeding or tender gums, easy bruising, nosebleeds, slow wound-healing, red pimples on skin.

How much?
RDA 60mg
ODA 2,000mg
SUPPLEMENTARY RANGE 800–2,800mg
TOXICITY May cause bowel looseness in excess, but this is not a sign of toxicity and stops rapidly when dose is reduced.

Best food sources Peppers (100mg), watercress (60mg), cabbage (60mg), broccoli (110mg), cauliflower (60mg), strawberries (60mg), lemons (50mg), kiwi fruit (55mg), peas (25mg), melons (25mg), oranges (50mg), grapefruit (40mg), limes (29mg), tomatoes (60mg).

Best supplement Vitamin C is ascorbic acid. This is mildly acidic in the digestive tract and in large doses (5g plus) does not suit everyone. The ascorbate form (e.g. calcium ascorbate, magnesium ascorbate) is mildly alkaline and more easily tolerated. However, if you take large amounts during a meal you may neutralise stomach acidity necessary for protein digestion. The ascorbate form is good if you also want to supplement the mineral it is bound to. Vitamin C works with bioflavonoids. Best supplements include these. Ester C is also a good form to take.

Helpers Bioflavonoids in fruit and vegetables increase its effect. Works with B vitamins to produce energy. Works with vitamin E as an antioxidant.

Robbers Smoking, alcohol, pollution, stress, fried food.

● Vitamin D (ergocalciferol, cholecalciferol)

What it does Helps maintain strong and healthy bones by retaining calcium.

Deficiency signs Joint pain or stiffness, backache, tooth decay, muscle cramps, hair loss.

How much?
RDA 5mcg
ODA 11mcg
SUPPLEMENTARY RANGE 3–5mcg
TOXICITY 1,250mcg is potentially toxic.

Best food sources Herrings (22.5mcg), mackerel (17.5mcg), salmon (12.5mcg), oysters (3mcg), cottage cheese (2mcg), eggs (1.75mcg).

Best supplement Cholecalciferol (animal origin), ergocalciferol (yeast origin).

Helpers Sufficient exposure to sunlight, as vitamin D is made in the skin. Under these conditions dietary vitamin D may not be necessary. Vitamins A, C and E protect D.

Robbers Lack of sunlight, fried foods.

● Vitamin E (d-alpha tocopherol)

What it does Antioxidant, protecting cells from damage, including against cancer. Helps body use oxygen, preventing blood clots, thrombosis, atherosclerosis. Improves wound-healing and fertility. Good for the skin.

Deficiency signs Lack of sex drive, exhaustion after light exercise, easy bruising, slow wound-healing, varicose veins, loss of muscle tone, infertility.

How much?
RDA 10mg
ODA 300mg
SUPPLEMENTARY RANGE 150–400mg
TOXICITY None reported below 2,000mg d-alpha tocopherol long-term use and 35,000mg short-term use.

Best food sources Unrefined corn oils (53mg), sunflower seeds (52.6mg), peanuts (11.5mg), sesame seeds (22.7mg), other seed foods, e.g. beans (7.7mg), peas (2.3mg), wheat germ (27.5mg), tuna (6.3mg), sardines (2.0mg), salmon (1.5mg), sweet potatoes (4.0mg).

Best supplement D-alpha tocopherol (not synthetic dl-alpha tocopherol).

Helpers Works with vitamin C and selenium.

Robbers High-temperature cooking, especially frying. Air pollution, birth-control Pill, excessive intake of refined or processed fats and oils.

● K (phylloquinone)

What it does Controls blood-clotting.

Deficiency signs Haemorrhage (easy bleeding).

How much?
RDA None established; sufficient amounts made by beneficial bacteria in the gut.
ODA None established; sufficient amounts made by beneficial bacteria in the gut
SUPPLEMENTARY RANGE Not necessary to supplement.
TOXICITY Not a concern.

Best food sources Cauliflower (3,600mcg), Brussels sprouts (1,888mcg), lettuce (135mcg), cabbage (125mcg), beans (290mcg), broccoli (200mcg), peas (260mcg), watercress (56mcg), asparagus (57mcg), potatoes (50mcg), corn oil (50mcg), tomatoes (5mcg), milk (1mcg).

Best supplement Not necessary to supplement.

Helpers Healthy intestinal bacteria – then no need for dietary source.

Robbers Antibiotics. In babies, lack of breastfeeding.

Minerals

● Calcium

What it does Promotes a healthy heart, clots blood, promotes healthy nerves, contracts muscles, improves skin, bone and teeth health, relieves aching muscles and bones, maintains the correct acid–alkaline balance, reduces menstrual cramps and tremors.

Deficiency signs Muscle cramps or tremors, insomnia or nervousness, joint pain or arthritis, tooth decay, high blood pressure.

How much?
RDA 800mg
ODA 1,000mg
SUPPLEMENTARY RANGE 0–400mg
TOXICITY Problems of excessive calcium arise from other factors such as excessive vitamin D intake (above 625mcg per day). Excess will interfere with absorption of other minerals, especially if their intake is slightly low. May lead to calcification of kidneys, heart and other soft tissue, e.g. kidney stones.

Best food sources Swiss cheese (925mg), Cheddar cheese (750mg), almonds (234mg), brewer's yeast (210mg), parsley (203mg), corn tortillas (200mg), globe artichokes (51mg), prunes (51mg), pumpkin seeds (51mg), cooked dried beans (50mg), cabbage (4mg), winter wheat (46mg).

Best supplement Calcium is reasonably well absorbed in any form. The best forms of calcium to supplement are calcium amino acid chelate or citrate, which are approximately twice as well absorbed as calcium carbonate.

Helpers Works well in ratios of 3:2 calcium:magnesium and 2:1 calcium:phosphorous. Vitamin D and boron. Exercise.

Robbers Hormone imbalances, alcohol, lack of exercise, caffeine, tea. Lack of hydrochloric acid and excess fat or phosphorus hinders absorption. Stress causes increased excretion.

● Chromium

What it does Forms part of glucose-tolerance factor (GTF) to balance blood sugar, helps to normalise hunger and reduce cravings, improves lifespan, helps protect DNA and RNA, essential for heart function.

Deficiency signs Excessive or cold sweats, dizziness or irritability after six hours without food, need for frequent meals, cold hands, need for excessive sleep or drowsiness during the day, excessive thirst, addiction to sweet foods.

How much?
RDA None established
ODA 125mcg
SUPPLEMENTARY RANGE 25–200mcg
TOXICITY There is a wide range of safety between the helpful and harmful doses of chromium. Toxicity occurs only above 1,000mg, which is five thousand times the top therapeutic level.

Best food sources Brewer's yeast (112mcg), wholemeal bread (42mcg), rye bread (30mcg), oysters (26mcg), potatoes (24mcg), wheat germ (23mcg), green peppers (19mcg), eggs (16mcg), chicken (15mcg), apples (14mcg), butter (13mcg), parsnips (13mcg), cornmeal (12mcg), lamb (12mcg), Swiss cheese (11mcg).

Best supplement Chromium polynicotinate/picolinate, brewer's yeast.

Helpers Vitamin B3 and three amino acids – glycine, glutamic acid and cystine – combine to form glucose-tolerance factor (GTF). Improved diet and exercise.

Robbers High intake of refined sugars and flours, obesity, additives, pesticides, petroleum products, processed foods, toxic metals.

● Iron

What it does As a component of haemoglobin, iron transports oxygen and carbon dioxide to and from cells. Component of enzymes, vital for energy production.

Deficiency signs Anaemia, e.g. pale skin, sore tongue, fatigue, listlessness, loss of appetite, nausea, sensitivity to cold.

How much?
RDA 14mg
ODA 20mg
SUPPLEMENTARY RANGE 5–15mg
TOXICITY None below 1,000mg.

Best food sources Pumpkin seeds (11.2mg), parsley (6.2mg), almonds (4.7mg), prunes (3.9mg), cashew nuts (3.6mg), raisins (3.5mg), Brazil nuts (3.4mg), walnuts (3.1 mg), dates (3.0mg), pork (2.9mg), cooked dried beans (2.7mg), sesame seeds (2.4mg), pecan nuts (2.4mg).

Best supplement Amino acid-chelated iron is three times more absorbable than iron sulphate or oxide.

Helpers Vitamin C (increases iron absorption), vitamin E, calcium but not in excess, folic acid, phosphorus, stomach acid.

Robbers Oxalates (spinach and rhubarb), tannic acid (tea), phytates (wheat bran), phosphates (soft fizzy drinks, food additives), antacids, high zinc intake.

● Magnesium

What it does Strengthens bones and teeth, promotes healthy muscles by helping them to relax, so important for PMS, important for heart muscles and nervous system. Essential for energy production. Involved as a co-factor in many enzymes in the body.

Deficiency signs Muscle tremors or spasms, muscle weakness, insomnia or nervousness, high blood pressure, irregular heartbeat, constipation, fits or convulsions, hyperactivity, depression, confusion, lack of appetite, calcium deposited in soft tissue, e.g. kidney stones.

How much?
RDA 300mg
ODA 500mg
SUPPLEMENTARY RANGE 50–250mg
TOXICITY None below 1,000mg.

Best food sources Wheat germ (490mg), almonds (270mg), cashew nuts (267mg), brewer's yeast (231mg), buckwheat flour (229mg), Brazil nuts (225mg), peanuts (175mg), pecan nuts (142mg), cooked beans (37mg), garlic (36mg), raisins (35mg), green peas (35mg), potato skin (34mg), crab (34mg).

Best supplement Amino acid chelate and citrate are twice as well absorbed as magnesium carbonate or sulphate.

Helpers Vitamins B1, B6, C and D, zinc, calcium, phosphorus.

Robbers Large amounts of calcium in milk products, proteins, fats, oxalates (spinach, rhubarb), phytate (wheat bran, bread).

● Manganese

What it does Helps to form healthy bones, cartilage, tissues and nerves, activates more than twenty enzymes including an antioxidant enzyme system, stabilises blood sugar, promotes healthy DNA and RNA, essential for reproduction and red blood cell synthesis, important for insulin production, reduces cell damage, required for brain function.

Deficiency signs Muscle twitches, childhood growing pains, dizziness or poor sense of balance, fits, convulsions, sore knees, joint pain.

How much?
RDA None established
ODA 10mg
SUPPLEMENTARY RANGE 1–9mg
TOXICITY Not a concern.

Best food sources Watercress (0.5mg), pineapple (1.7mg), okra (0.9mg), endive (0.4mg), blackberries (1.3mg), raspberries (1.1mg), lettuce (0.15mg), grapes (0.7mg), lima beans (1.3mg), strawberries (0.3mg), oats (0.6mg), beetroot (0.3mg), celery (0.14mg).

Best supplement Amino acid chelate, manganese citrate or gluconate.

Helpers Zinc, vitamins E, B1, C, K.

Robbers Antibiotics, alcohol, refined foods, calcium, phosphorus.

● Molybdenum

What it does Helps rid the body of the protein breakdown products, e.g. uric acid, strengthens teeth and may help reduce the risk of dental caries, detoxifies the body from free radicals, petrochemicals and sulphites.

Deficiency signs Deficiency signs are not known unless excess copper or sulphate interferes with its utilisation. Animals show signs of breathing difficulties and neurological disorders.

How much?
RDA None established
ODA None established
SUPPLEMENTARY RANGE 100–1,000mcg (1mg)
TOXICITY Intakes of 10–15mg/day cause a high incidence of gout-like symptoms associated with high uric acid.

Best food sources Tomatoes, wheat germ, pork, lamb, lentils, beans.

Best supplement Amino acid-chelated molybdenum.

Helpers Protein including sulphur-containing amino acids, carbohydrates, fats.

Robbers Copper, sulphates.

● Phosphorus

What it does Forms and maintains bone and teeth, needed for milk secretion, builds muscle tissue, is a component of DNA and RNA, helps maintain pH of the body, aids metabolism and energy production.

Deficiency signs Dietary deficiencies are unlikely since it is present in almost all foods. May occur with long-term antacid use or with stresses such as bone fracture. Signs include general muscle weakness, loss of appetite and bone pain, rickets, osteomalacia (softening of bones).

How much?
RDA 800mg
ODA 800mg
SUPPLEMENTARY RANGE Not necessary to supplement
TOXICITY No known cases; however, it may result in deficiency of calcium, increased neuroexcitability and convulsions.

Best food sources Present in almost all foods.

Best supplement Calcium phosphate, lecithin, monosodium phosphate.

Helpers Correct calcium: phosphorus ratio, lactose, vitamin D.

Robbers Too much iron, magnesium, aluminium.

● Potassium

What it does Enables nutrients to move into and waste products to move out of cells, promotes healthy nerves and muscles, maintains fluid balance in the body, relaxes muscles, helps secretion of insulin for blood sugar control to produce constant energy, involved in metabolism, maintains heart functioning, stimulates gut movements to encourage proper elimination.

Deficiency signs Rapid irregular heartbeat, muscle weakness, pins and needles, irritability, nausea, vomiting, diarrhoea, swollen abdomen, cellulite, low blood pressure resulting from an imbalance of potassium: sodium ratio, confusion, mental apathy.

How much?
RDA 2,000mg
ODA 2,000mg

SUPPLEMENTARY RANGE Not necessary to supplement

TOXICITY At an intake of around 18,000mg cardiac arrest may occur.

Best food sources Watercress (329mg), endive (316mg), cabbage (251mg), celery (285mg), parsley (540mg), courgettes (248mg), radishes (231mg), cauliflower (355mg), mushrooms (371mg), pumpkin (339mg), molasses (2,925mg).

Best supplement Potassium gluconate/chloride, slow-releasing potassium, seaweed, brewer's yeast.

Helpers Magnesium helps to hold potassium in cells.

Robbers Excess sodium from salt, alcohol, sugar, diuretics, laxatives, corticosteroid drugs, stress.

● Selenium

What it does Antioxidant properties help to protect against free radicals and carcinogens, reduces inflammation, stimulates immune system to fight infections, promotes a healthy heart and helps vitamin E's action, required for male reproductive system, needed for metabolism.

Deficiency signs Family history of cancer, signs of premature ageing, cataracts, high blood pressure, frequent infections.

How much?
RDA None established
ODA 100mcg
SUPPLEMENTARY RANGE 25–150mcg
TOXICITY None below 750mcg; when it interferes with normal structure and functions of proteins in hair, nails and skin, garlic breath may occur.

Best food sources Tuna (0.116mg), oysters (0.65mg), molasses (0.13mg), mushrooms (0.13mg), herrings (0.61mg), cottage cheese (0.023mg), cabbage (0.003mg), beef liver (0.049mg), courgettes (0.003mg), cod (0.029mg), chicken (0.027mg).

Best supplement Selenomethionine, selenocysteine.

Helpers Vitamins E, A and C.

Robbers Refined food, modern farming techniques.

● Sodium

What it does Maintains body's water balance, preventing dehydration, helps nerve functioning, used in muscle contraction including heart muscle, utilised in energy production, helps move nutrients into cells.

Deficiency signs Dizziness, heat exhaustion, low blood pressure, rapid pulse, mental apathy, loss of appetite, muscle cramps, nausea, vomiting, reduced body weight, headache.

How much?

RDA 2,400mg

ODA 2,400mg

SUPPLEMENTARY RANGE Not necessary to supplement

TOXICITY May occur with high intake from processed foods and restricted water intake, oedema, high blood pressure, kidney disease.

Best food sources Sauerkraut (664mg), olives (2,020mg), shrimps (2,300mg), miso (2,950mg), beetroot (282mg), ham (1,500mg), celery (875mg), cabbage (643mg), crab (369mg), cottage cheese (405mg), watercress (45mg), red kidney beans (327mg).

Best supplement None needed. Plentiful in food.

Helpers Vitamin D.

Robbers Potassium and chloride counteract sodium, to keep a balance in the body.

● Zinc

What it does Component of over 200 enzymes in the body, component of DNA and RNA, essential for growth, important for healing, controls hormones which are messengers from organs such as testes and ovaries, aids ability to cope with stress effectively, promotes healthy nervous system and brain especially in the growing foetus, aids bone and teeth formation, helps hair to bloom, essential for constant energy.

Deficiency signs Poor sense of taste or smell, white marks on more than two fingernails, frequent infections, stretch marks, acne or greasy skin, low fertility, pale skin, tendency to depression, loss of appetite.

How much?

RDA 15mg

ODA 20mg

SUPPLEMENTARY RANGE 5–20mg

TOXICITY 2g or more can result in gastrointestinal irritation, vomiting, anaemia, reduced growth, stiffness, depraved appetite and death. Zinc has been administered to patients in ten-fold excess of the dietary allowances for years without adverse reactions, but copper levels should be monitored.

Best food sources Oysters (148.7mg), ginger root (6.8mg), lamb (5.3mg), pecan nuts (4.5mg), dry split peas (4.2mg), haddock (1.7mg), green peas (1.6mg), shrimps (1.5mg), turnips (1.2mg), Brazil nuts (4.2mg), egg yolks (3.5mg), wholewheat grain (3.2mg), rye (3.2mg), oats (3.2mg), peanuts (3.2mg), almonds (3.1mg).

Best supplement Amino acid chelate, zinc citrate and picolinate are better than zinc sulphate or oxide.

Helpers Stomach acid, vitamins A, E and B6, magnesium, calcium, phosphorus.

Robbers Phytates (wheat), oxalates (rhubarb and spinach), high calcium intake, copper, low protein intake, excess sugar intake, stress; alcohol prevents uptake.

Essential fats

● Omega 3 (EPA, DHA)

What it does Promotes a healthy heart, thins the blood, reduces inflammation, improves functioning of the nervous system, promotes neurotransmitter balance and reception, relieves depression, schizophrenia, attention deficit, hyperactivity and autism, improves sleep, improves skin condition, helps balance hormones, reduces insulin resistance.

Deficiency signs Dry skin, eczema, dry hair or dandruff, excessive thirst, excessive sweating, poor memory or learning difficulties, inflammatory health problems, e.g. arthritis, high blood lipids, depression, PMS or breast pain, water retention.

How much?
RDA None established
ODA 350mg of EPA, 350mg of DHA
SUPPLEMENTARY RANGE EPA 150–550mg, DHA 100–500mg
TOXICITY None established. Substantial excess can lead to oily skin and loose bowels.

Best food sources Mackerel, swordfish, marlin, tuna, salmon, sardines, flax seeds, sunflower seeds.

Best supplement While ALA (alpha-linolenic acid) is the actual essential nutrient found in seeds and nuts, from which EPA and DHA can be made in the body, EPA and DHA are a much more potent form of Omega 3.

Helpers Niacin, vitamin B6, vitamin C, zinc, magnesium and manganese help convert ALA to EPA/DHA and then prostaglandins. Antioxidant nutrients help to protect them.

Robbers Frying, storage, food processing, e.g. hydrogenation, smoking, alcohol.

● Omega 6 (GLA)

What it does Promotes a healthy heart, thins the blood, reduces inflammation, improves functioning of the nervous system, promotes neurotransmitter balance and reception, relieves depression, schizophrenia, attention deficit, hyperactivity and autism, improves skin condition, helps balance hormones, reduces insulin resistance.

Deficiency signs Dry skin, eczema, dry hair or dandruff, excessive thirst, excessive sweating, PMS or breast pain, water retention.

How much?
RDA None established
ODA 150mg
SUPPLEMENTARY RANGE 110–260mg
TOXICITY None established. Substantial excess can lead to oily skin and loose bowels.

Best food sources Safflower oil, sunflower oil, corn oil, sunflower seeds, pumpkin seeds, walnuts, wheat germ, sesame seeds.

Best supplement While linoleic acid is the actual essential nutrient found in seeds and nuts, from which GLA can be made in the body, GLA is a much more potent form of Omega 6. This can also be converted to arachidonic acid, another very important essential fatty acid.

Helpers Niacin, vitamin B6, vitamin C, zinc, magnesium and manganese help convert linoleic acid into GLA and then prostaglandins. Antioxidant nutrients help to protect them.

Robbers Frying, storage, food processing, e.g. hydrogenation, smoking, alcohol.

Semi-essential nutrients

● Bioflavonoids

What they do Help vitamin C to work, strengthen capillaries, speed up healing of wounds, sprains and muscle injuries, antioxidant.

Deficiency signs Easy bruising, varicose veins, frequent sprains.

How much?
RDA None

ODA None
SUPPLEMENTARY RANGE 50–1,000mg
TOXICITY None known.

Best food sources Berries, cherries, citrus fruit.

Best supplement Citrus bioflavonoids, rosehip extract, berry extracts.

Helpers Vitamin C.

Robbers Free radicals.

● Choline

What it does Component of lecithin which helps break down fat in liver, facilitates movement of fats into cells and synthesis of cell membranes in nervous system, protects lungs.

Deficiency signs Developmental abnormalities in newborn babies, high blood cholesterol and fat, fatty liver, nerve degeneration, high blood pressure, atherosclerosis, senile dementia, reduced resistance to infection.

How much?
RDA None established
ODA None established
SUPPLEMENTARY RANGE 25–150mg
TOXICITY None known.

Best food sources Lecithin, eggs, fish, liver, soya beans, peanuts, whole grains, nuts, pulses, citrus fruits, wheat germ, brewer's yeast.

Best supplement Lecithin.

Helpers Vitamin B5, lithium.

Robbers Alcohol, birth-control Pill.

● Co-enzyme Q10

What it does Central role in energy metabolism, improves heart function and other functions, helps to normalise blood pressure, increases exercise tolerance, antioxidant, boosts immunity.

Deficiency signs Lack of energy, heart disease, poor exercise tolerance, poor immune function.

How much?
RDA None

ODA None
SUPPLEMENTARY RANGE 10–90mg
TOXICITY None known.

Best food sources Sardines (6.4mg), mackerel (4.3mg), pork (2.4–4.1mg), spinach (1.0mg), soya oil (9.2mg), peanuts (2.7mg), sesame seeds (2.3mg), walnuts (1.9mg).

Best supplement Co-enzyme Q10 in a lipid base (aids absorption).

Helpers B complex, iron.

Robbers Stimulants, sugar.

● Inositol

What it does Needed for cell growth, required by brain and spinal cord and for formation of nerve sheath, mild tranquilliser, maintains healthy hair, reduces blood cholesterol.

Deficiency signs Irritability, insomnia, nervousness, hyper-excitability, reduction in nerve growth and regeneration, low HDL level.

How much?
RDA None established
ODA None established
SUPPLEMENTARY RANGE 25–150mg
TOXICITY None known.

Best food sources Lecithin granules, pulses, soya flour, eggs, fish, liver, citrus fruits, melon, nuts, wheat germ, brewer's yeast.

Best supplement Lecithin granules or capsules.

Helpers Choline.

Robbers Phytates, antibiotics, alcohol, tea, coffee, birth-control Pill, diuretics.

Part 9

Food Fact File

WHICH PROTEIN FOODS?

The protein in foods varies in both its quantity and quality. The table opposite shows you how much protein is in the listed foods (percentage of calories as protein), how much of the food you would need to eat to obtain 20 grams of protein, and how 'usable' is the protein, which is a measure of its quality in isolation. Less 'usable' protein sources may become highly usable when combined with other foods (see page 56). Most people need no more than 35 grams a day, so two of any of the servings below would suffice. If the quality of the protein is high, one and a half servings may be enough. Pregnant women, people recovering from surgery, athletes and anyone who does heavy manual work may need three servings a day.

■ Protein Quantity and Quality

Food	Percentage of calories as Protein	Amount required for 20g of Protein	Quality of Protein
Grains/pulses			
Quinoa	16%	100g/1 cup dry weight	Excellent
Com	4%	500g/3 cups	Reasonable
White rice	8%	338g/2.5 cups	Reasonable
Brown rice	5%	400g/3 cups	Excellent
Kidney beans	26%	99g/0.66 cup	Poor
Chick peas	22%	109g/0.66 cup	Reasonable
Soya beans	54%	60g/1 cup	Reasonable
Tofu	40%	275g/1 packet	Excellent

Baked beans	18%	430g/1 large tin	Reasonable
Wheat germ	24%	132g/2 cups	Reasonable
Lentils	28%	92g/⅓ cup	Poor

Fish/meat

Tuna, canned in oil	61%	84g/1 small tin	Excellent
Cod	60%	35g/1 small piece	Excellent
Sardines, canned	49%	100g/1 serving	Excellent
Scallops	15%	133g/1 serving	Excellent
Oysters	11%	182g/0.5 cup	Excellent
Lamb chop	24%	110g/1 small	Reasonable
Beef	52%	80g/2 slices	Excellent
Chicken	63%	71g/1 small breast roast	Excellent

Nuts/seed

Sunflower seeds	15%	188g/1 cup	Reasonable
Pumpkin seeds	21%	70g/0.5 cup	Reasonable
Cashew nuts	12%	112g/1 cup	Reasonable
Peanuts	17%	90g/0.5 cup	Reasonable
Almonds	13%	110g/1 cup	Reasonable

Eggs/dairy

Eggs	34%	169g/2 medium	Excellent
Yoghurt, natural	22%	440g/3 small pots	Excellent
Cheddar cheese	25%	84g/0.33 oz	Excellent
Cottage cheese	49%	120g/1 small pot	Excellent
Milk, whole	20%	600ml/2 cups	Excellent
Edam cheese	28%	70g/2.5oz	Excellent
Camembert cheese	25%	110g/2 wedges	Excellent

Vegetables

Peas, frozen	26%	259g/2 cups	Reasonable
Green beans	20%	200g/2 cups	Reasonable
Broccoli	50%	600g/large bag	Reasonable
Spinach	49%	390g/large bag	Reasonable
Potatoes	11%	950g/4 large	Reasonable

WHICH FATS AND OILS?

Foods vary in the quality and quantity of fat they contain. The perfect diet provides no more than 20 per cent of its calories from fat, However, more important is the kind of fat, Polyunsaturated fats, or rather oils as they are always liquid, are essential, while monounsaturated and saturated fats are not. So in an ideal food more of the fat is polyunsaturated. The table opposite shows which fat-containing foods to avoid and which to increase, Those in bold type are best avoided, or limited, because they contain few essential fats, are high in saturated fat and have an overall high fat percentage.

There are different families of unsaturated fats. The Omega 6 and Omega 3 families are essential. Ideally your diet should provide roughly equal amounts of these. The Omega 9 family derive from the monounsaturated fat oleic acid, of which olive oil is a good source. These are not essential, but not harmful, except in excess. The table below shows which cold-pressed oils contain which unsaturated fats.

☐ % polyunsaturated   ▨ % monounsaturated   ■ % saturated

% of calories as fat

		% poly	% mono	% sat
Butter	100	10%	29%	61%
Olive oil	100	13%	73%	14%
Vegetable margarine	98	55%	20%	25%
Cod	8	57%	16%	27%
Haddock	7	45%	21%	34%
Tuna	32	40%	40%	20%
Plaice	22	34%	38%	28%
Mackerel	63	32%	41%	27%
Salmon	42	30%	43%	27%
Sardines	62	22%	57%	21%
Brazil nuts	85	40%	35%	25%
Peanuts	73	30%	50%	20%
Almonds	74	20%	72%	8%
Sunflower seeds	73	67%	21%	12%
Sesame seeds	73	45%	40%	15%
Avocados	80	8%	80%	12%
Cottage cheese	40	63%	11%	25%
Cheddar cheese	74	33%	21%	47%
Camembert	73	33%	21%	46%
Milk, whole	49	5%	30%	65%
Milk, skimmed	5	5%	30%	65%
Milk chocolate	36	3%	34%	63%
Chocolate biscuits	47	8%	39%	53%
Chicken	71	17%	48%	35%
Pork	65	10%	48%	42%
Bacon	80	9%	48%	43%
Sausages	77	9%	48%	43%
Lamb	76	7%	41%	52%
Beef	32	6%	49%	45%

Fat composition of foods

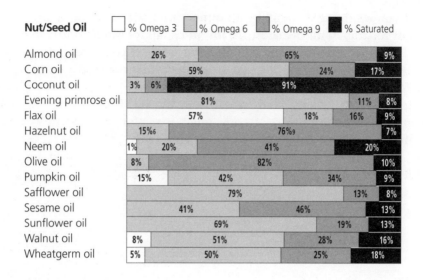

Nut/Seed Oil □ % Omega 3 ▦ % Omega 6 ▨ % Omega 9 ■ % Saturated

Almond oil	26%	65%	9%
Corn oil	59%	24%	17%
Coconut oil	3% 6%	91%	
Evening primrose oil	81%	11%	8%
Flax oil	57%	18% 16%	9%
Hazelnut oil	15% 6	76% 9	7%
Neem oil	1% 20%	41%	20%
Olive oil	8%	82%	10%
Pumpkin oil	15%	42% 34%	9%
Safflower oil	79%	13%	8%
Sesame oil	41%	46%	13%
Sunflower oil	69%	19%	13%
Walnut oil	8%	51% 28%	16%
Wheatgerm oil	5%	50% 25%	18%

Fats and oils – which omega?

WHICH CARBOHYDRATES?

Carbohydrates should make up the major part of your diet, accounting for two-thirds of the calories you consume. Since there are more calories per gram of both protein and fat this means that, by weight, carbohydrates should make up more than two-thirds of your diet.

The type of carbohydrate is as important as the amount. Some carbohydrates, such as sugar, are 'fast releasing', which means that they raise your blood sugar level quickly. Others, such as oats, are 'slow releasing'. The most accurate way to gauge whether or not you should eat a food is by checking the Glycemic Load (GL) of a food, which is a calculation based on both the *quantity* of carbohydrate in a food, and the *quality* of that carbohydrate.

A GL of 10 or less is good, shown in bold
A GL of 11–14 is OK, shown in normal text
A GL of 15 or more is bad, *shown in italics*

However, even this is a guide only because the amount you eat of a food will obviously alter its effect on your blood sugar, and hence your weight. So, while I generally say liberally eat the bold foods with a low GL, limit the normal text foods and avoid the italics foods, what is most important is to limit the *total* GL of your diet. **Eat no more than 50 GL points a day, or 15 with each meal.**

If you want to lose weight eat no more than 40 GL points a day. This means roughly10 for breakfast, 10 for lunch, 10 for dinner and 5 in each of two snacks, mid-morning and mid-afternoon. If you choose the good, low GL foods you'll be able to eat more food. If you choose the bad high GL foods you'll have to eat much less.

In the chart below mainly select from the **bold** foods then use the right-hand column to work out how much to eat for 10 GL points. Foods containing no carbohydrate, composed entirely of protein or fat (meat, fish, eggs, cheese, mayonnaise) have, in effect, a GL of 0, and are not included in this chart.

GLYCEMIC LOAD (GL) OF COMMON FOODS

Item	Serving size (in g)	GLs per serving	10GLs	5GLs	5GLs
BAKERY PRODUCTS					
Muffin – apple, made without sugar	**60**	**9**	**1 muffin**	**Half muffin**	**33g**
Muffin – apple muffin, made with sugar	60	13	1 small muffin	½ small muffin	23g
Crumpet	50	13	1 crumpet	½ crumpet	19g
Muffin – apple, oat, sultana, made from packet mix	50	14	1 small muffin	½ small muffin	18g
Muffin – bran	57	15	½ muffin	¼ muffin	18g
Muffin – blueberry	57	17	½ muffin	¼ muffin	17g
Muffin – banana, oat and honey	50	17	½ muffin	¼ muffin	15g
Muffin – carrot	57	20	½ muffin	¼ muffin	14g
Banana cake, made without sugar	80	16	1 small slice	½ small slice	25g
Croissant	57	17	½ croissant	¼ croissant	17g
Doughnut	47	17	½ doughnut	¼ doughnut	14g
Sponge cake, plain	63	17	½ slice	¼ slice	19g
BREADS					
Rye kernel (pumpernickel) bread	**30**	**6**	**2 slices**	**1 slice**	**25g**
Sourdough rye	**30**	**6**	**2 slices**	**1 slice**	**25g**
Volkenbrot, wholemeal rye bread	**30**	**7**	**2 slices**	**1 slice**	**21g**

Item	Serving size (in g)	GLs per serving	10GLs	5GLs	5GLs
Rice bread, high-amylose	30	7	2 small slices	1 small slice	21g
Rice bread, low-amylose	30	8	2 thin slices	1 thin slice	19g
Wholemeal rye bread	30	8	2 thin slices	1 thin slice	19g
Wheat tortilla (Mexican)	50	8	1½ tortillas	Less than 1 tortilla	31g
Chapatti, white wheat flour, thin, with green gram	50	8	1½ chapattis	1 chapatti	31g
White, high-fibre	30	9	1 thick slice	1 thin slice	17g
Wholemeal (whole wheat) wheat flour bread	30	9	1 thick slice	1 thin slice	17g
Gluten-free fibre-enriched,	30	9	1 thick slice	½ thick slice	17g
Gluten-free multigrain bread	30	10	1 slice	½ slice	15g
Light rye	30	10	1 slice	½ slice	15g
White wheat flour bread	30	10	1 slice	½ slice	15g
Pita bread, white	30	10	1 pitta	½ slice	15g
Wheat flour flatbread	30	10	1 slice	½ slice	15g
Gluten-free white bread,	30	11	1 slice	½ slice	14g
Corn tortilla	50	12	1 tortilla	½ tortilla	21g
Middle Eastern flatbread	30	15	⅔ slice	⅓ slice	10g
Baguette, white, plain	30	15	¹⁄₂₀ baton	¹⁄₄₀ baton	10g
Bagel, white, frozen	70	25	½ bagel	¼ bagel	14g

Item	Serving size (in g)	GLs per serving	10GLs	5GLs	5GLs
BREAKFAST CEREALS					
Porridge made from rolled oats	**30**	**2**	**As much as you like**	**1 v.large bowl**	**75g**
Get Up & Go with strawberries and ½ pint of milk (E)	**30**	**5**	**½ pint drink**	**¼ pint drink**	**5fl oz/ 150ml**
All-Bran ™	**30**	**6**	**2 small servings**	**1 small serving**	**25g**
Muesli, gluten-free	**30**	**7**	**2 small servings**	**1 small serving**	**21g**
Muesli (Alpen)	**30**	**10**	**1 serving**	**½ serving**	**15g**
Muesli, Natural	**30**	**10**	**1 serving**	**½ serving**	**15g**
Raisin Bran™ (Kellogg's)	30	12	1 small serving	⅓ serving	13g
Weetabix™	30	13	2 biscuits	1 biscuit	12g
Bran Flakes™	30	13	1 small serving	⅓ serving	12g
Sultana Bran™ (Kellogg's)	30	14	1 small serving	⅓ serving	11g
Special K™ (Kellogg's)	30	14	1 small serving	⅓ serving	11g
Shredded Wheat	30	15	1 biscuit	⅓ serving	10g
Cheerios™	30	15	1 v.small serving	⅓ serving	10g
Frosties™, sugar-coated cornflakes (Kellogg's)	30	15	1 v.small serving	⅓ serving	10g
Grapenuts™	30	15	1 v.small serving	⅓ serving	10g
Golden Wheats™ (Kellogg's)	30	16	1 v.small serving	⅓ serving	9g
Puffed Wheat	30	16	1 v.small serving	⅓ serving	9g
Honey Smacks™ (Kellogg's)	30	16	1 v.small serving	⅓ serving	9g
Cornflakes, Crunchy Nut™ (Kellogg's)	30	17	1 v.small serving	⅓ serving	9g
Coco Pops™ (cocoa flavoured puffed rice)	30	20	½ serving	¼ serving	8g

Item	Serving size (in g)	GLs per serving	10GLs	5GLs	5GLs
Rice Krispies™ (Kellogg's)	30	21	½ serving	¼ serving	7g
Cornflakes™ (Kellogg's)	30	21	½ serving	¼ serving	7g
CEREAL GRAINS					
Semolina	**150**	**6**	**A v.large serving**	**Small serving**	**125g**
Taco shells, cornmeal-based, baked (Old El Paso)	**20**	**8**	**2 shells**	**1 shell**	**13g**
Quinoa	**150**	**8**	**1½ cups**	**⅔ cup**	**94g**
Cornmeal	**150**	**9**	**A v.large serving**	**Small serving**	**83g**
Kamut (E)	**150**	**9**	**A v.large serving**	**Small serving**	**83g**
Pearl Barley	150	11	1 serving	½ serving	68g
Cracked wheat (bulgur/bourghul)	150	12	1 serving	½ serving	63g
Brown basmati rice	150	13	1 small serving	½ serving	58g
Buckwheat	150	16	1 small serving	⅓ serving	47g
Rice, brown	150	18	1 small serving	⅓ serving	42g
Long grain, white, pre-cooked microwaved 2 min (Express Rice Uncle Ben's)	150	19	½ serving	¼ serving	39g
Basmati, white, boiled	150	22	½ serving	¼ serving	34g
Couscous	150	23	½ serving	¼ serving	33g
Rice, white	150	23	½ serving	¼ serving	33g
Long grain, boiled	150	23	½ serving	¼ serving	33g

Item	Serving size (in g)	GLs per serving	10GLs	5GLs	5GLs
Millet, porridge	*150*	*25*	*½ serving*	*¼ serving*	*30g*
CRISPBREADS/CRACKERS					
Oatcake	**25**	**8**	**4 oatcakes**	**2 oatcakes**	**16g**
Digestive	**25**	**10**	**1 biscuit**	**½ biscuit**	**13g**
Cream Cracker	25	11	2 biscuits	1 biscuit	11g
Rye crispbread	25	11	2 biscuits	1 biscuit	11g
Water cracker	25	13	2 biscuits	1 biscuit	11g
Puffed rice cakes	*25*	*17*	*2 biscuits*	*1 biscuit*	*7g*
DAIRY PRODUCTS AND ALTERNATIVES					
Plain yoghurt (no sugar)	**200**	**3**	**3 small pots**	**1½ small pots**	**333g**
Non-fat yoghurt (plain,no sugar)	**200**	**3**	**3 small pots**	**1½ small pots**	**333g**
Milk, full-fat	**250**	**3**	**833ml**	**416ml**	**416ml**
Milk, skim (Canada)	**250**	**4**	**625g**	**312g**	**312g**
Soya yoghurt (Provamel)	**200**	**7**	**2 small pots**	**1 small pots**	**150g**
Soy milk (no sugar)	**250**	**7**	**2 small cups**	**1 small cup**	**178ml**
Custard, home made from milk	**100**	**7**	**1 small cup**	**½ cup**	**71g**
Ice cream, Regular	**50**	**8**	**2 scoops**	**1 scoop**	**31ml**
Soy milk, (sweetened with apple juice concentrate),	**250**	**8**	**2 small cups**	**1 small cup**	**156ml**
Soy milk, reduced-fat (1.5%), 120 mg calcium	**250**	**8**	**2 small cups**	**1 small cup**	**156ml**
Soy milk (sweetened with sugar)	**250**	**9**	**1½ cups**	**⅔ small cup**	**138ml**
Low-fat yoghurt, fruit, sugar, (Ski TM)	**200**	**10**	**1½ small pots**	**⅔ of small pot**	**100g**

Item	Serving size (in g)	GLs per serving	10GLs	5GLs	5GLs
Rice milk,E	250	14	1 small cup	½ cup	90g
Milk, condensed, sweetened (Nestlé)	50	17	1 tsp	½ tsp	14g

FRUIT AND FRUIT PRODUCTS

Item	Serving size (in g)	GLs per serving	10GLs	5GLs	5GLs
Blackberries E	120	1	2 large punnets	1 large punnet	600g
Blueberries E	120	1	2 large punnets	1 large punnet	600g
Raspberries E	120	1	2 large punnets	1 large punnet	600g
Strawberries, fresh, raw	120	1	2 large punnets	1 large punnet	600g
Cherries, raw, NS	120	3	2 punnets	1 punnet	200g
Grapefruit, raw	120	3	1 large	1 small	200g
Pear, raw	120	4	2 large pears	1 large pear	150g
Melon/Cantaloupe, raw	120	4	1 small melon	½ small melon	150g
Watermelon, raw	120	4	2 big slices	A big slice	150g
Peaches raw (or canned in natural juice)	120	5	2 peaches	1 peach	120g
Apricots, raw	120	5	8 apricots	4 apricots	120g
Oranges, raw	120	5	2 large	1 large	120g
Plum, raw	120	5	8 plums	4 plums	120g
Apples, raw	120	6	2 small	1 small	100g
Kiwi fruit, raw	120	6	2 kiwis	1 kiwi	100g
Pineapple raw	120	7	2 thin slices	1 thin slice	85g
Grapes, raw	120	8	20 grapes	10 grapes	75g
Mango, raw	120	8	½ mango	1 slice	75g

Item	Serving size (in g)	GLs per serving	10GLs	5GLs	5GLs
Apricots, dried	**60**	**9**	**6 apricots**	**3 apricots**	**33g**
Fruit Cocktail, canned (Delmonte)	**120**	**9**	**1 small can**	**½ small can**	**66g**
Paw paw/papaya, raw	**120**	**10**	**½ small papaya**	**1 slice**	**60g**
Prunes, pitted	**60**	**10**	**6 prunes**	**3 prunes**	**30g**
Apple, dried	**60**	**10**	**6 rings**	**3 rings**	**30g**
Banana raw	120	12	1 banana	½ banana	50g
Apricots, canned in light syrup	120	12	Less than 1 small tin	½ small tin	50g
Lychee, canned in syrup and drained	120	16	½ can	¼ × 200g can	37g
Figs, dried, tenderised, Dessert Maid brand	60	16	2 figs	1 fig	19g
Sultana	60	25	20	10	12g
Raisins	60	28	20	10	11g
Dates, dried	60	42	2 dates	1 date	7g
Jams/Spreads					
Pumpkin seed butter E	**16**	**1**	**3 large pots**	**1½ large pots**	**765g**
Peanut butter (no sugar) E	**16**	**1**	**3 large pots**	**1½ large pots**	**765g**
Blueberry spread (no sugar) E	**30**	**4**	**6 dsp**	**3 dsp**	**21g**
Apricot fruit spread, reduced sugar	**30**	**7**	**4 dsp**	**2 dsp**	**21g**
Orange Marmalade, (Australia)	**30**	**9**	**4 dsp**	**2 dsp**	**17g**
Strawberry jam	**30**	**10**	**3 dsp**	**1 heaped dsp**	**15g**
LEGUMES AND NUTS					
Hummus (chickpea dip)	**30**	**1**	**4 large tubs**	**4 small tubs**	**765g**
Soya beans	**150**	**1**	**6 cups**	**3 cups**	**750g**

Item	*Serving size (in g)*	*GLs per serving*	*10GLs*	*5GLs*	*5GLs*
Peas, dried, boiled	**150**	**2**	**3 cups**	**1½ cups**	**375g**
Pinto beans, boiled in salted water	**150**	**4**	**2 cups**	**1 cup**	**187g**
Borlotti beans, boiled, canned	**150**	**4**	**1½ cans**	**⅔ can**	**187g**
Lentils	**150**	**5**	**2 cups**	**1 cup**	**150g**
Butter Beans	**150**	**6**	**1½ cups**	**⅔ cup**	**125g**
Split peas, yellow, boiled 20 min	**150**	**6**	**1½ cups**	**⅔ cup**	**125g**
Baked Beans, canned	**150**	**7**	**½ tin**	**¼ tin**	**107g**
Kidney beans	**150**	**7**	**¾ tin**	**⅓ tin**	**107g**
Chickpeas (Garbanzo beans, Bengal gram), boiled	**150**	**8**	**1½ cups**	**⅔ cup**	**94g**
Chickpeas, canned in brine	**150**	**9**	**¾ tin**	**⅓ tin**	**83g**
Chestnuts, cooked E	**150**	**8**	**1½ cups**	**⅔ cup**	**94g**
Flageolet beans, canned in brine E	**150**	**8**	**¾ tin**	**⅓ tin**	**83g**
Haricot/Navy beans	150	12	½ tin	¼ tin	62g
Blackeyed beans, boiled	150	13	1 cup	½ cup	58g
PASTA and NOODLES					
Ravioli, durum wheat flour, meat filled, boiled	**90**	**7.5**	**½ packet**	**1 small serving**	**60g**
Vermicelli, white, boiled	**90**	**8**	**A large serving**	**½ large serving**	**56g**
Spaghetti, wholemeal, boiled	**90**	**8**	**A large serving**	**½ large serving**	**56g**
Pasta, wholemeal, boiled	**90**	**8**	**A large serving**	**½ serving**	**56g**

Item	Serving size (in g)	GLs per serving	10GLs	5GLs	5GLs
Fettucine, egg	**90**	**9**	**1 serving**	**½ serving**	**50g**
Spirali, durum wheat, white, boiled to al dente texture	**90**	**9**	**1 serving**	**½ serving**	**47g**
Spaghetti, white, boiled	**90**	**9**	**1 serving**	**½ serving**	**47g**
Instant noodles	**90**	**9**	**1 serving**	**½ serving**	**47g**
Spaghetti durum wheat boiled 10-15 min,	**90**	**10**	**1 serving**	**½ serving**	**43g**
Gluten-free pasta, maize starch, boiled 8 min	90	11	1 small serving	½ small serving	41g
Macaroni, plain,	90	11	1 v.small serving	½ v.small serving	39g
Rice noodles, dried, boiled	90	11	1 v. small serving	½ v.small serving	39g
Udon noodles, plain, (buckwheat/wheat)	*90*	*15*	*⅔ serving*	*⅓ serving*	*30g*
Corn pasta, gluten-free (62.5g serving size)	*90*	*16*	*1 small serving*	*½ small serving*	*28g*
Gnocchi	*90*	*16*	*1 v.small serving*	*½ small serving*	*27g*
Rice pasta, brown, boiled 16 min	*90*	*17*	*1 v.small serving*	*½ small serving*	*26g*
SNACK FOODS (SAVOURY)					
Olives, in brine E	**50**	**1**	**4 cups**	**2 cups**	**270g**
Peanuts	**50**	**1**	**1 large pack**	**1 medium or 2 small packs**	**250g**
Cashew nuts, salted	**50**	**3**	**1½ small packs**	**Less than 1 small pack**	**83g**
Popcorn, salted, no sugar	**20**	**8**	**1 small pack**	**½ small pack**	**12g**
Potato crisps, plain, salted	50	11	1½ small packs	⅔ small pack	23g

Item	Serving size (in g)	GLs per serving	10GLs	5GLs	5GLs
Pretzels, oven-baked, traditional wheat flavour	30	16	8	4	9g
Corn chips plain, salted	50	17	13 chips	7 chips	15g
SNACK FOODS (SWEET)					
Fruitus apple cereal bar E	**35**	**5**	**2 bars**	**1 bar**	**35g**
Rebar fruit and veg bar E	**50**	**8**	**1 bar**	**½ bar**	**25g**
Muesli bar containing dried fruit	30	13	Less than 1 bar	Less than ½ bar	12g
Chocolate, milk, plain (Mars/Cadburys/Nestle)	50	14	Less than ½ bar	Less than ¼ bar	18g
Apricot fruit bar (dried apricot filling in wholemeal pastry)	50	17	1 bar	½ bar	15g
Twix ® Cookie Bar, caramel (M&M/Mars, USA)	60	17	1 stick	½ stick	18g
Snickers Bar ®	60	19	⅔ bar	⅓ bar	16g
Polos – peppermint sweets	30	21	8	4	7g
Jelly beans assorted colours	30	22	4 jellybeans	2 jellybeans	7g
Pop Tarts™, double choc	50	24	21g	10g	10g
Mars Bar ®	60	26	½ bar	¼ bar	13g
SOUPS					
Tomato soup	**250**	**6**	**1 can**	**½ can**	**208g**
Minestrone	**250**	**7**	**1 can**	**½ can**	**179g**
Lentil, canned	**250**	**9**	**⅔ can**	**½ can**	**139g**

Item	Serving size (in g)	GLs per serving	10GLs	5GLs	5GLs
Split Pea	250	16	½ can	¼ can	78g
Black Bean	250	17	½ can	¼ can	74g
Green Pea, canned	250	17	½ can	¼ can	74g
SUGARS					
Xylitol	**20**	**2**	**6 tbsp**	**3 tbsp**	**50g**
Blue Agave cactus nectar (liquid sweetener in drinks)	**20**	**2**	**100ml**	**50ml**	**50g**
Fructose	**20**	**4**	**3 tbsp**	**5 tsp**	**25g**
Sucrose	20	14	3 tsp	1½ tsp	7g
Honey	20	16	2 tsp	1 tsp	6g
Glucose	20	20	2 tsp	1 tsp	5g
Maltose(malt)	20	22	2 tsp	1 tsp	5g
VEGETABLES					
Tomato E	**70**	**2**	**5 medium**	**2½ medium**	**175g**
Broccoli E	**100**	**2**	**5 handfuls**	**2½ handfuls**	**250g**
Kale E	**75**	**1**	**10 handfuls**	**5 handfuls**	**375g**
Avocado E	**190**	**1**	**10**	**5**	**950g**
Onion E	**180**	**2**	**5 medium**	**2½ medium**	**450g**
Asparagus E	**125**	**2**	**5 handfuls**	**2½ handfuls**	**315g**
Green beans E	**75**	**1**	**10 handfuls**	**5 handfuls**	**375g**
Carrots	**80**	**3**	**2 carrots**	**1 carrot**	**133g**
Green peas	**80**	**3**	**5 tbsp**	**2–3 tbsp**	**133g**
Pumpkin	**80**	**3**	**267**	**1½ servings**	**133g**
Beetroot	**80**	**5**	**4 small**	**2 small**	**80g**

Item	Serving size (in g)	GLs per serving	10GLs	5GLs	5GLs
Swede	**150**	**7**	**½ swede**	**1 small serving**	**107g**
Banana/plantain, green	**120**	**8**	**1 small**	**½ small**	**75g**
Broad beans	**80**	**9**	**2 tbsp**	**1 tbsp**	**44g**
Sweet corn	**80**	**9**	**1 serving**	**½ serving**	**44g**
Parsnips	80	12	1 small	½ small	33g
Yam	150	13	1 small serving	½ small serving	58g
Boiled potato	150	14	2 small	1 small	53g
Microwaved potato	150	14	2 small	1 small	53g
Mashed potato	150	15	2 tbsp	1 tbsp	50g
New Potato unpeeled and boiled 20 min	150	16	4 very small	2 very small	47g
Instant mashed potato	150	17	88	1 dsp	44g
Sweet potato	150	17	1 small	½ small	44g
Baked potato white, baked in skin	150	18	83	⅔ medium	42g
French Fries	150	22	68	4–5	34g
Baked potato, baked without fat	150	26	½ medium	¼ medium	29g

GLYCEMIC LOAD (GL) OF COMMON DRINKS

Item	*Serving size (in g)*	*GLs per serving*	*10GLs*	*5GLs*	*5GLs*
DRINKS					
Tomato juice, canned, no added sugar	**250**	**4**	**625**	**½ pint**	**315**
Yakult®, fermented milk drink with Lactobacilus casei	**65**	**6**	**108**	**⅔ 65ml bottle**	**30**
Smoothie drink, soy, banana	**250**	**7**	**357**	**⅔ 250ml carton**	**175**
Smoothie drink, soy, chocolate hazelnut	**250**	**8**	**313**	**⅗ 250ml carton**	**150**
Carrot juice, freshly made	**250**	**10**	**250**	**⅕ pint or ⅓ cup**	**125**
Grapefruit juice, unsweetened	250	11	227	⅕ pint or ⅓ cup	115
Apple juice, pure, unsweetened,	250	12	208	⅙ pint or ⅓ cup	105
Orange Juice	250	13	192	⅙ pint or ⅓ cup	95
Cordial, orange, reconstituted	250	13	192	⅙ pint or ⅓ cup	95
Smoothie, raspberry	250	14	179	⅖ 250ml carton or ⅓ cup	90
Pineapple juice, unsweetened	*250*	*16*	*156*	*¼ pint or ½ cup*	*80*
Cranberry juice drink, Ocean Spray ®	*250*	*16*	*156*	*¼ pint or ½ cup*	*80*
Coca Cola ®, soft drink/soda	*250*	*16*	*156*	*⅕ 330ml can*	*80*
Fanta ®, orange soft drink	*250*	*23*	*109*	*⅙ pint or ½ cup*	*50*
Lucozade ®, original	*250*	*40*	*63*	*⅛ pint or ¼ cup*	*30*

The GI and GL values of foods listed here are derived from research published by Foster-Powell K, Holt SH, Brand-Miller JC 'International table of glycemic index and glycemic load values, *American Journal of Clinical Nutrition*, 76(1), pp. 5–56 (2002).

Foods marked 'E' are estimated values, while other foods have measured values. As the GIs of more foods are calculated this table is updated on www.theholforddiet.com

NOTES

Serving size notes:

All pasta serving sizes are for cooked food. For the equivalent of dry weight halve the score. Ie if you're cooking spaghetti and the serving size is 120g that means you put 60g in the saucepan.

Portion guide at a glance

All servings provide 7GLs.

Food	Dry weight (gm)	Looks like	Looks like when cooked
Rice	40	1 ½ tbsp	2 ½ tbsp
Pasta	40	2 handfuls	4 handfuls
Quinoa	65	3 tbsp	4 rounded tbsp
Potato (boiled new)	70	¾ small	¾ small
Cous cous	25	1 tbsp	3 handfuls

HOW MUCH FIBRE?

Foods vary in both the amount of fibre they contain and its quality. One measure of quality is the amount of water that the fibre absorbs, which indicates to what extent it can make foecal matter lighter, bulkier and easier to move through the digestive tract. The ideal intake of fibre is not less than 35 grams a day. The following table shows you how much of given foods provides 10 grams of fibre (or the equivalent effect of 10 grams of grain fibre if the type of fibre is substantially more absorbent and therefore the amount you need in comparison is less). All measures are based on raw or dry foods. Please note that cooking decreases the fibre content of foods. So four servings of any of these foods will provide an ideal intake of fibre. All foods are raw, unless otherwise stated.

Amount of food required to supply 109 of fibre	Food Amount (for equivalent of 109 grain fibre)
Wheatbran	23g/0.5 cup
All-Bran	37g/0.5 cup
Apricots, dried	42g/1 cup
Figs, dried	54g/0.3 cups
Oats	5g/1 cup
Peas	83g/1 cup
Cornflakes	91g/3.5 cups
Almonds	107g/0.8 cups
Wholemeal bread	115g/5 slices
Peanuts	125g/1 cup
Baked beans	137g/small can
Prunes	146g/1 cup
Sunflower seeds	147g/1 cup
Rye bread	160g/6 slices
Rice crispies	222g/8 cups
Oatcakes	250g/1 0 biscuits
Lentils, cooked	70g/2 cups
Carrots	310g/3 carrots
Broccoli	358g/1 large head
White bread	370g/15 slices
Baked potato (skin on)	400g/11 large
Coleslaw	400g/11 large serving
Oranges	415g/3 oranges
Cabbage	466g/1 medium
Cauliflower	475g/1 large
Apple	500g/3–4 apples
New potatoes, boiled	500g/7 potatoes
Bananas	625g/3 bananas
Peaches	625g/6 peaches

BALANCING ACID/ALKALINE FOODS

When foods are metabolised by the body, a residue is left which can alter the body's acidity and alkalinity. Depending on the chemical composition of the 'ash', the food is called 'acid forming' or 'alkaline forming'. This is not to be confused with the immediate acidity of a food. Oranges, for example, are acid due to their citric acid content. However, citric acid is completely metabolised and the net effect of eating an orange is to alkalise the body, hence it is classified as alkaline forming. Roughly 80 per cent of our diet should come from alkaline-forming foods, and 20 per cent from acid-forming foods. The table below shows which foods are which.

▪ Which foods are Acid, Alkaline and Neutral

ACID		NEUTRAL	ALKALINE	
High	Medium		Medium	High
	Brazil nuts		Almonds	
	Walnuts		Coconut	
Edam	Cheddar cheese	Butter	Milk	
Eggs	Stilton cheese	Margarine		
Mayonnaise			Beans	Avocado
		Coffee	Cabbage	Beetroot
Fish	Herrings	Tea	Celery	Carrots
Shellfish	Mackerel	Sugar	Lentils	Potatoes
		Syrup	Lettuce	Spinach
Bacon	Rye		Mushrooms	
Beef	Oats		Onions	
Chicken	Wheat		Root vegetables	
Liver	Rice		Tomatoes	
Lamb				
Veal	Plums		Apricots	Dried fruit
	Cranberries		Apples	Rhubarb
	Olives		Banana	
			Berries	
			Cherries	
			Figs	
			Grapefruit	
			Grapes	
			Lemon	
			Melon	
			Oranges	
			Peaches	
			Pears	
			Raspberries	
			Tangerines	
			Prunes	

WHICH FOODS ARE RICH IN PHYTO-ESTROGENS?

Phyto-oestrogens are plant-based oestrogen-like chemicals that appear to protect against hormone-related cancers. There are many types of phyto-oestrogen – more than 800 in total. One of the most potent forms that is used in a lot of the cancer research is called isoflavones – in particular compounds called genistein and daidzein – and these are found in highest concentrations in soya products. Others called ligands are rich in linseeds, black/green tea, coffee, fruit and vegetables, split peas, lentils and beans. And another common category called coumestans are found in alfalfa, beans, split peas and lentils.

Cultures whose diets include such foods have much lower risk for prostate cancer, breast cancer and menopausal symptoms. I recommend you aim for around 15mg (15,000mcg) a day, which is equivalent to an Asian diet, ideally eating a phyto-oestrogen-rich food source twice a day, as they are only in circulation for about six hours. This is easily achieved by a small portion of tofu (100g serving provides 78mg), a 100mg glass of soya milk or soya yoghurt (11mg) or a portion of chickpeas, perhaps as hummus (2mg). Eating rye bread, beansprouts, beans, lentils, nuts and seeds all helps.

The table below is adapted from the Phyto-oestrogen Database 2004, compiled by Dr Margaret Ritchie, Bute Medical School at the University of St Andrews and reproduced with her kind permission. It provides a measure of the isoflavone phyto-estrogen level in common foods per 100g, which is roughly per serving.

■ Phyto-oestrogen content of commonly eaten foods

	mcg per 100g
Soya flour, full fat	166700
Soya beans	142100
Miso	126500
Soya mince	121100
Tofu	78700
Soya cheese	33000
Vegetarian sausages	26300
Vegeburger	26200
Tofu burger	24200
Soya milk, plain	11815
Soya yogurt, plain	11815
Chickpea channa dahl	1960
Soy sauce	1800
Multigrain crispbread	1187.30
Wholemeal bread	829.80
Beansprouts	758.20
Rye bread	757.20
Frankfurter sausages	676
Premium sausages	620
Currant bread	547
Granary bread	369.60
Pitta bread	320.70
Malt loaf	293
Currants	250

Runner beans	221.90
Nut and seed roast	162
Brown rice	132.60
Chick peas	124.10
Mixed nuts and raisins	100
Fruit cake, wholemeal	96.43
Fruit loaf	93.89
Ice cream, dairy	91
Sage and onion stuffing	90
Sausage and bean hotpot	85
Nut cutlets	61.60
Muesli, Swiss style	51.70
Red kidney beans	40
Turkey burgers, breaded	40
Green beans/French beans	38.40
Blackeye beans	32
Hazelnuts	24
Haricot beans	23.60
Peanuts, plain	23.50
Noodles, wheat	23.30
Lentils, green and brown	22.30
Mung bean dahl	20.62
Mung beans	20.62
Aubergine, stuffed with lentils and vegetables	19
Passion fruit	17.40
Prunes, ready to eat	12.79
Apples	12
Brown rice and red kidney beans	12
Hummus	11

WHICH ANTIOXIDANT-RICH FOODS?

The total antioxidant power of a food can be measured by a test developed at Tufts University in Boston, which determines a food's 'oxygen radical absorbance capacity', known as ORAC for short. Each food can now be assigned a certain number of ORAC units. Foods that score high in these units are especially helpful in countering oxidant, or free-radical, damage in your body.

We should all obtain 3,500 ORAC units a day, although 5,000 to 6,000 will give you even more protection against ageing. You'll also be better protected against many diseases, including cancer and heart disease. What this means in practice is eating a cup of blueberries (3,240 ORAC units), a quarter of a cup of raisins, and three prunes; or a half pint of strawberries and two servings of kale, tenderstem or broccoli. Alternatively, you could eat five servings of fresh fruit and vegetables every day.

■ FRUITS AND VEGETABLES WITH ANTIOXIDANT POWER

Per 100 grams units	ORAC units	Per item or serving	ORAC units
Prunes	5770	1 pitted prune	462
Raisins	2830	¼ cup	1019
Blueberries	2234	½ cup	1620
Blackberries	2036	½ cup	1466
Kale	1770	½ cup cooked	1150
Strawberries	1536	½ cup	1144
Spinach, raw	1210	1 cup	678
Raspberries	1227	½ cup	755
Tenderstem	1183	½ cup cooked	1159
Plums	949	1 plum	626
Alfalfa sprouts	931	1 cup	307
Spinach, steamed	909	½ cup cooked	1089
Broccoli	888	½ cup cooked	817
Beets	841	½ cup cooked, sliced	715
Avocado	782	½ Florida	149
Orange	750	1 orange	982
Grape, red	739	10 grapes	177
Pepper, red	731	1 medium pepper	540
Cherry	670	10 cherries	455
Kiwi fruit	602	1 fruit	458
Beans, baked	503	½ cup	640
Grapefruit, pink	483	½ fruit	580
Beans, kidney	460	½ cup cooked	400
Onion	449	½ cup chopped	360
Grapes, white	446	10 grapes	107
Corn	402	½ cup cooked	330
Aubergine	386	½ cup cooked	185
Cauliflower	377	½ cup cooked	234
		½ cup raw	188
Peas, frozen	364	½ cup cooked	291
Potatoes	313	½ cup cooked	244
Potatoes, sweet	301	½ cup cooked	301
Cabbage	298	½ cup raw	105
Leaf lettuce	262	10 leaves	200
Cantaloupe	252	½ melon	670
Banana	221	1 banana	252
Apple	218	1 medium apple	300

Tofu	213	½ cup	195
Carrots	207	½ cup raw	115
		½ cup cooked	160
Beans, string	201	½ cup cooked	125
Tomato	189	1 medium	233
Zucchini	176	½ cup raw	115
Apricots	164	3 raw	175
Peach	158	1 medium	137
Squash, yellow	150	½ cup cooked	183
Beans, lima	136	½ cup	115
Lettuce, iceberg	116	5 large leaves	116
Pear	134	1 medium	222
Watermelon	104	¹⁄₁₆ 10" diametre	501
Melon, honeydew	97	¹⁄₁₀ melon	125
Celery	61	½ cup diced	60
Cucumber	54	½ cup slices	28

THE BEST FRUIT AND VEGETABLES

The charts below show the best five fruits and vegetables, based on five key health factors: the ORAC rating, glucosinolate content (a key phytonutrient), zinc, folic acid and vitamin C. Make sure these are a staple food in your diet.

■ The Top Five Vegetables

	Zinc	Folic Acid	ORAC	Glucosinolates	Vitamin C	Total Score
Tenderstem	5	3	4	5	4	21
Broccoli	3	3	2	3	3	14
Asparagus	4	5	2	3	1	16
Curly Kale	3	4	5	3	5	20
Spinach	5	5	4	3	2	19

■ The Top Five Fruits

	Zinc	Folic Acid	ORAC	Glucosinolates	Vitamin C	Total Score
Strawberries	5	3	4	4	5	21
Blueberries	4	5	5	5	5	21
Raspberries	3	3	4	4	5	19
Oranges	3	4	3	3	5	18

Recommended Reading

Chapter 2
Eat Right for Your Type, Dr P. D'Adamo: G. P. Putnam's Sons, 1997
What is Optimum?, Dr E. Cheraskin: ION Press, 1994

Chapter 3
Biochemical Individuality, Professor R. Williams: Texas University Press,
    1969

Chapter 4
Nutrition and Evolution, Professor M. Crawford and O. Marsh: Keats,
    1995

Chapter 6
How to Protect Yourself from Pollution, P. Holford and Dr P. Barlow: ION
    Press, 1990
Our Stolen Future, T. Colborn, J. P. Myers and D. Dumanoski: Little,
    Brown, 1996

Chapter 9
Fats That Heal, Fats That Kill, Dr U. Erasmus: Alive Books, 1987/1994

Chapter 11
The Vitamin Controversy, Institute of Optimum Nutrition: ION Press,
1987

Chapter 12
Elemental Health, P. Holford: ION Press, 1983

Chapter 14
Living Food – The Key to Health and Vitality, P. Holford: ION Press, 1996

Chapter 16
The H Factor, J. Braly and P. Holford: Piatkus Books, 2003

Chapter 17
Improve Your Digestion, P. Holford: Piatkus Books, 1999

Chapter 18
Say No to Heart Disease, P. Holford: Piatkus Books, 1998
Unified Theory on the Cause and Treatment of Cardiovascular Disease
(video), Dr L. Pauling: ION Press, 1995

Chapter 19
Boost Your Immune System, J. Meek and P. Holford: Piatkus Books, 1998

Chapter 20
Balancing Hormones Naturally, K. Neil and P. Holford: Piatkus Books,
1998
What Your Doctor May Not Tell You about the Menopause, Dr J. Lee with
V. Hopkins: Warner Books, 1996

Chapter 22
Say No to Arthritis, P. Holford: Piatkus Books, 1999

Chapter 26
Stopping the Clock, Dr R. Klatz and Dr R. Goldman: Keats, 1996

Chapter 27
Cancer Prevention and Nutritional Therapies, Dr R. Passwater: Keats, 1996
The Plant Programme, Professor J. Plant and G. Tidey: Virgin Books, 2003
What Your Doctor May Not Tell You About Breast Cancer, Dr J. Lee, Dr D.
Zara and V. Hopkins: Warner Books, 2003

Chapter 28
Boost Your Immune System, J. Meek and P. Holford: Piatkus Books, 1998

Chapter 29
The Holford Diet, P. Holford: Piatkus Books, 2004

Chapters 30 and 31
Optimum Nutrition for the Mind, P. Holford: Piatkus Books, 2003

Chapters 32 and 33
Optimum Nutrition Before, During and After Pregnancy, P. Holford and
    S. Lawson: Piatkus Books, 2004

Chapter 34
The Male Menopause, Dr M. Carruthers: HarperCollins, 1996
What Your Doctor May Not Tell You about the Menopause, Dr J. Lee with
    V. Hopkins: Warner Books, 1996

Chapter 35
The 20-Day Rejuvenation Diet Program, Dr J. Bland: Keats, 1997

Chapter 37
Nutrition Counselling in the Treatment of Eating Disorders, M. Herrin:
    Brunner-Routledge, 2003

Chapter 38
What is Optimum?, Dr E. Cheraskin: ION Press, 1994

Chapter 42
Vitamins and Minerals – How Much Is Safe?: ION Press, 1991

Part 7
Nutritional Influences on Illness, Dr M. Werbach: Keats, 1987/1988

Resources

Brain Bio Centre

The Brain Bio Centre is an out-patient clinical treatment centre, specialising in the 'optimum nutrition' approach to mental health problems. The centre offers comprehensive assessment of biochemical imbalances that can contribute to mental health problems, and advice on how to correct these imbalances as a means to restore health. For more information visit www.foodforthebrain.org or call +44 (0)20 8332 9600.

British Society for Allergy Environmental and Nutritional Medicine

The organisation for medical doctors working with allergies (including chemical sensitivities) and nutritional problems. Full members are all doctors; associate membership and other categories exist for related professions. Holds regular meetings and supports the publication of the *Journal of Nutritional and Environmental Medicine*. For further information visit www.jnem.demon.co.uk or call +44 1547 550 380.

Eating disorders

If you have a concern about eating disorders I recommend you contact BEAT, 103 Prince of Wales Road, Norwich NR1 1DW. Adult helpline: +44 (0)845 634 1414. Youthline: +44 (0)845 634 7650. Website: www.b-eat.co.uk.

Institute for Optimum Nutrition (ION)

ION runs courses from a Home Study to a Foundation Degree in Nutritional Therapy and regularly organises lectures for health professionals and the general public. Services and facilities include a membership scheme, subscription to *Optimum Nutrition* magazine, a library and information centre, nutritional therapy clinics and a printed directory listing DipION Nutritional Therapists across the UK and overseas.

For a free information pack email reception@ion.ac.uk. Fax: +44 (0)870 979 1133. Tel: +44 (0)20 8614 7800. Website: www.ion.ac.uk.

Mental Health Project

The Mental Health Project is a voluntary action group that exists to inform the public about the role of nutrition in mental health, to promote the nutrition connection to health professionals, policy-makers and sufferers, and to provide resources to encourage more research and implementation of nutritional strategies. For more details visit www.foodforthebrain.org.

The Natural Progesterone Information Service (NPIS)

NPIS provides women and their doctors with details on how to obtain natural progesterone information packs for the general public and health practitioners, and books, tapes and videos relating to natural hormone health. Website: www.npis.info. For an order form and prescribing details (for doctors) please write to NPIS, P.O. Box 24, Buxton, SK17 9FB.

Nutrition consultations

For a personal referral by Patrick Holford to a nutritional therapist in your area, visit www.patrickholford.com and select 'consultations' for an immediate online referral. This service gives details on whom to see in the UK as well as internationally. If there is no one available nearby you can always do an online assessment – see below.

Nutrition assessment online

You can have your own personal health and nutrition assessment online using the My Nutrition questionnaire. Visit www.patrickholford.com and go to 'consultations'.

Nutritional therapy training

Institute for Optimum Nutrition (ION) runs courses including a home-study course and a three-year Nutritional Therapists Diploma course. It also has a directory of nutritional therapists throughout the UK. Contact ION at Avalon House, 72 Lower Mortlake Road, Richmond, Surrey, TW9 2JY. Tel: +44 (0)20 8614 7800. Website: www.ion.ac.uk.

Psychocalisthenics®
Psychocalisthenics is an excellent exercise system that takes less than twenty minutes a day, and develops strength, suppleness and stamina and generates vital energy. The best way to learn it is to do the Psychocalisthenics training. See www.patrickholford.com (seminars) for details on this or call +44 (0)1252 782 661. Also available in the book *Master Level Exercise: Psychocalisthenics* and on the *Psychocalisthenics* CD and DVD. For further information please see www.metafitness.com.

Salt alternatives
The average person gets far too much sodium because we eat too much salt (sodium chloride) and salted foods, and not enough potassium and magnesium, found in fruit and vegetables. The net result is water retention and weight gain, anxiety, insomnia, high blood pressure and muscle cramps. Not all salt, however, is bad for you. Solo Low Sodium Sea Salt contains 60 per cent less sodium and is high in the essential minerals magnesium and potassium. Their 200g reusable shaker is sold in the UK, Ireland, Spain, Netherlands, Singapore, Hong Kong, Japan, Bahrain, Saudi Arabia, United Arab Emirates, Jordan, Baltic states and United States of America. Visit their website: www.soloseasalt.com for more information or call: +44 (0)20 8464 1665.

Skin-care products
Environ products were developed by cosmetic surgeon Dr Des Fernandes to prevent skin cancer and address the damaging effects of the environment on our skin. Formulated with scientifically proven active ingredients including Vitamin A and antioxidant vitamins C, E and betacarotene, which are used in progressively higher concentrations, Environ will maintain a normal healthy skin, especially when there are signs of ageing, pigmentation, problem skin and scarring.

To purchase Environ products contact Totally Nourish on: +44 (0)800 085 7749, or go to www.totallynourish.com. For international enquiries call Environ (in Cape Town) on +2721 671 1467, or go to factory@environ.co.za.

Water filters
There are many water filters on the market. One of the best is offered by the Fresh Water Filter Company. For details visit www.freshwaterfilter.com, or call +44 (0)20 8558 7495.

Tests

General tests

Laboratory tests are available for all the tests mentioned in this book, through qualified nutrition consultants and doctors. Leading laboratories include:

- Biolab Medical Unit (doctor's referral only): Tel: +44 (0)20 7636 5959/5905

- Genova Diagnostics Europe Headquarters, Parkgate House, 356 West Barnes Lane, New Malden, Surrey KT3 6NB. Tel: +44 (0)20 8336 7750. Fax: +44 (0)20 8336 7751. Website: www.gdx.uk.net.

- YorkTest Laboratories, Freepost RLUC-GYTE-SGTU Yorktest, York YO10 5DQ, Freephone: 0800 074 6185. Website: www.yorktest.com.

Adrenal stress index or DHEA hormone testing

An adrenal stress profile (ASP) test measures cortisol and DHEA in saliva, while the DHEA test measures just this single hormone. You can arrange testing via a nutritional therapist or via Individual WellBeing in London. The cost, at the time of going to press, is £70 for the ASP and £45 for DHEA. Tel: +44 (0)20 8336 7750. Website: www.gdx.uk.net.

Food or chemical allergy and intolerance

YorkTest laboratories will test you for sensitivity to all foods including gluten, gliadin, wheat and yeast. They also sell a home test kit for food and chemical allergies that requires a pinprick blood sample. Call them for a FoodScan home test kit on freephone: 0800 074 6185. Visit www.yorktest.com for more information and prices.

Hair-mineral analysis test

To determine the presence of any toxic metals, a hair analysis can be arranged via your local nutritional therapist (see www.patrickholford.com for a referral).

Homocysteine test

YorkTest Laboratories produce a home test kit enabling you to take your own pinprick blood sample and return it to the lab for analysis. If your homocysteine level is high, full instructions are provided to help you reduce it. At the time of going to press, the test costs £75. Tel: 0800 458 2052. Website: www.yorktest.com. Also see www.thehfactor.com for details of other labs and supplements and to order *The H Factor* (see Recommended Reading, page 522).

Parasite and digestive stool analysis test

This helps to identify causes of digestive disorders. Such a test can be arranged through your local nutritional therapist (see www.patrickholford.com for a referral).

Supplement, remedy and supplier directory

Finding your own perfect supplement programme can be confusing, but my website www.patrickholford.com offers useful guidance.

The backbone of a good supplement programme is:

- A high-strength multivitamin

- Additional vitamin C

- An all-round antioxidant complex

- An essential-fat supplement containing Omega 3 and Omega 6 oils

In this section I list some of my favourite herbal, food and nutritional supplements. The addresses of the companies whose products I've referred to are given at the end.

Herbal, food and nutritional supplements

Adaptogenic herbs

These include ashwagandha, Asian and American ginseng (Panax), Siberian ginseng (Eleutherococcus), reishi, rhodiola and liquorice. These herbs are available in supplements. The amino acids tyrosine and phenylalanine are also important as the building material for dopamine, adrenalin and noradrenalin. Biocare's Awake contains these amino acids, plus ginseng and reishi. Take two in the morning. Liquorice provides adrenal support. Try Solgar's DGL Root Extract, morning only.

Aloe vera

This plant from the cactus family has many healing properties and supports healthy digestion, skin and immunity. As such it is a good all-round tonic. Aloe vera juices vary considerably in strength or dilution. What you should look for is the amount of MPS (mucopolysaccharide precipitating solids) per litre. You want more than 10,000 MPS for a high-quality product. My favourite is Aloe Vera from BioCare. Take two capsules daily.

Antioxidants

A good all-round antioxidant complex should provide vitamin A (betacarotene and/or retinol), vitamins C and E, zinc, selenium, glutathione or cysteine, anthocyanidins of berry extracts, lipoic acid and co-enzyme Q10. My favourite is BioCare's AGE Antioxidant followed by Solgar's Advanced Antioxidant Nutrients. Complexes of bioflavonoids, often found together with vitamin C, are available from both companies.

Bone health

Minerals such as calcium, magnesium, boron, zinc and silica plus vitamin C and D all help support bone health. My two favourite supplements are Solgar's Advanced Calcium Complex and BioCare's Osteoplex.

Brain support and phospholipid supplements

The brain needs essential fats (see below), phospholipids such as phosphatidyl choline and phosphatidyl serine, plus other key nutrients to function optimally. These include pyroglutamate and DMAE, from which the brain can make phosphatidyl choline. BioCare's Essential Omegas contains all these, plus some ginkgo.

Phosphatidyl serine is available in 100mg capsules from BioCare, Solgar and other companies. Phosphatidyl choline (PC) can be found in lecithin granules.

Calming nutrients and herbs

The contraction and relaxation of nerves and muscles is controlled by calcium and magnesium. BioCare's Chill formula contains amino acids, magnesium and herbs.

Hops, passion flower and valerian are traditionally classified as 'calming' herbs. Valerian, in fact, is more soporific. Try Solgar's Standardised Valerian Root Extract. BioCare's Chill provides hops, passion flower, glutamine and taurine, precursor of the neurotransmitter GABA, plus B vitamins.

Colon-cleansing and detox supplements

Various herbs and fibres help to cleanse the digestive tract and are a great support for a detox programme. My favourite is BioCare's ColonGuard.

Digestive enzymes and support

Any decent digestive enzyme needs to contain enzymes to digest protein (protease), carbohydrate (amylase) and fat (lipase). Some also contain amyloglucosidase (also called glucoamylase), which digests glucosides founds in certain beans and vegetables noted for their flatulent effects. One of my favourites is Solgar's Vegan Digestive Enzymes. BioCare's DigestPro is excellent.

Some people have low levels of betaine hydrochloride (stomach acid). You can supplement this on its own and, if it helps digestion, then lack of this may be your problem. Solgar's Digestive Aid supplement contains betaine HCL, plus other digestive enzymes. It is not vegetarian.

Essential fats and fish oil supplements

The most important Omega 3 fats are DHA and EPA, the richest source being cod liver oil. The most important Omega 6 fat is GLA, the richest source being borage (also known as starflower) oil. My favourite supplement is BioCare's Essential Omegas, which provides a highly concentrated mix of EPA, DHA and GLA. They also produce an Omega 3 Fish Oil supplement – good value, as is Seven Seas Extra High Strength Cod Liver Oil. Both these products have consistently proven the purest when tested for PCB residues, which are in almost all fish. Cod liver oil also contains vitamin A. BioCare's GLA Emulsion and Solgar's One-A-Day GLA are good value if you want only Omega 6 fats.

Eye support

Eyes need antioxidants and a good supply helps support healthy eyesight. Solgar's Bilberry, BioCare's EyeCare Plus and Solgar's Bilberry Ginkgo Eyebright Complex also provide vitamin A and other antioxidants such as vitamin C and E and selenium, which also protect against radiation from computer screens. BioCare's EyeCare Plus also has lutein, zeaxanthin and bilberry anthocyanidins which are powerful eye-friendly antioxidants.

Get Up and Go!

This tasty breakfast shake that you blend with some milk or juice, plus a banana or other fruit, provides significant amounts of vitamins and minerals plus protein from a blend of rice, soya and quinoa, plus fibre from rice and oat bran, plus essential fatty acids from sesame, sunflower and pumpkin seeds. At less than 500 calories, this adds up to a substantial and sustaining healthy breakfast. Tel: +44 (0)20 7499 4022.

Hair and skin

Particularly for women who are losing their hair, Nature's Best NutriHair (mail order on +44 (0)1892 552118), best taken three times a day, is excellent. MSM, the highly bioavailable form of sulphur, is great for the skin. MSM 1,000mg tablets are available from BioCare.

Hormone-friendly supplements

There are many herbs, vitamins, minerals and phytonutrients, such as isoflavones, that influence hormonal health. For the thyroid try BioCare's Thyro Complex. For women with periods try BioCare's Female Balance, which contains isoflavones. If you are menopausal, also try Female Balance. For men, try Saw Palmetto & Pygeum Bark, and Muira Puama & Damiana Aphrodisiaca.

Supplements containing isoflavones include Solgar's Super Concentrated Isoflavones and Novagen, which is derived from red clover.

Immune support and vitamin C supplements

Vitamin C is the nutrient most vital for keeping your immune system healthy. Also important are zinc, bioflavonoids and anthocyanidins which are found in berries, the best being elderberry and bilberry. Of the herbs, echinacea and cat's claw (*Uncaria tomentosa*) offer the best immune support. BioCare's ImmuneC provides vitamin C, bilberry extract, black elderberry extract and zinc. Grapefruit seed extract, known as citricidal, is another important part of a natural immune protection programme, and is also available through BioCare.

Joint support supplements and balms

Combinations of boswellia, curcumins, hop extract, glucosamine, MSM, plus Omega 3 fats all help to keep inflammation in check. For stiff or injured muscles or joints I recommend the herb boswellia, as well as ginger, capsaicin and peppermint. For skin-healing, ascorbyl palmitate (vitamin C) and aloe vera are excellent, as is MSM, a form of sulphur. BioCare's MSM Plus contains MSM, glucosamine and vitamin B6.

Multivitamin and mineral supplements

Supplementing the right multivitamin is the most important supplement decision you make. Most multivitamins are based on RDA levels of nutrients, which are not the same as optimum nutrition levels. The best multivitamin, based on optimum nutrition levels, is BioCare's Advanced Optimum Nutrition Formula. The second best is Solgar's VM2000. Both of these recommend 2 tablets a day. Advanced Optimum Nutrition Formula has better mineral levels, especially for calcium and magnesium. Ideally, both should be taken with an extra 1g of vitamin C. BioCare also do an excellent children's multivitamin called Optimum Nutrition for Children.

Probiotics

Probiotics are supplements of beneficial bacteria, the two main strains being *Lactobacillus acidophilus* and *Bifidobacterium bifidus*. There are various types of strain within these two, some more important in children, others in adults. There is quite some variability in amounts of bacteria (some labels say things like 'a billion viable organisms per capsule') and quality. I consider the following supplements to be high quality and well formulated: BioCare's Bifidoinfantis can be taken from birth to being weaned; once weaned, babies and children can take BioCare's Banana or Strawberry Acidophilus powder, plain Bioacidophilus capsules or Solgar's ABCDophilus. Adults can also try BioCare's DigestPro or BioCare's Bio-Acidophilus.

Supplements for snoring

A great supplement for snorers is available from Snore Away (mail order on +44 (0)1355 243091).

Weight-loss support

There are three supplements worth considering to support proper metabolism while you are on a weight-loss diet. These are 200 mcg of chromium, 750mg HCA (hydroxycitric acid) and 1,000mg CLA (conjugated linoleic acid). I recommend BioCare's Cinnachrome and GL Support. Solgar also have HCA and Chromium supplements.

Supplement resources

The following companies produce good-quality supplements that are widely available in the UK:

BioCare Available in most health food shops. Tel: +44 (0)121 433 3727. Website: www.BioCare.co.uk.

Seven Seas Specialise in cod liver oil, rich in omega-3 fats. Available in health food stores and pharmacies. Website: www.seven-seas.ltd.uk.

Solgar Available in most health food shops. Contact Solgar on +44 (0)1442 890355 for your nearest supplier. Website: www.solgar.co.uk.

Totally Nourish offer a wide range of health products, which I recommend, from supplements to water filters, by mail and online. But you can also order by phone on +44 (0)800 085 7749, or visit www.totallynourish.com.

And in other regions

South Africa Bioharmony produce a wide range of products in South Africa and other African countries. For details of your nearest supplier call 0860 888 339 or visit www.bioharmony.co.za.

Australia Solgar supplements are available in Australia. Website: www.solgar.com.au. Another good brand is Blackmores.

New Zealand BioCare products are available in New Zealand. Contact Aurora Natural Therapies, 12A Battys Road, Springlands, Blenheim 7201 or visit www.aurora.org.nz.

Singapore BioCare and Solgar products are available in Singapore. Contact Essential Living on 6276 1380 for your nearest supplier or visit www.essliv.com.

References

Part 1

1. Stephens, N. et al., 'Randomised controlled trial of vitamin E in patients with coronary disease: Cambridge Heart Antioxidant Study (CHAOS)', *Lancet*, vol 347 (9004), pp. 781–6 (1996).

2. Braly J. and Holford P., *The H Factor*, Piatkus Books (2003).

3. Bergkvist, L. et al., 'The risk of breast cancer after estrogen and estrogenprogestin replacement', *New England Journal of Medicine*, vol 32, pp. 293–7 (1989).

4. Rodriguez, C. et al., 'Estrogen replacement therapy and fatal ovarian cancer', *American Journal of Epedemiology*, vol 141:9, pp. 828–35 (1995).

5. Million Women Study collaborators, 'Breast cancer and hormone-replacement therapy in the Million Women Study', *Lancet*, vol 362, pp. 419–27 (2003).

6. 'The Aquatic Ape', *Nutrition and Health*, vol 9:3 (1993).

7. Ibid.

8. Willatts, P. et al., 'Effects of long-chain polyunsaturated fatty acid supplementation in infancy on cognitive function in later childhood', Maternal and Infant LCPUFA Workshop, Meeting of the American Oil Chemists Society, Kansas City, April 2003.

9. Cheraskin, E., 'The breakfast/lunch/dinner ritual,' *Journal of Orthomolecular Medicine*, vol 8, pp. 6–10 (1993).

10. Braly J. and Hoggan R., *Dangerous Grains: Why Gluten Cereal Grains May Be Hazardous to Your Health*, Avery Publishing Group, UK (2002).

11. Popper, H. and Steigmann, F. J., *American Medical Association*, vol 123, pp.1108–14 (1943).

12. Hoffer, A. and Osmond, H., 'Treatment of schizophrenia with nicotinic acid', *Acta Psychiatrica Scandinavia*, vol 40, pp. 171–89 (1964); Hoffer, A., 'Chronic schizophrenic patients treated ten years or more', *Journal of Orthomolecular Medicine*, vol 9:1, pp. 1–37 (1994).

13. Barker, H., MRC Environmental Epidemiology Unit, Southampton, UK.

14. Bryce-Smith, D., 'Pre-natal zinc deficiency', *Nursing Times*, pp. 44–6 (1986).

15. Schoenthaler, S. et al., 'Controlled trial of vitamin-mineral supplementation on intelligence and brain function', *Personality and Individual Differences,* vol 12:4, pp. 343–50 (1991); Schoenthaler, S. et al., 'Controlled trial of vitamin-mineral supplementation: effects on intelligence and performance', ibid. pp. 351–62.

16. Gesch, B., 'The SCASO Project', *International Journal of Biosocial Medical Research*, vol 12(1), pp. 41–68 (1990).

17. Koyama, K. et al., 'Efficacy of methylcobalamin on lowering total homocysteine plasma concentrations in haemodialysis patients receiving high-dose folate supplementation', *Nephrology, Dialysis, Transplantation: Official Publication of the European Dialysis and Transplant Association*, vol 17, pp. 916–22 (2002).

18. Schectman, G. et al., 'Ascorbic acid requirements for smokers: analysis of a population survey', *American Journal of Clinical Nutrition*, vol 53:6, pp. 1466–70 (June 1991).

19. Ash, J., 'Investigation into the mechanisms of the effects of 220 dyes on hyperactive children', final-year project, School of Biological Sciences, University of Surrey, Guildford, UK. Copy held by Dr Neil Ward.

20. Heaton, S. A. A., *Organic Farming, Food Quality and Human Health: A review of the evidence,* Soil Association, Bristol, UK (2001).

21. MAFF, *Annual Report of the Working Party on Pesticide Residues 1998*, Health and Safety executive, MAFF Publications, London (1999).

22. Abou-Donia, M. B. et al., 'Neurotoxicity resulting from coexposure to pyridostigmine bromide, DEET and permethrin: implications for gulf war chemical exposures', *Journal of Toxicology and Environmental Health*, vol 48, pp. 35–65 (1996).

23. Nott, T., 'Washing aid for fruit and vegetables', *Pesticides News*, vol 35 (1997) and 'Pesticides in fruit and veg', *Health Which?*, pp. 8–11 (June 1998).

24. Benbrook, C. M., *Impacts of Genetically Engineered Crops on Pesticide Use in the United States: The First Eight Years*, BioTech InfoNet, Technical Paper No 6 (November 2003).

Part 2

1. BMA 'The impact of genetic modification on agriculture', *Food & Health Report*, BMA (1999).

2. Dickerson, J.W.T. et al., 'Disease patterns in individuals with different eating patterns', *Journal of the Royal Society of Health*, vol 105, pp. 191–4 (1985).

3. *American Journal of Public Health* (1997).

4. Knight, E. et al., *Annals Internal Medicine*, vol 138(6), pp. 460–7 (18 March 2003).

5. Feskanich, D. et al, 'Protein consumption and bone fractures in women', *American Journal of Epedemiology*, vol 143, 472–9 (1996).

6. Reddy, S. et al., 'Effect of low-carbohydrate, high-protein diets on acid-base balance, stone-forming propensity', *American Journal of Kidney Diseases*, vol 40, pp. 265–74 (2002).

7. Murata, K. et al., 'Delayed brainstem auditory evoked potential latencies in 14 year old children exposed to methylmercury', *Journal of Pediatrics* (2004); Grandjean, P. et al, 'Cardia autonomic activity in methylmercury neurotoxicity: 14 year follow-up of Faroese birth cohort', ibid.

8. Anderson et al., 'Breast-feeding and cognitive development: a meta-analysis', *American Journal of Clinical Nutrition*, vol 70, pp. 525–35 (1999).

9. Moss, M. and Freed, D., 'The cow and the coronary', *International Journal of Cardiology*, vol 87, pp. 203–16 (2003).

10. Malin, A. et al., 'Evaluation of the synergistic effect of insulin resistance and IGF on the risk of breast carcinoma', *Cancer*, vol 100(4), pp. 694–700 (2004).

11. Oliver, S. E. et al., 'Screen-detected prostate cancer and IGF', *International Journal of Cancer*, vol 108(6), pp. 887–92 (2004).

12. *The Immunology Review*, vol 2:3 (Spring 1994).

13. Granfeldt, Y., Byorck, I. and Hagander, B., 'On the importance of processing conditions, product thickness and egg addition for the glycaemic and hormonal responses to pasta: a comparison of bread made with "pasta ingredients",' *European Journal of Clinical Nutrition*, vol 45, pp. 489–99 (1991).

14. Richardson, N. J., Rogers, P.J. et al., 'Mood and performance effects of caffeine in relation to acute and chronic caffeine deprivation', *Pharmacology, Biochemistry and Behavior*, vol 52(2), pp. 313–20 (1995).

15. Gilliland, K. and Andress, D., 'Ad lib caffeine consumption, symptoms of caffeinism, and academic performance', *American Journal of Psychiatry*, vol 138(4), pp. 512–14 (1981).

16. See full references at http://www.doctoryourself.com/caffeine_allergy.html.

17. Davies, S., 'The myth of the balanced diet', Power of Prevention Conference 1993. Available from the Institute of Optimum Nutrition (cassette T16, 'The myth of the balanced diet').

18. Bateman Catering Organisation, 'A square meal for Britain?' (1981).

19. Seal, E. C., Metz, J., Flicker, L. and Melny, J., 'A randomized, double-blind, placebo-controlled study of oral vitamin B12 supplementation in older patients with subnormal or borderline serum vitamin B12 concentrations', *Journal of the American Geriatric Society*, vol 50(1), pp. 146–51 (2002).

20. *The Vitamin Controversy*, ION Press (1987).

21. Cheraskin, E. et al., 'Establishing a suggested optimum nutrition allowance (SONA)', (1994); 'What is optimum?', *Optimum Nutrition Magazine*, vol 7.2, pp. 46–7 (1994).

22. Milunsky, A. et al., 'Multivitamin/folic acid supplementation in early pregnancy reduces the prevalence of neural tube defects', *Journal of the American Medical Association*, vol 262:20, pp. 2847–52 (1989).

23. Chandra, R. K., 'Effect of vitamin and trace-element supplementation on cognitive function in elderly subjects', *Nutrition*, vol 17(9), pp. 709–12 (2001).

24. Chandra, R. K., 'Study of multivitamin/mineral supplementation in elderly', *Lancet*, vol 340, pp. 1124–7 (1992).

25. Hemila, H. et al., 'Vitamin C and the common cold: a retrospective analysis of Chalmers' review', *Journal of American College Nutrition*, vol 14:2, pp. 116–23 (1995).

26. Stephens, N. et al., 'Randomised controlled trial of vitamin E in patients with coronary disease: Cambridge Heart Antioxidant Study (CHAOS)', *Lancet*, vol 347 (9004), pp. 781–6 (1996).

27. Geleijnse, J. et al., 'Reduction of blood pressure with a low sodium, high potassium, high magnesium salt in older subjects with mild to moderate hypertension', *British Medical Journal*, vol 309, pp. 436–40 (1994).

28. Salonen, J. T., Nyyssonen, K., Korpela, H. et al., 'High stored iron levels are associated with excess risk of myocardial infarction in Eastern Finnish men', *Circulation*, vol 86, pp. 803–11(1992).

29. Lodge Rees, E., 'Aluminium toxicity as indicted by hair analysis', *Journal of Orthomolecular Psychiatry*, vol 8:1, pp. 37–43 (1979).

30. Cowdry, Quentin and Stokes, 'Aluminium in the water causes senile dementia', *Daily Telegraph* (13 January 1989).

31. Rifat, L. et al., 'Effect of exposure of miners to aluminium powder', *Lancet*, vol 336, pp. 1162–5 (1990).

32. Suay Llopis, L. and Ballester Diez, F., 'Review of studies on exposure to aluminium and AD',

Revista Espana Salud Publica, 76(6), pp. 645–58 (2002); Campbell, A., 'The potential role of aluminium in AD', *Nephrology Dialysis Transplantation*, vol 17 Suppl 2, pp. 17–20 (2002).

33. Becaria, A., Bondy, S. C. and Campbell, A., 'Aluminum and copper interact in the promotion of oxidative but not inflammatory events: implications for AD', *Journal of Alzheimer's Disease*, vol 5(1), pp. 31–8 (2003).

34. Holford, P. and Pfeiffer, C., *Mental Health and Mental Illness – The Nutrition Connection*, ION Press (1996). Also see www.mentalhealthproject/features for feature on copper and schizophrenia.

35. Needleman, H. L. and Gatsonis, C. A., 'Low level lead exposure and the IQ of children', *Journal of the American Medical Association*, vol 263(5), pp. 673–8 (1990).

36. Yule, Q., Lansdown, R. et al., 'The relationship between blood lead concentrations, intelligence and attainment in a school population: a pilot study', *Developmental Medicine and Child Neurology*, vol 23(5), pp. 567–76 (1981).

37. Ward, N. I. and Bryce-Smith, D., 'Lead, cadmium and zinc levels in relation to fetal development and abnormalities', *Heavy Metals in the Environment*, vol 2, pp. 280–4 (1995).

38. Smith, L. H., MD, with Hattersley, J. G., MA, *The Infant Survival Guide: Protecting Your Baby from the Dangers of Crib Death, Vaccines and Other Environmental Hazards*, Smart Publications, Petaluma, CA (2002).

39. Mercola, Dr J., 'What you must know before eating fish', www.mercola.com (2002).

40. *Journal of the American Medical Association*, vol 289, pp. 1667–74 (2003).

41. Wenstrup, D. et al., 'Trace element imbalances in isolated subcellular fractions of AD patients', *Brain Research*, vol 553, pp. 125–31 (1990).

42. Hock, C. et al., 'Increased blood mercury levels in patients with AD', *Journal of Neural Transmission*, vol 105(1), pp. 59–68 (1998).

43. Leong, C. C. et al., 'Retrograde degeneration of neurite membrane structural integrity of nerve growth cones following in vitro exposure to mercury', *Neuroreport*, vol 12(4), pp. 733–7 (2001). See also www.commons.ucalgary.ca/mercury.

44. Goyer, R. and Cherian, M.G., 'Ascorbic acid and EDTA treatment of lead toxicity in rats', *Life Science*, vol 24(5), pp. 433–8 (1979).

45. O'Flaherty, E. J., 'Modeling normal aging bone loss, with consideration of bone loss in osteoporosis', *Toxicological Sciences*, vol 55(1), pp. 171–88 (2000).

46. Aaman, Z. et al., 'Plasma concentrations of vitamins A and E and carotenoids in Alzheimer's Disease', *Age and Aging*, vol 21:2, pp. 91–4 (March 1992).

47. Morris, M. et al., 'Vitamin E and vitamin C supplement use and risk incident Alzheimer disease', *Alzheimer Disease and Associated Disorders*, vol 12, pp. 121–6 (1998).

48. Morris, M. et al., 'Dietary intake of antioxidant nutrients and the risk of incident AD', *Journal of the American Medical Association*, vol 284(24), pp. 3230–7 (2002). Also see pp. 3223–61.

49. Jacques, P. F., 'Relationship of vitamin C status to cholesterol and blood pressure', *Annals of the New York Academy of Sciences*, vol 669, pp. 205–14 (1992).

50. Bond, G. et al., 'Dietary vitamin A and lung cancer: Results of a case control study among chemical workers', *Nutrition and Cancer*, vol 9, pp. 109–21 (1987).

51. Robertson, J. M. et al., 'Vitamin E intake and risk of cataracts in humans', *Annals of the New York Academy of Sciences*, vol 570, pp. 372–82 (1989).

52. Mayne, S. T., 'Dietary beta carotene and lung cancer risk in US nonsmokers', *Journal of the National Cancer Institute*, vol 86(1), pp. 33–8 (1994).

53. Garwal, H. S. et al., 'Response of oral leukophakia to beta carotene', *Journal of Clinical Oncology*, vol 8, pp. 1715–20 (1990).

54. Manson, J. E. et al., 'A prospective study of antioxidant vitamins and incidence of coronary heart disease in women', *Abstract in Circulation*, vol 84:4, pp. 11–546 (1991).

55. Osilesi, O. et al., 'Blood pressure and plasma lipids during ascorbic acid supplementation in borderline hypertensive and normotensive adults', *Nutrition Research*, vol 11, pp. 405–12 (1991).

56. Wald, D. S and Morris, J. K., *British Medical Journal*, vol 325, pp. 1202 (2002).

57. Clerk, M. et al., 'MTHFR 677C>T Polymorphism and Risk of Coronary Heart Disease', *Journal of the American Medical Association*, vol 288(16), pp. 2023–31 (2002).

58. Lichtenstein, P. et al., 'Environmental and heritable factors in the causation of cancer', *New England Journal of Medicine*, vol 343(2), pp. 135–6 (2000).

59. Toshifumi, M. et al., 'Elevated plasma homocysteine levels and risk of silent brain infarction in elderly people', *Stroke,* vol 32, p. 1116 (2001).

60. Seshadri, S. et al., 'Plasma homocysteine as a risk factor for dementia and Alzheimer's disease', *New England Journal of Medicine*, vol 346(7), pp. 476–83 (2002).

61. Vollset, S. E. et al., 'Plasma total homocysteine and cardiovascular and noncardiovascular mortality: the Hordaland Homocysteine Study', *American Journal of Clinical Nutrition*, vol 74(1), pp. 130–6 (2001).

62. Koyama, K. et al., 'Efficacy of methylcobalamin on lowering total homocysteine plasma concentrations in haemodialysis patients receiving high-dose folate supplementation', *Nephrology Dialysis Transplantation*, vol 17, pp. 916–22 (2002).

63. McGregor et al., 'Betaine supplementation decreases post-methionine hyperhomocysteinemia in chronic renal failure', *Kidney International*, vol 61(3), pp. 1040–6 (2002).

64. You, W. C. et al., *Journal of the National Cancer Institute*, vol 81(2), pp. 162–4 (1989).

65. Steinmetz et al., *American Journal of Epidemiology*, vol 139(1), pp. 1–15 (1994).

66. Carper, J., *Stop Ageing Now*, pp.162 and 325 Thorsons, (1997).

67. Chung, M. J., Lee, S. H. and Sung, N. J., 'Inhibitory effect of whole strawberries, garlic juice or kale juice on endogenous formation of N-nitrosodimethylamine in humans', *Cancer Letters*, vol 182(1), pp. 1–10 (2002).

68. Xue, H. et al., 'Inhibition of cellular transformation by berry extracts', *Carcinogenesis,* vol 22(5), pp. 831–3 (2001).

69. Loarca-Pina, G. et al., 'Antimutagenicity of ellagic acid against aflatoxin B1 in the Salmonella microsuspension assay', *Mutation Research*, 360(1), pp.15–21 (1996).

70. Narayanan, B. A. et al., 'p53/p21 (WAF1/CIP1) expression and its possible role in G1 arrest and apoptosis in ellagic acid treated cancer cells', *Cancer Letters*, vol 136(2), pp. 215–21 (1999).

71. Stoner, G. D. et al., 'Isothiocyanates and freeze-dried strawberries as inhibitors of esophageal cancer', *Toxicological Sciences*, vol 52 Suppl 2, pp. 95–100 (1999).

72. Casto, B. C. et al., 'Chemoprevention of oral cancer by black raspberries', *Anticancer Research*, vol 22(6C), pp. 4005–15 (2002).

73. Gerster, H., 'The potential role for lycopene in human health', *Journal of American College Nutrition*, vol 16, pp. 109–26 (1997).

74. Goel, R. K. et al., 'Anti-ulcerogenic effect of banana powder (Musa sapientum var. paradisiaca) and its effect on mucosal resistance', *Journal of Ethnopharmacology*, vol 18(1), pp. 33–44 (1986).

75. *American Journal of Clinical Nutrition*, vol 65 (1997).

76. Thomas, B. (ed.), *Manual of Dietetic Practice*, 3rd edn, Blackwell (2001).

77. Kleiner, S. M., 'Water: an essential but overlooked nutrient', *Journal of the American Dietary Association*, vol 99(2), pp. 200–6 (1999).

78. Batmanghelidj, F., *Your Body's Many Cries for Water*, Tagman Press (1992).

79. Grandjean, A. C. et al., 'The effect of caffeinated, non-caffeinated, caloric and non-caloric beverages on hydration', *Journal of American College Nutrition*, vol 19(5), pp. 591–600 (2000).

Part 3

1. Niedzielkin, K. and Kordecki, H., 'The treatment of irritable bowel syndrome: probiotics in the modification of bacteria in the colon', *Gastroenterologia Polska*, vol 5 Suppl 1, p. 26 (1998).

2. King, T. et al., 'Abnormal colonic fermentation in irritable bowel syndrome', *Lancet*, vol 352, pp. 1187–9 (1998).

3. Peltonen, R. et al., 'Changes of faecal flora in rheumatoid arthritis during fasting and one-year vegetarian diet', *British Journal of Rheumatology*, vol 33, pp. 638–43 (1994).

4. Majamaa, H. and Isolaui, E., 'Probiotics: a novel approach in the management of food allergy', *Journal of Allergy and Clinical Immunology*, vol 99, pp. 179–85 (1997).

5. Hunter, J. O., 'Food allergy – or enterometabolic disorder?' *Lancet*, vol 338, pp. 495–6 (1991).

6. Stephens, N. et al. 'Randomised controlled trial of vitamin E in patients with coronary disease: Cambridge Heart Antioxidant Study (CHAOS)', *Lancet*, vol 347 (9004), pp. 781–6 (1996).

7. Stampfer, M. J. et al, 'Vitamin E consumption and the risk of coronary disease in women', *New England Journal of Medicine*, vol 328(20), pp. 1444–9 (1993).

8. Rimm, E. B., et al., 'Vitamin E consumption and the risk of coronary heart disease in men', *New England Journal of Medicine*, vol 328(20), pp. 1450–6 (1993).

9. Heart Protection Study collaborative group, 'MRC/BHF Heart Protection Study', *Lancet*, vol 360, pp. 23–3 (2002).

10. Din, N. et al., 'Omega 3 fats and cardiovascular disease', *British Medical Journal*, vol 328, pp. 30–5 (2004).

11. Holmquist, C., Larsson, S., Wolk, A. and de Faire, U., 'Multivitamin supplements are inversely associated with risk of myocardial infarction in men and women – Stockholm Heart Epidemiology Program (SHEEP)', *Journal of Nutrition*, vol 133(8), pp. 2650–4 (2003).

12. Mullins, K., 'The Blood Pressure Project' (1990). Copy held at ION library, London.

13. As reported in *The New Super-Nutrition* by Richard Passwater, Pocket Books (1991).

14. Kritchevsky, S. and Kritchevsky, D., *Journal of American College Nutrition*, vol 19 Suppl 5, pp. 5495–555 (2000).

15. *Optimum Nutrition* magazine, vol 8:2, pp. 8–9 (Autumn 1995).

16. Cheraskin, E., 'If high blood cholesterol is bad – is low good?', *Journal of Orthomolecular Medicine*, vol 1:3, pp. 176–83 (1986).

17. Colgan, M., 'Effects of nutrient supplements on athletic performance', paper given to the US Navy Research and Development Center, San Diego (April 1983).

18. Saynor, R. et al., 'The long-term effect of dietary supplementation with fish lipid concentrate on serum lipids, bleeding time, platelets and angina', *Atherosclerosis*, vol 50, pp. 3–101 (1984).

19. Pauling, L. and Rath, M., 'A unified theory of human cardiovascular disease leading the way to the abolition of this disease as a cause for human mortality', *Journal of Orthomolecular Medicine*, vol 7:1, pp. 5–12 (1992).

20. *Newsweek*, 11 August 1997.

21. Selhub, J. et al., 'Association between plasma homocysteine concentrations and extracranial carotid artery stenosis', *New England Journal of Medicine*, vol 332(5), pp. 286–91 (1995).

22. Graham, I. et al., 'Plasma homocysteine as a risk factor for vascular disease', *Journal of the American Medical Association*, vol 277(22), pp. 1775–81 (1997).

23. These 'in vitro' studies on human T-cells show that vitamin C suppresses the HIV virus in both chronically and latently infected cells, while AZT has no significant effect. It is a tragedy that this simple, non-toxic treatment hasn't been further tested. Harakeh, S., and Jariwalla, R.J., 'Ascorbate effect on cytokine stimulation of HIV production' *Nutrition*, vol 11(5 Suppl), pp. 684–7 (September–October 1995). Also see Harakeh, S., and Jariwalla, R.J., 'NF-kappa B-independent suppression of HIV expression by ascorbic acid', *AIDS Research and Human Retroviruses*, vol 13(3), pp. 235–9 (February 1997); Harakeh, S., Niedzwiecki, A., and Jariwalla, R.J., 'Mechanistic aspects of ascorbate inhibition of human immunodeficiency virus', *Chemico-Biological Interactions*, vol 91(2–3), pp. 207–15 (June 1994); Harakeh, S., Jariwalla, R.J., 'Comparative study of the anti-HIV activities of ascorbate and thiol-containing reducing agents in chronically HIV-infected cells', *American Journal of Clinical Nutrition*, vol 54(6 Suppl), pp. 1231S–1235S (December 1991); Harakeh, S., Jariwalla, R.J., and Pauling, L., 'Suppression of human immunodeficiency virus replication by ascorbate in chronically and acutely infected cells', *Proceedings of the National Academy of Sciences USA*, vol 87(18), pp. 7245–9 (September 1990).

24. Geoffrey Cannon, *Superbug*, Virgin (1995).

25. Kiecolt-Glaser, J. K. et al., 'Modulation of cellular immunity in medical students', *Journal of Behavioural Medicine*, vol 9, pp. 5–21 (1986).

26. Chandra, R. K., 'Study of multivitamin/mineral supplementation in elderly', *Lancet*, vol 340 (8828), pp. 1124–7 (1992).

27. *New Scientist*, 17 December 1994.

28. Hilton, E. et al., 'Ingestion of yoghurt containing *Lactobacillus acidophilus* as prophylaxis for candidal vaginitis', *Annals of Medicine*, vol 116, pp. 353–7 (1992).

29. Ginty, F., 'Dietary protein and bone health', *Proceedings of the Nutrition Society*, vol 62(4), pp. 867–76 (2003).

30. Kremer et al, *Lancet*, vol 1, pp. 184–7 (1985).

31. Caterson, B. et al., Kennedy Institute of Rheumatology Conference report (awaiting publication), (2004).

32. Singh, G. B. et al, 'New phytotherapeutic agent for treatment of arthritis and allied disorders with novel mode of action', IV and Int. Congress on Phytotherapy, Abstract SL74, Munich, Germany; Gupta, V. et al., 'Chemistry and pharmacology of gum resin of Boswellia Serrata', *Indian Drugs*, vol 24(5), pp. 221–31 (1986).

33. Kulkarni, R. et al., 'Treatment of osteoarthritis with a herbal formulation: a double-blind, placebo controlled, crossover study', *Journal of Ethnopharmacology*, vol 33, pp 91–5 (1991); also see same author, *Indian Journal of Pharmacology*, vol 24, pp 98–101 (1992).

34. Ibid.

35. Towhead, T. et al., 'Glucosamine therapy for treating osteoarthritis', *Cochrane Database of Systematic Reviews* 2001, 1: CD002946.

36. Houpt, J. et al., *Journal of Rheumatology*, vol 26, pp. 2423–30 (1999).

37. Schallreuter, K. and Wood, J., 'Free radical reduction in the human epidermis', *Free Rad Biol Med* vol 6, pp. 519–32 (1989).

Part 4

1. Benton, D. and Roberts, G., 'Effect of vitamin and mineral supplementation on intelligence of school children', *Lancet*, vol 1(8578), pp. 140–3 (1988).

2. Chandra, R. K., 'Effect of vitamin and trace-element supplementation on cognitive function in elderly subjects', *Nutrition*, vol 17(9), pp. 709–12 (2001).

3. Medical Reseach Council, research on higher IQ and premature babies (see www.mrc.ac.uk).

4. Harrel, R., 'Can nutritional supplements help mentally retarded children? An exploratory study', *Proceedings of the National Academy of Sciences*, vol 78:1, pp. 574–8 (1981).

5. Gesch, B., 'Influence of supplementary vitamins, minerals and essential fatty acids on the anti-social behaviour of young adult prisoners', *British Journal of Psychiatry*, vol 181, pp. 22–8 (2002).

6. Nemets, B. et al., 'Addition of omega-3 fatty acid to maintenance medication treatment for recurrent unipolar depressive disorder', *American Journal of Psychiatry*, vol 159, pp. 477–9 (2002).

7. Puri, B. et al., 'Eicosapentaenoic acid in treatment-resistant depression', *Archives of General Psychiatry*, vol 59(1), Letters to the Editor (2002).

8. Pyapali, G. et al., 'Prenatal dietary choline supplementation', *Journal of Neurophysiology*, vol 79(4), pp. 1790–6 (1998); Meck, W. H. et al., *Neuroreport*, vol 8, pp. 2831–5 (1997).

9. Crook, T. et al., 'Effects of phosphatidyl serine in age-associated memory impairment', *Neurology*, vol 41(5), pp. 644–9 (1991).

10. Pepeu, G. et al., 'Neurochemical actions of "Nootropic Drugs"', *Advances in Neurology* vol 51: *Alzheimer's Disease*, Raven Press, New York (1990).

11. Bartus, R. T. et al., 'Profound effects of combining choline and piracetam on memory enhancement and cholinergic function in aged rats', *Neurobiology of Ageing*, vol 2, pp. 105–11 (1981).

12. Shauss, A.G., 'Nutrition and behavior', *Journal of Applied Nutrition*, vol 35(1), pp. 30–5 (1983); MIT Conference Proceedings on Research Strategies for Assessing the Behavioural Effects of Foods and Nutrients (1982).

13. Benton, D. et al., 'Mild hypoglycaemia and questionnaire measures of aggression', *Biological Psychology*, vol 14(1–2), pp. 129–35 (1982); Roy, A. et al., 'Monoamines, glucose metabolism, aggression toward self and others', *International Journal of Neuroscience*, vol 41(3–4), pp. 261–4 (1988); Schauss, A.G., *Diet, Crime and Delinquency*, Parker House (1980); Virkkunen, M., 'Reactive hypoglycaemic tendency among arsonists', *Acta Psychiatrica Scandinavica*, vol 69(5), pp. 445–52 (1984); Virkkunen, M. and Narvanen, S., 'Tryptophan and serotonin levels during the glucose tolerance test among habitually violent and impulsive offenders', *Neuropsychobiology*, vol 17(1–2), pp. 19–23 (1987); Yaryura-Tobias, J. and Neziroglu F., 'Violent behaviour, brain dysrythmia and glucose dysfunction. A new syndrome', *Journal of Orthomolecular Psychiatry*, vol 4, pp. 182–5 (1975).

14. Bruce, M. and Lader, M., 'Caffeine abstention and the management of anxiety disorders', *Psychological Medicine*, vol 19, pp. 211–14 (1989); Wendel, W. and Beebe, W., 'Glycolytic activity in schizophrenia', in *Orthomolecular Psychiatry: Treatment of schizophrenia*, Hawkins, D. and Pauling, L. (eds) (1973).

15. Prinz, R. and Riddle, D., 'Associations between nutrition and behaviour in 5 year old children', *Nutrition Review*, vol 43, suppl (1986).

16. Christensen, L., 'Psychological distress and diet – effects of sucrose and caffeine', *Journal of Applied Nutrition*, vol 40(1), pp. 44–50 (1988).

17. Fullerton D. et al., 'Sugar, opionoids and binge eating', *Brain Research Bulletin*, vol 14(6), pp. 273–80 (1985).

18. Christensen, L., 'Psychological distress and diet', *Journal of Applied Nutrition*, vol 40, pp 44–50 (1988).

19. Colgan, M. and Colgan L, 'Do nutrient supplements and dietary changes affect learning and emotional reactions of children with learning difficulties? A controlled series of 16 cases', *Nutritional Health*, vol 3, pp. 69–77 (1984); Goldman, J. et al., 'Behavioural effects of sucrose on preschool children', *Journal of Abnormal Child Psychology*, vol 14(4), pp. 565–77 (1986); Lester, M. et al., 'Refined carbohydrate intake, hair cadmium levels and cognitive functioning in children', *Nutrition and Behaviour*, vol 1, pp. 3–13 (1982); Schoenthaler, S. et al., 'The impact of low food additive and sucrose diet on academic performance in 803 New York City public schools', *International Journal of Biosocial Research*, vol 8(2), pp. 185–95 (1986).

20. Ichazo, O., *The Arican*, vol 2:2 (Spring 1990). Also see, on www.patrickholford.com, the report entitled 'How Drugs Deplete Vital Energy' – an interview with Oscar Ichazo.

21. Colgan, M., 'Effects of nutrient supplements on athletic performance', paper given to the US Navy Research and Development Center, San Diego (April 1983).

22. Kotulak, R. and Gomer, P., *Aging On Hold – Secrets of Living Younger Longer*, Chapter 5 by Walford, R., pp. 51–73, Tribune Publishing, USA (1992).

23. Hagen, T. M. et al., *Proceedings of the National Academy of Science* (USA), vol 99, pp. 1870–5, pp. 1876–81 and 2356–61 (2002).

24. *American Journal of Clinical Nutrition*, vol 64, pp. 190–6 (1996).

25. Vollset, S. E. et al, 'Plasma total homocysteine and cardiovascular and noncardiovascular mortality: the Hordaland Homocsyteine Study', *American Journal of Clinical Nutrition*, vol 74(1), pp. 130–6 (2001).

26. Waller, R., 'The Diseases of Civilisation,' *The Ecologist*, vol 1(2) (1970).

27. World Cancer Research Fund, 'Food, Nutrition and the Prevention of Cancer: A global perspective', 1997.

28. Epstein, S., 'Winning the War against Cancer – are we even fighting it?' *The Ecologist*, vol 28(2), pp. 69–80 (1998).

29. Huang, L. A. et al., 'Treatment of acute promyelocytic leukemia with all trans retinoic acid: a five-year experience', *Chinese Medical Journal*, vol 106:10, pp. 743–8 (1993).

30. Lippman, S. M. et al., 'Molecular epidemiology and retinoid chemoprevention of head and neck cancer', *Journal of the National Cancer Institute.*, vol 89:3, pp. 199–21 (5 Feb 1997); Lippman, S. M. and Hong, W. K., '13-cis-retinoic acid plus interferon-alpha in solid tumors: keeping the cart behind the horse', *Annals of Oncology* (Netherlands), vol 5:5, pp. 391–3 (May 1994).

31. Hirayama, T., 'A large scale cohort study on cancer risks by diet – with special reference to the risk reducing effects of green-yellow vegetable consumption', *Princess Takamatsu Symposium* (USA), vol 16, pp. 41–53 (1985).

32. Omenn, G. et al., 'The Beta-Carotene and Retinol Efficacy Trial (CARET)', *New England Journal of Medicine*, vol 334, pp. 1150–5 (1996).

33. Albanes, D. et al., 'Alpha-tocopherol and beta-carotene supplements and lung cancer', *Journal of the National Cancer Institute*, vol 88, pp. 1560–70 (1996); 'The effect of vitamin E and beta carotene on the incidence of lung cancer', *New England Journal of Medicine*, vol 330(15), pp. 1029–35 (1994).

34. Baron, J. et al., 'Neoplastic and antineoplastic effects of beta-carotene on colorectal adenoma', *Journal of the National Cancer Institute*, vol 95(10), pp. 717–22 (2003).

35. Mannisto S, et al., 'Dietary carotenoids and risk of lung cancer in a pooled analysis of seven cohort studies', *Cancer Epidemiology Biomarkers and Prevention*, vol 13(1), pp. 40–8 (2004).

36. Cameron, E. and Pauling, L., 'Supplemental ascorbate in the supportive treatment of cancer: prolongation of survival times in terminal human cancer', *Proceedings of the National Academy of Sciences*, vol 73, pp. 3685–9 (1976); Cameron, E. and Pauling, L., 'Supplemental ascorbate in the supportive treatment of cancer: a re-evaluation of prolongation of survival times in terminal human cancer', ibid., vol 75, pp. 4538–42 (1978).

37. Block, G., 'Epidemiologic evidence regarding vitamin C and cancer', *American Journal of Clinical Nutrition*, vol 54, Suppl 6, pp. 1310–14 (1991).

38. *American Journal of Clinical Nutrition*, vol 64, pp. 190–6 (1996).

39. Salonen, J. T., 'Risk of cancer in relation to serum concentrations of selenium and vitamin A and E', *British Medical Journal*, vol 209, pp. 417–20 (1985).

40. Yu, S. Y. et al., 'Chemoprevention trial of human hepatitis with selenium supplementation in China', *Biological Trace Element Research*, vol 1–2, pp. l5–22 (1989).

41. See http://news.bbc.co.uk/go/em/fr/-/1/hi/health/3122033.stm.

42. Chang, K-J. et al., 'Influences of percutaneous administration of estradiol and progesterone on human breast epithelial cell cycle in vivo', *Fertility and Sterility*, vol 63:4, p. 785 (April 1995).

43. Emery University School of Public Health.

44. Beral, V.; Million Women Study collaborators, 'Breast cancer and hormone-replacement therapy in the Million Women Study', *Lancet*, vol 362, pp. 414–15 (2003).

45. Lee, J., Zava, D. and Hopkins, V., *What Your Doctor May Not Tell You About Breast Cancer*, Thorsons (2002).

46. Wu, L. L. and Wu, J. T., 'Hyperhomocysteinemia is a risk factor for cancer and a new potential tumor marker', *Clinica Chimica ACTA*, vol 322, pp. 21–8 (2002).

47. Prinz-Langenohl, R., Fohr, I. and Pietrzik, K., 'Beneficial role for folate in the prevention of colorectal and breast cancer', *European Journal of Nutrition*, vol 40, pp. 98–105 (2001).

48. Hirayama, T., 'A large scale cohort study on cancer risks by diet – with special reference to the risk reducing effects of green-yellow vegetable consumption', *Princess Takamatsu Symposium* (USA), vol 16, pp. 41–53 (1985).

49. You, W. C. et al., *Journal of the National Cancer Institute*, vol 81(2), pp. 162–4 (1989); Abdullah, T. H. et al., *Journal of the National Medical Association*, vol 80(4), pp. 439–45 (1988).

50. Peters, R. K. et al., 'Cancer Causes and Control', vol 3, pp. 457–73 (1992); Gollein, B. R. and Gorbach, S. L., *Journal of the National Cancer Institute*, vol 64, pp. 255–61 (1980).

51. Douglas, R. M., Chalker, E. B. and Treacy B., 'Vitamin C for preventing and treating the common cold', *Cochrane Database of Systematic Reviews*. 2000;(2):CD000980.

52. Zakay-Rones, Z. et al., 'Inhibition of several strains of influenza virus in vitro and reduction of symptoms by an elderberry extract (Sambucus nigra L.) during an outbreak of influenza B Panama', *Alternative and Complementary Medicine*, vol 1:4, pp. 361–9 (1995).

53. Royal College of Physicians special report, 'Containing the Allergy Epidemic' (June 2003).

54. US News and World Report, vol 106(7), 77(2) (20 Feb. 1989).

55. Fasano, A. and Catassi, C., 'Current Approaches to Diagnosing and Treating Celiac Disease', *Gastroenterology*, vol 120, pp. 636–51 (2001); also see http://www.celiaccenter.org.

56. Brand-Miller, J. et al., 'Glycemic Index and obesity', *American Journal of Clinical Nutrition*, vol 76, suppl, pp. 2815–55 (2002).

57. Slabber, M. et al., 'Effects of a low-insulin-response, energy restricted diet on weight loss and plasma insulin concentrations in hyperinsulinemic obese females', *American Journal of Clinical Nutrition*, vol 60(1), pp. 48–53 (1994).

58. Cangiano, C., Ceci, F., Cascino, A., Del Ben, M., Laviano, A., Muscaritoli, M., Antonucci, F. and Rossi-Fanelli, F., 'Eating behavior and adherence to dietary prescriptions in obese adult subjects treated with 5-hydroxytryptophan', *American Journal of Clinical Nutrition*, vol 56(5), pp. 863–7 (1992); Cangiano, C. et al., 'Effects of oral 5-hydroxy-tryptophan on energy intake and macronutrient selection in non-insulin dependent diabetic patients', *International Journal of Obesity and Related Metabolic Disorders*, vol 22(7), pp. 648–54 (1998).

59. Clouatre, D. and Rosenbaum, M., *The Diet and Health Benefits of HCA*, Keats (1994).

60. Samaha, F. F. et al., 'A low-carbohydrate as compared with a low-fat diet in severe obesity', *New England Journal of Medicine*, vol 348(21), pp. 2074–81 (2003); Foster, G.D. et al., 'A randomized trial of a low-carbohydrate diet for obesity', *New England Journal of Medicine*, vol 348(21), pp. 2082–90 (2003).

61. Bravata, D. M., et al., 'Efficacy and safety of low-carbohydrate diets: a systematic review', *Journal of the American Medical Association*, vol 289(14), pp. 837–50 (2003).

62. Maconaghie, P., 'A comparison of the metabolic diet with the Unislim diet for industry weight loss', ION (1988).

63. Feskanich, D., *American Journal of Epidemiology*, 'Protein consumption and bone fractures in women', vol 143, p. 472 (1996).

64. Knight, E. et al., *Annals of Internal Medicine*, vol 138(6), pp. 460–7 (2003); Reddy, S. et al., *American Journal of Kidney Diseases*, vol 40, pp. 265–74 (2002).

65. Fairburn, C. G. and Harrison, P. J., 'Eating Disorders', *Lancet,* vol 361, pp. 407–16 (2003).

66. Vos, T. et al., 'The burden of mental disorders in Victoria', *Social Psychiatry Psychiatric Epidemology,* vol 36, pp. 53–62 (2001).

67. National Institute for Clinical Excellence (NICE), 'Eating Disorders: Core interventions in the treatment and management of anorexia nervosa, bulimia nervosa and related eating disorders', NICE (2004).

68. Johnson, W. G. et al., 'Repeated binge/purge cycles in bulimia nervosa: role of glucose and insulin', *International Journal of Eating Disorders,* vol 15:4, pp. 331–4 (1994).

69. Wurtman, R. J. and Wurtman, J. J., 'Brain serotonin, carbohydrate-craving, obesity and depression', *Advances in Experimental Medicine and Biology,* vol 398, pp. 35–41 (1996).

70. Goodwin, G. M. et al., 'Plasma concentrations of tryptophan and dieting', *British Medical Journal,* vol 300, pp. 1499–500 (1990); Wolfe, B. E., Metzger, E. D. and Stollar, C., 'The effects of dieting on plasma tryptophan concentration and food intake in healthy women', *Physiological Behaviour,* vol 61 (4), pp. 537–41 (1997).

71. *New York Times* re Fava, M., MD, Massachusetts, General Hospital Study, Boston, 28 May 1993.

72. Smith, K. A., Fairburn, C. G. and Cowen, P. J., 'Symptomatic relapse in bulimia nervosa following acute tryptophan depletion', *Archives of General Psychiatry,* vol 56, pp. 171–6 (1999).

73. Laessle, R. G. et al, 'A comparison of nutritional management with stress management in the treatment of bulimia nervosa', *British Journal of Psychiatry,* vol 159, pp. 250–61 (1991); Brambilla, G. et al., 'Combined cognitive-behavioural, psychopharmalogical and nutritional therapy in bulimia nervosa', *Neuropsychobiology,* vol 32(2), pp. 64–7 (1995).

74. World Health Organization, The World Health Report 2001 – Mental Health: New Understanding, New Hope, see www.who.int/whr/2001.

Part 5

1. Hargreave, T. B. et al., 'Randomised trial of mesterolone versus vitamin C for male infertility', *British Journal of Urology,* vol 56:6, pp. 740–4, (1984); Abel, B. J. et al., 'Randomised trial of clomiphene citrate treatment and vitamin C for male infertility', *British Journal of Urology,* vol 54:6, pp. 780–4 (1982).

2. Milunsky, A. et al., 'Multivitamin/folic acid supplementation in early pregnancy reduces the prevalence of neural tube defects', *Journal of the American Medical Association,* vol 262:20, pp. 2847–52 (1989).

3. Huff, R., *US State Department of Developmental Services report on Autism* (1999).

4. Colquhon, I. and Bunday, S., 'A lack of essential fatty acids as a possible cause of hyperactivity in children', *Medical Hypotheses,* vol 7, pp. 673–9 (1981).

5. Richardson, A. J. et al., 'A randomized double-blind, placebo-controlled study of the effects of supplementation with highly unsaturated fatty acids on ADHD-related symptoms in children with specific learning difficulties', *Progress in Neuro-Psychopharmacology and Biological Psychiatry,* vol 26(2), pp. 233–9 (2002).

6. Megson, M., 'Is autism a G-Alpha protein defect reversible with natural vitamin A?', *Medical Hypotheses,* vol 54(6), pp. 979–83 (2000).

7. Megson, M., 'The biological basis for perceptual deficits in autism: vitamin A and G-Proteins', lecture at Ninth International Symposium on Functional Medicine, May 2002.

8. Prinz, R. J. et al., 'Dietary correlates of hyperactive behaviour in children', *Journal of Consulting and Clinical Psychology,* vol 48, pp. 760–9 (1980).

9. Schoenthaler, S. J., 'The Northern California diet-behaviour program: An empirical evaluation of 3,000 incarcerated juveniles in Stanislaus County juvenile hall', *International Journal of Biosocial Research,* vol 5(2), pp. 99–106 (1983); Schoenthaler, S. J., 'The Los Angeles probation

department diet-behaviour program: An empirical analysis of six institutional settings', ibid., pp. 107–17 (1983).

10. Langseth, L. and Dowd, J., 'Glucose tolerance and hyperkinesis', *Food and Cosmetics Toxicology*, vol 16, p. 129 (1978).

11. Whiteley, P., Autism Research Unit at Sunderland University, speaking at Autism Unravelled conference, 11 May 2001, London.

12. Whitely et al., 'A gluten free diet as an intervention for autism and associated disorders: preliminary findings', *Autism: International Journal of Research and Practice*, vol 3, pp. 45–65 (1999).

13. Brush, M. G., 'Nutritional approaches to the treatment of pre-menstrual syndrome', *Nutrition and Health*, vol 2:3/4, pp. 203–9 (1983).

14. Abraham, G. E. et al., 'Effect of vitamin B6 on pre-menstrual symptomatology in women with pre-menstrual tension syndromes: a double-blind crossover study', *Infertility*, vol 3, pp. 155–65 (1980).

15. Horrobin, D. F., 'Gamma linolenic acid: an intermediate in essential fatty acid metabolism with potential as an ethical pharmaceutical and as a food', *Reviews in Contemporary Pharmacotherapy*, vol 1, pp. 1–45 (1990).

16. Flynn, A. M. and Brooks, M., *A Manual of Natural Family Planning*, Thorsons/HarperCollins (1990).

17. Sun, J., 'Morning/evening menopausal formula relieves menopausal symptoms: a pilot study', *Journal of Alternative and Complementary Medicine*, vol 9(3), pp. 403–9 (2003).

18. Seal, E. C., Metz, J., Flicker, L., and Melny J., 'A randomized, double-blind, placebo-controlled study of oral vitamin B12 supplementation in older patients with subnormal or borderline serum vitamin B12 concentrations', *Journal of the American Geriatric Society*, vol 50(1), pp. 146–51 (2002).

19. Holford, P., 'Alzheimer's and dementia: the nutrition connection', *Primary Care Mental Health*, vol 2, pp. 5–12 (2004).

20. Strassman, R., *DMT – the Spirit Molecule*, Park Street Press (1999).

Part 6

1. *Vitamins and Minerals – How Much Is Safe?*, ION Press (1991).

2. Food Standards Agency, 'Safety of vitamins and minerals', *Report of the Expert Group on Vitamins and Minerals (EVM)* (2003); Shrimpton, D. and Richardson, R., 'Vitamins and Minerals: An overview of benefits and safety', Health Food Manufacturers' Association, www.hfma.co.uk (2003).

3. Lazarou, J. et al., 'Incidence of Adverse Drug Reactions in Hospitalised Patients', *Journal of the American Medical Association*, vol 279(15), pp. 1200–10 (1998).

4. Pirmohamed, M. et al., 'Adverse Drug Reactions as cause of Admission to Hospital', *British Medical Journal*, vol 329, pp. 15–19 (2004).

5. See www.healthyoptions.co.nz/Australia.pdf

6. Stearns, D. M., Wise, J. P., Sr, Patierno, S. R. and Wetterhahn, K. E., 'Chromium(III) picolinate produces chromosome damage in Chinese hamster ovary cells', *The Federation of American Societies for Experimental Biology Journal*, vol 9, pp. 1643–8 (1995).

7. Anderson, R. A., Bryden, N. A. and Polansky, M. M., 'Lack of toxicity of chromium chloride and chromium picolinate in rats', *Journal of American College Nutrition*, vol 16, pp. 273–9 (1997).

Index

Note: page numbers in *italics* refer to information contained in tables, page numbers in **bold** refer to diagrams.

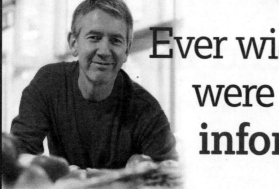

100%Health®
Weekend Intensive
The workshop that works.

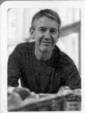